More Praise for *Wild Nights*

"A fascinating look at a phenomenon we have taken for granted. Benjamin Reiss pulls the bedcovers off of sleep, revealing a deep and significant history of Western culture and politics. It turns out that nothing escapes the tendrils of somnolence—race, gender, capitalism, and technology are all culprits or agents in creating our restless nights. Written with subtlety and provocation, this is a must-read for anyone whose head ever hit a pillow."

—Lennard J. Davis, author of *Enabling Acts* and
Obsession: A History

"Through impressive research and beautiful writing, Benjamin Reiss brings readers on a scientific, literary, and historical voyage, exploring our complicated relationship with sleep in an active world."

—Lauren Hale, editor in chief of *Sleep Health*

"Ranging widely across time and cultures, *Wild Nights* offers a rich perspective on Americans' present-day expectations about a good night's sleep. With Thoreau's *Walden* as his ballast, Benjamin Reiss examines the ways that religious thought, economic change, medical prescriptions, and big business have pushed sleep for those in the middle class into a single mold, while the rest of the world serves and goes without. This smart and engaging book is an ideal companion for that middle-of-the-night break, as well as for serious thought in the bright light of day."

—Helen Lefkowitz Horowitz, author of
A Taste for Provence and *Wild Unrest*

"A lively, astute, wide-ranging reconnaissance of the attempted reengineering of modern humanity's sleep habits. Benjamin Reiss pointedly and persuasively questions whether today's 'sleep science' delivers better results than what seemed second nature to our preindustrial forebears."

—Lawrence Buell, Harvard University

Wild Nights

Also by Benjamin Reiss

The Showman and the Slave

Theaters of Madness

The Cambridge History of the American Novel
(co-editor)

Keywords for Disability Studies
(co-editor)

Wild Nights

How Taming Sleep Created Our
Restless World

BENJAMIN REISS

BASIC BOOKS

New York

Designed by Amy Quinn

Library of Congress Cataloging in Publication Data

Names: Reiss, Benjamin, author.

Title: Wild nights : how taming sleep created our restless world / Benjamin Reiss.

Description: New York : Basic Books, [2017] | Includes bibliographical references and index.

Identifiers: LCCN 2016043568 | ISBN 9780465061952 (hardback) ISBN 978-0-465-09485-1 (ebook)

Subjects: LCSH: Sleep disorders. | Sleep. | BISAC: HISTORY / Social History. | SOCIAL SCIENCE / Anthropology / General. | HISTORY / United States / General. | SOCIAL SCIENCE / Disease & Health Issues.

Classification: LCC RC547 .R446 2017 | DDC 616.8/4982—dc23 LC record available at https://lccn.loc.gov/2016043568

10 9 8 7 6 5 4 3 2 1

For Devora, Isaac, Sophie—
and Pepper, goddess of the nap

CONTENTS

INTRODUCTION   *The Gates of Sleep*   1

Part I: The Invention of Normal Sleep
CHAPTER ONE   *Before Sleep Was Normal*   23
CHAPTER TWO   *A Different Drummer*   57

Part II: Taming Sleep
CHAPTER THREE   *Lady Macbeth's Doctor; or,*
                 Sleepwalkers and Lunatics   91
CHAPTER FOUR   *Sleeping Slaves, Waking Masters*   119

Part III: Rocking the Cradle
CHAPTER FIVE   *Wild Things*   141
CHAPTER SIX   *Utopian Sleepers*   171

Part IV: Global Weirding
CHAPTER SEVEN   *Beyond Normal*   199

EPILOGUE   *Three Chairs*   223

ACKNOWLEDGMENTS   231
NOTES   235
BIBLIOGRAPHY   273
INDEX   293

Wild nights—Wild nights!
Were I with thee
Wild nights should be
Our luxury!

Futile—the winds—
To a Heart in port—
Done with the Compass—
Done with the Chart!

Rowing in Eden—
Ah—the Sea!
Might I but moor—tonight—
In thee!

—Emily Dickinson

In wildness is the
preservation of the world.

—Henry David Thoreau

The Gates of Sleep

Sleep is both a universal need and a freely available resource for all societies and even species. So why is it the source of frustration for so many people today? Why do we spend so much time trying to manage it and medicate it, and training ourselves—and our children—how to do it correctly? And why do so many of us feel that, despite all our efforts to tame our sleep, it's fundamentally beyond our control?

The answers have more to do with the world we've built for ourselves over time—and the strangely restrictive place within it that we've reserved for sleep—than with any deficiency in our bodies. Our culture prides itself on variety and choice: what we buy, how we vote, what we eat, what we believe, whom we love, and how we lead our lives are all supposed to be matters of individual inclination—at least for those who can afford to choose. And yet of all the major daily human activities in much of North America and Europe, and increasingly elsewhere in the world, the topic of sleep inspires a numbing conformity to a one-size-fits-all standard-issue package. Sleeping in one straight shot through the night—"consolidated" sleep—has become a near-universal expectation, even for those whose bodies and minds seem naturally inclined to shut down and switch back on differently. Would-be sleepers are encouraged to develop rigid bedtime routines, regardless of season or setting. Sleep is supposed to occur in a private and almost neurotically sealed space, with, at most, two consenting adults sharing a bed. Children are to be trained from a very early age to reproduce these features of "normal" sleep, and we insist that they do so in isolation from adults. Should any of us fail to achieve the expected results, we call our sleep disordered and resort to medication or reprogramming, or we just resign ourselves to feeling miserable.

What is strangest about these expectations and social rules is that for all their power today, at most times and in most places in human history, practically no one followed any of them. And we now cling to them neurotically even as our world throws up new challenges to regular sleep: "flexible" work times, distracting and hyperstimulating electronic devices, ever more powerful caffeinated beverages, high-speed travel across time zones, and an unsleeping world of commerce, information, and entertainment that beckons us across the digital highway at every moment. The poor fit between the rules for "normal" sleep and the lives so many of us lead induces a self-perpetuating pattern of worry and micromanagement. Battering our sleep with rules, training manuals, rituals, and commercial sleep products like anti-snoring pillows and memory foam mattresses only leads us to be more intolerant of small changes to routine and environment, creating a society of fussy, stressed-out sleepers. And for those who, for reasons of biology or circumstance, can't sleep by the rules, the consequences are worse.

That is because, like all rules, the ones that govern sleep create conflicts: between the body and the mind, between bodies and the sleeping environment, and among social groups who are differently affected by the rules. For those who can't adapt to the rules, those who refuse, or those who are denied the time and space to sleep normally, sleep becomes an ordeal. These conflicts, in a sense, are as much the source of our current sleep troubles as purely medical issues are. Or rather, by some strange alchemy, the social and psychological problems created by our attempts to define and enforce what is normal are often interpreted as medical problems.

On a sultry night in New Orleans in late August 2005, I found myself unwillingly enrolled in a crash course on both the tenacity and the fragility of the rules that govern sleep. On that night, my wife, Devora, and I packed up our car with suitcases, some books, snacks, CDs, and toys for the kids, then caught a few hours of sleep before heading out at four in the morning. Like virtually everyone else who had a car, enough money to reserve hotel space, and no serious physical infirmities or essential obligations in the city, we were taking part in a mass exodus. Hurricane Katrina was bearing down, and suddenly we were rudely cast outside the gates of normal sleep, trying to find our way back in.

Yet we were fortunate. Our two children were young enough not to be overly anxious about the storm—for them it was an adventure. We had a car and some money in the bank. We had devoted family and friends far from the storm's path who were ready to help in whatever way they could. I had professional connections to people who could help me get back on my feet if disaster struck. But what we thought most about in the hours leading up to our evacuation was where we would *sleep.*

Shelter is an obvious human need, one that grows most intense during slumber. Our defenses are down, our responsiveness to stimuli dramatically reduced, and our need for protection therefore increased. Every species has a way of dealing with this vulnerability: ducks sleep in a row, with the ones on the edge keeping an outer eye open; dolphins and some whales sleep with only half the brain at a time; and the sleeping parrot fish secretes a packet of foul-tasting slime around its body to ward off predators. Human defenses against the vulnerability of sleep have involved more complicated controls: caves at first, but now locked homes, alarm and surveillance systems, and police to protect against threats to physical safety along with a host of sanitary measures to make sleep restorative rather than unhealthful. Many of these defenses broke down during Hurricane Katrina, as the mad scramble for shelter made clear to everyone. With some effort capped by a grueling slow-motion highway exodus, those with enough resources could find safe sleep; those who lacked them found wretched sleeping conditions in the New Orleans Superdome or the Convention Center, where heat, hunger, noise, stench, and fear made sleep all but impossible.

The need to find safe sleeping accommodations made our trek understandable, even inevitable. But much of our effort went toward something else, toward fulfilling a "need" that was culturally conditioned rather than biologically dictated: Devora and I were intent on finding a hotel spread out of harm's way that would allow the kids their own sleeping spaces apart from their parents and from each other. Part of this desire was rational: we wanted a space large enough that we could shelter the kids from our own anxious conversations. But on another, semiconscious level we simply wanted to re-create, on the fly, the aspects of "normal" sleep that bear most directly on children. Like so many other parents, we had spent countless painful nights trying first one method and then another to teach our children to sleep on their own, apart from us, in one straight shot through the night, at regularly scheduled times. We had achieved the sleep schedule and configuration of a typical middle-class American family, and we didn't want the storm to put all that effort to waste.

The rules we were trying to uphold have little to do with innate needs; in fact, they would seem strange to most societies across human history. In most times and places, sleep was social, with families, and sometimes even strangers, sharing common sleeping spaces; it was generally distributed in several chunks throughout the day and night; and its duration and patterning varied greatly depending on the season, patterns of natural lighting, the availability of resources, and other environmental cues. Only over the past few hundred years did sleep come to be privatized, packaged into one standard time slot, and removed from nature's great rhythmic cycles of temperature and light. Wrenching sleep out of these patterns, putting it in a box, shutting it off from social life, and making it conform to a set of demands that have little to do with circadian and other natural forces are all hallmarks of modern sleep. As a society, most of us assent to these rules without seeing them *as* rules but rather as part of nature itself.

Disasters have a way of laying bare all that we take for granted: what we assume is normal, natural, or even necessary suddenly appears to be a flimsy construction, part of our desire to maintain a particular way of life rather than a requirement for maintaining life itself. Surveying a scene of Katrina evacuees huddled on the floor in a Houston arena, former First Lady Barbara Bush, the mother of President George W. Bush, cast the evacuees' abnormal sleeping arrangements as natural—for *them*: "So many of the people in the arena here, you know, were underprivileged anyway. So this is working out very well for them." The rules, it seems, apply only to *us*. For the comfortable and the privileged, the obsession with maintaining the rules defining normal sleep is more about securing a place in the established social order than about basic physical well-being. Bush's comments were part of a centuries-long script in which those who can control their own sleeping conditions define what a proper, civilized way of life is supposed to look like, in part by distinguishing their own sleep from that of the uncivilized and the downtrodden.

Except that the rules don't seem to be working very well, even for those who can afford to play by them, and even when they aren't disrupted by disasters. A significant part of the contemporary obsession with sleep is the sense that we're somehow doing it *wrong*. Despite all of the sleep-related medical, scientific, and technological advances over the past two centuries, and despite the billions of dollars poured into what one journalist called the "sleep-industrial complex"—in the form of pills, mattresses, apps, wearable electronics, self-help books, breathing machines, and even "smart beds" that monitor our every move at night—a nagging culture-wide anxiety that we're in the midst of a sleep crisis persists. Popular books and magazine articles proclaim a war on sleep; over 2,500 sleep clinics in the United States alone treat millions of patients; and in general the weirdest person at a dinner party is the one who says she sleeps like a baby every night. (Not that babies sleep well.)

But are we sleeping less than our ancestors—or are we just more anxious about it? Attempts to answer this question have been inconclusive, if not contradictory. Twenty percent of American adults responding to a National Sleep Foundation poll reported sleeping less than six hours per night in 2009; about a decade earlier, it had been only 12 percent, indicating a sharp increase. More systematic research published in the journals *Sleep* and *Sleep Medicine Reviews* called that finding into question, with two teams of researchers concluding that there had been little change in average sleep duration over recent decades.

The lack of clear consensus might lead one to be skeptical of the notion of a raging epidemic of sleep deprivation, especially when one considers the advantages that contemporary, middle-class sleepers have over their ancestors and over less fortunate people worldwide today. Advances in hygiene, fireproofing, policing, and overall standard of living arguably make sound sleep available to a larger number of people than ever before. Labor laws in the most economically dominant nations protect most citizens from the brutal assaults on their circadian rhythms that were common in the peak era of industrialization in the West—and that have now been directed at workers in nations that are trying to catch up to Western economic standards. But whether or not our society is suffering a significant decline in the quantity of sleep, we seem to be experiencing an erosion in the *quality* of sleep.

This is not to deny the reality of what we medically label "sleep disorders," the genuine distress they cause, or the efficacy of some of the medical and other solutions we propose for them—far from it. Yet in a time when more than seventy recognized sleep disorders are being treated in thousands of clinics, and billions are spent annually on sleeping pills, we might question what produced all the trouble, and whether our frenzied attempts to tame sleep have made the problem better or worse. The obsessiveness and even panic attending much contemporary discussion of sleep, as well as our frantic and overwrought attempts to tame it and make it play by the rules, correspond to a feeling that sleep simply won't bend to our collective will, rather than to a quantifiable reduction in sleeping hours across contemporary society. Because sleep is one of the great psychosomatic enterprises—meaning that it's a physiological state that is powerfully affected by psychological factors—the panic and obsessiveness may well be creating a spike in genuine sleep disorders rather than the other way around.

Media reports of a "sleep crisis" are correct to identify an alarming state of affairs, but by suggesting simply that "we"—usually an economically secure readership—don't get enough sleep, they misidentify the crisis and so may only feed it. In reality our society is undergoing two sleep crises: a psychological struggle, in which those who live in relative states of comfort try to wrestle their sleep into submission, and a more existential struggle experienced by those who are expected to sleep by the rules of others yet are denied the time, space, and security to do so. What links these two sets of struggles is the growing economization of sleep, a process begun in the industrial revolution and accelerating today. On the one hand, sleep is made to work for profit; on the other, a host of commercial products (from pills to wearable sleep-tracking devices) promise the illusion of sleep on demand.

This book recovers some of sleep's hidden history—one that leads to our present, sleep-obsessed society, its tacitly accepted rules, and their consequences. It tries to answer the riddle of why, at a time in human history when comfortable and hygienic sleeping conditions are more widely available than ever, and our medical and scientific understanding of sleep's functions and inner workings has advanced exponentially, sleep has become such a battleground. While doing so, it keeps an eye on the social divisions underlying our rules for standard-issue sleep, as well as the consequences for those who can't, or won't, sleep by the rules.

, What this book *won't* do is tell you the correct, or best, or most natural way to sleep. The search for "natural" sleep patterns, which has preoccupied sleep researchers from the nineteenth century onward, has paradoxically played a role in sleep's growing disconnection from natural systems. Human sleep patterns are remarkably flexible, which is part of what has allowed our species to flourish in so many different climates and circumstances. This flexibility helps to explain the extreme diversity of sleeping arrangements around the world and through history: some societies nap while some don't; some sleep in large groups, others more or less alone; some naked, some clothed; some in public, some hidden. Instead of proposing a "new normal"—an idea about sleep that is supposedly the most natural or healthful way to do it—I want to move beyond the idea that there is a correct way to sleep, a single healthy way to sleep, a natural or restorative way to sleep. Instead, this book is a testament to sleep's amazing diversity—and an account of how that diversity has become restricted in a way that disadvantages certain sleepers: those whose bodies seem to be wired to sleep differently, or who lack the resources and amenities needed to sleep "normally."

Wild Nights explains how we inherited rules that put extreme pressure on sleep, the impact these rules and our frantic responses to them have had on different groups of people through history (especially over the past two hundred years or so), and—following historical trajectories forward—the future versions of sleep that might be emerging.

———

Although there is no single historical cause for the contemporary obsession with taming sleep, its thickest roots—especially in North America and Europe—reach back to the massive changes in technology and the organization of labor that took place in the late eighteenth and especially the nineteenth centuries. Taken together, these developments fundamentally altered the human experience of *time* and expectations for how bodies should move through it.

What we now think of as "time" is largely an invention of the industrial age. Factories and the economic system that grew around them in the nineteenth century depended on disconnecting workers' sense of time from the natural rhythms of day changing into night and season into season. Instead of waking more or less when the sun rose and dropping off not long after it set, sleeping more in the lean winter months and less in harvest times, and punctuating their days with naps, workers had to learn to rise consistently to the sound of a factory bell and organize their downtime accordingly. Schedules for travel, school, and commerce followed these industrial patterns of uniform clock time: a time newly homogeneous across season, region, or profession. When employers demanded too much of the workers' time, depriving them of adequate sleep, the workers advocated for sleep that was *more* standardized, rather than less. What they pictured was a time that was reserved exclusively for sleep, a time both demanded by industry and made impossible by it. The eight-hour ideal as we know it is largely a result of this push and pull between management and labor.

In order for the system to work, with workers getting to the factory floor at the appropriate time, so that the factories could be productive throughout the year, sleep had to be subjected to increasing levels of control. For this to happen, sleep had to be understood as a medical issue that could be empirically observed, manipulated, and corrected. Much of the biomedical research into sleep from the late nineteenth century until the present day has been underwritten by businesses with an interest in understanding how to manipulate or exploit body rhythms to make workers more efficient—as well as by the military, which wants to create armies of flexibly alert fighters. Sleep science emerged as a profound response to the industrial age, in which the rhythms of daily life came unstuck from the internal rhythms of workers, and experts were needed to understand what was happening in order to repair the damage.

This industrial manipulation of time was intensified by the spread of electricity and powerful artificial lighting, from the widespread use of gaslight early in the nineteenth century to electric lighting at the turn of the twentieth—and now the ubiquitous flood of blue light emanating from electronic screens. Historians and anthropologists, as well as many scientific sleep researchers, have begun to explore the profound effects of artificial lighting and the electrification of domestic spaces on sleep patterns. Even today, most societies that have not experienced the widespread introduction of electricity into homes tend to distribute sleep in several segments throughout the day and night; yet in Western Europe and North America, across the nineteenth and twentieth centuries, packaging one's sleep in one bundle quickly became the norm. Historian Roger Ekirch's influential argument is that before the industrial age, most societies practiced "segmented sleep" at night, in which sleep came in two installments, with an interval of quiet wakefulness. As powerful new light sources pushed back the boundaries of night, however, people were induced to stay up later, pushing the first installment of sleep forward until that interval was lost. Sleep now had to be stuffed into one package. This novel arrangement put extreme pressure on those whose circadian rhythms simply couldn't adapt to this historically novel expectation, leading to a spike in medical complaints about poor sleeping.

Industrialization, powerful lighting, and electrification also brought with them a parade of gadgets and devices with which nineteenth- and twentieth-century westerners could amuse themselves, increasingly with little regard for time of day. We are all familiar with the inducements to fall into social media and streamed entertainments well past bedtime; but people have been complaining about being tempted to keep unseasonable hours since cities and homes were first lit up by gaslight in the late eighteenth century. Reading a book or magazine at night, listening to a phonograph or viewing a magic lantern or stereograph, or even walking down a well-lit street to a tavern or theater: these quaint-sounding activities hardly seem like disruptive forces today, but they were as novel and (over)stimulating for many in the nineteenth century as surfing the Web was at the turn of the twenty-first. And just as the Internet seems to overwhelm our circuits with its constant news feeds and status updates, so nineteenth-century Americans and Europeans complained about the ubiquity of a news cycle driven by telegraphy, cheap print, and rapid delivery via trains and canals. Information overload has been connected to sleep loss for centuries.

Electricity and artificial light also affected the spatial arrangements associated with sleep, especially within middle-class families, which were acquiring larger and more autonomous homes as industrial wealth spread through society in the nineteenth and twentieth centuries. The key development—so obvious that many of us can barely see it as anything other than natural—was the spatial separation of parents or other adult caretakers from children throughout the night. Why, given that virtually no society anywhere before the nineteenth-century West insisted on children sleeping alone, did this bizarre ideal take hold? One factor is that parents, given access to new entertainment technologies in the home, wanted a space of their own to stay up late once children went to bed.

The deeper issue was their society's emphasis on privacy, a value that is most dear at night. The sociologist Norbert Elias argued in 1939 that for bourgeois European families, sleeping in private, out of view of others, became a hallmark of "civilization" across the eighteenth and nineteenth centuries. As with other manners, one needed to be taught how to do this from an early age. Accordingly, each child had to be trained to go to bed in his or her own room and stay there through the night. And so the child's bed became a central training ground for a society of sturdy, solitary sleepers—people who attended to their bodily needs out of view of others. As I explain in Chapter Five, sleep dogma—reinforced across the nineteenth and twentieth centuries by health reformers, psychologists, and pediatricians—promoted the idea of consolidated nighttime sleep for children in their own rooms: a very weird arrangement by historical and cross-cultural measures. The goal was the creation of hearty, autonomous, self-willed adults who could march off confidently into the workforce, in full possession of their powers to sleep and wake when instructed, and careful not to let themselves drop off in public. But as any parent can attest, no young child *wants* to sleep alone through the night: most have to be trained according to a very strict routine. The expectation for solitary childhood sleep thus has tended to produce finicky young sleepers who are easily disturbed by changes in routine or environment: the snoring of others, ticking sounds in the wall, fluctuations in temperature, the wrong firmness of mattress or pillow, the absence of a favorite stuffed animal, and the like. Enforced solitary sleep for children, then, likely fed a culture-wide obsessiveness about sleep, magnifying problems that might not seem so bad in other times and places.

Learning to sleep "normally" means being trained to sleep by the rules of this system as a child, then outfitting yourself with enough space and gear to reproduce it when you're an adult. Those who can't pay their way into normal sleep are left outside the gates, scrambling through odd jobs, undiagnosed health problems, and vulnerable nighttime conditions in which restful slumber is almost unthinkable.

And those who, by virtue of inclination or cultural background, sleep differently come to be regarded as backward or even perverse. The sociologist Elias's observation that Europeans defined themselves as civilized in part by doing their sleeping in private also implied that non-Europeans whose sleep did not conform to this standard were defined as "other," somehow primitive or in need of reform; this judgment also applied to Europeans who couldn't afford to do all of their sleeping in private. Scenes of naked "savages" lying on communal sleeping mats (similar to those primarily black and brown bodies that Barbara Bush saw sprawled out after Katrina), African slaves bundled in the holds of slave ships, or poor urban whites sleeping ten or twelve to a room in rickety tenements came to represent all that an ideal white European or American should *not* be. Accordingly, health reformers and moralizers set about convincing the laboring classes to sleep more privately—as did missionaries and colonial authorities in places where European and American power extended its reach.

And so, in the industrial age, sleeping became subject to novel demands that put pressure on sleep's rhythms, environments, and configurations. The pressures are felt in different ways by different groups—young, old, rich, poor, black, white, female, male—but we've all been dealing with the fallout from the invention of normal sleep in the nineteenth century ever since.

———

Few people leave detailed records of their sleeping habits and perceptions of sleep; fewer still are attuned to how sleep responds to social change. And so finding first-person accounts of sleep's historical transformation seemed a difficult task. What did it feel like to live through the changes that created modern sleep, to have one's body pushed and pulled by new demands and new distractions, to experience the loss of social sleep, to sense the rhythms of industrial life supplanting those of nature, to be woken by factory bells and train whistles rather than by one's own circadian rhythms or birdcall or sunlight or some elemental need, to be jolted into consciousness by powerful doses of caffeine rather than by the sensations of morning doing what it will to your body?

But seek, and ye shall find: as I was beginning to sketch out my ideas for a history of sleep, I had the good fortune to assign Henry David Thoreau's *Walden* to my undergraduate students as part of a survey of American literature. I was astonished to find that in all my years of reading and teaching that book, I had completely missed a major concern that was lying right on the surface of the text, in virtually every chapter—something that seemed not only to open a window onto Thoreau's time and place, but to provide a fascinating perspective on my own.

I now found in *Walden* an astonishing record of the conflict between natural and artificial rhythms, between human bodies and the industrialized world they were supposed to inhabit. From the first chapter onward, sleeping and waking on one's own schedule is one of Thoreau's great preoccupations. Finding one's own rhythm—or, as he put it, marching to the beat of a different drummer—is one of the rewards to be sought in nature and an essential part of liberating oneself from social expectations and economic indebtedness. "You could sit up as late as you pleased," he rhapsodized about life in his cabin in the woods, "and, whenever you got up, go abroad without any landlord or house-lord dogging you for rent." The last lines of the book have often been read metaphorically, as a call to higher consciousness; but they are, literally, also a summons to his readers to do what they need to wake up: "Only that day dawns to which we are awake. There is more day to dawn. The sun is but a morning star." The morning star, in Thoreau's imagination, was something like what the North Star was to runaway slaves: both a compass and a beacon of freedom. But one could only follow it if one was fully alert and fully rested. Certainly the book is meant as an inspiration to renounce materialism, to forswear war and brutality, to live life by one's own principles, and to better understand nature. But in addition, all of *Walden*, it suddenly seemed to me, could be read as the efforts of an exhausted man to wake up, to understand why he and his countrymen could never fully be rested, and to inspire the kinds of changes that would be necessary for his society to achieve alert wakefulness. In a sense, Thoreau went to Walden Pond to get a good night's sleep.

Thoreau's career might seem an unlikely source for understanding how our contemporary sleep troubles began. But in a way, his most famous literary achievement was also a significant record in the history of sleep. In the years leading up to his sojourn in the Concord woods, out of which he produced his masterpiece, Thoreau experienced a set of health and emotional crises that so unstrung him that getting a good night's sleep became almost impossible. He went off to Walden Pond in order to repair himself as well as to meditate upon the relationship between his own body and nature's great cycles: the passage of day to night, season to season.

He was also profoundly attentive to the jarring effects of industrial time on his countrymen, the famous "mass of men [who] lead lives of quiet desperation." In the pages of *Walden* and other writings, we can find surprising premonitions of our own contemporary sleep troubles: disruptions from sound pollution and sensationalistic 24/7 media; overreliance on caffeine and other artificial stimulation; anxiety about waking on time for work in a technology-driven economy; and the nervous exhaustion that follows from trying to adjust to the hectic pace of the waking world. The book he wrote about his experiences is one of the most profound meditations on time that we have in American literature. It's also a record of what was happening *to* time as he and his society experienced it: how it was altered by new technologies such as the railroad, the factory, and the telegraph, and how difficult it was in the frenetic pace of the "restless, nervous, bustling nineteenth century" to truly experience and savor the natural world.

One aspect of the natural world from which Thoreau felt most alienated was his own body, which had fallen out of sync with the great pulsing rhythms he heard and saw all around him at the pond. Recovering his balance, and his rest, on his own time—to the beat of his own drummer—was the subtext of his experiment in the woods. And in the midst of that pursuit, he began to connect his own nervous exhaustion to deeper social problems in the world that he temporarily left behind. Throughout his most famous work, Thoreau portrays his countrymen as permanently unawake, nearly zombified in their subservience to technology and the unnatural rhythms it induces. The reasons for this general somnolence sound surprisingly contemporary: addiction to stimulating substances and entertainments; the frantic pace of commerce and high-speed communications; noise pollution from onrushing trains, the clatter of factories, and the cries of newsboys; overstimulation from the scandals and sensational stories that were delivered by newsmen over the lightning-fast telegraph; the pressure to organize one's work and travel times on an exacting schedule; and fears of fatigue-related accidents at work or in travel. A century and a half before the first smartphone, Thoreau even saw some of the cultural patterns unfolding that would eventually lead us to reach compulsively for our electronic devices in the middle of the night: "Hardly a man takes a half-hour's nap after dinner, but when he wakes he holds up his head and asks, 'What's the news?' as if the rest of mankind had stood his sentinels." In short, Thoreau spoke back to an emerging 24/7 economy addicted to speed, commerce, and communication for its own sake, in which citizens were nonetheless expected to sleep efficiently, soundly, and normally.

Walden is known as a classic of nature writing, and Thoreau's environmental ethos helps us see that the forces damaging sleep over the past two centuries are the same ones despoiling our ecological system to this day. While shutting down at night is a way of pausing in our depletion of resources, our social expectations for sleep—involving economic imperatives and a desire for privacy—have hidden environmental consequences. Whereas some premodern societies apparently approached a state of human hibernation in winter when less food was available (as I explain in Chapter One), people in most highly technologically developed societies tend to wake as early in the winter as in the summer, thereby increasing both food and energy consumption. We train our children to sleep in separate bedrooms, thereby requiring larger homes with larger carbon footprints. We ingest chemicals to switch off or rev up our brains on a rigid schedule of work and schooling, and then we expel those same chemicals into the water supply. Beyond these phenomena, our sense that we can *conquer* sleep, tame it, make it conform, relies on the same environmentally devastating mindset that Thoreau decried: an attitude of dominion over nature (including our own bodies) through technology and consumerism. Taming sleep served an industrial society; and that society created unprecedented havoc for the natural world.

———

Henry David Thoreau is not the subject of this book so much as its guiding spirit and lead witness. Thoreau has his own chapter—Chapter Two—and makes cameos in a few more; but other writers' lives and works are central to the stories I tell about human sleep and its changes, too: among them are Marcel Proust, Charlotte Perkins Gilman, Frederick Douglass, Herman Melville, and George Orwell, as well as the great children's writers Maurice Sendak, Margaret Wise Brown, and—yes—Adam Mansbach of *Go the F**k to Sleep* fame. I see this gallery of writers partly as reporters from the outposts of sleep who can provide vivid illustrations of patterns of sleeping and waking in different times and places. But unlike most reporters, they offer a window onto the inner experience of what they chronicle. Since sleep is such an intimate, even hidden, aspect of human experience, it requires a literary focus on interior states to draw out its history.

Complementing these literary records, *Wild Nights* also presents a number of real-life stories of troubled sleepers, hibernating peasants, sleepwalking preachers, cave-dwelling sleep researchers, slaves who led nighttime rebellions, workers who stood up (or laid down) to their bosses, spectacularly frazzled parents, and utopian dreamers in order to flesh out sleep's hidden role in our history. And it takes us to some surprising locations: bedrooms, hospitals, clinics, and labs, to be sure, but also the streets of New York, London, and Delhi, utopian communes, battlefields, factories, the holds of slave ships and whalers, tenement houses, church pews, insane asylums, office cubicles, trains, planes, space ships, and a cabin by the shore of Walden Pond—all spaces where wild human sleep was tamed, and our restless world took shape. The title *Wild Nights* comes from the Emily Dickinson poem reprinted at the beginning of the book. It's about the night as a time to experience rapture and ecstasy, a notion that might serve as a powerful counterweight to our own tendency to try to batter our sleep, and the sleep of others, with tools and systems of taming. "Done with the compass!" she exults. "Done with the chart!" Any parent frustrated with training a child to be a normal sleeper might appreciate the sentiment.

In preparing to write this book, I had an unusual opportunity to work closely with a neurologist, David Rye, an expert on sleep disorders, in co-teaching an interdisciplinary class on "Sleep in Science and Culture" at Emory University. This experience not only offered me grounding in the scientific and medical aspects of human sleep, but gave me a profound appreciation for how multidimensional human sleep is. Rather than a niche concern, sleep touches nearly every aspect of life, and virtually every intellectual discipline has its own insights to contribute. Sleep science and medicine address the bodily mechanisms involved in sleep; anthropologists and sociologists study the cultural systems shaping the way different groups sleep; historians look at the broad forces that create changes in human behaviors; philosophers and scholars of religion tell us much of what sleep means.

I am a literary scholar by training, and a cultural historian by inclination. This means that I find careful reading of literary works to be the most illuminating way to think about how our world came to be as it is, and how people experienced their part in that unfolding story. Powerful literary writing addresses us not as medical patients, scientific objects, or representatives of historical periods or social groups, but as particular individuals who are shaped by all of these dimensions and have something to say about them.

Wild Nights, then, blends literature, the social and medical history of sleep, cross-cultural analysis, and some brief forays into science—as well as some occasional personal anecdotes where relevant. Each chapter explores the history of a different aspect of modern sleep and its costs: the suppression of premodern sleep customs in the nineteenth century; Thoreau as critic of his society's unnatural rhythms; the shift from religious to medical notions of sleep; the history of sleeping on slave plantations and its relevance to contemporary health disparities among racial minorities and the poor;

the emergence of children's sleep as a special problem; attempts to reform or revolutionize sleep; and new developments that point toward the possible demise of our two-centuries-old sleep regime. Rather than adding up to a singular linear history of modern sleep, the book's chapters use historical storytelling and literary interpretation to give a perspective both broad and intimate on particular aspects of disordered sleep and our obsessive attempts to tame it.

The topical structure of the book mirrors the biological complexity of sleep itself. Sleep science tells us that sleep is not one state but many. It comes in several stages, which are in some ways as different from each other as they are from waking: rapid eye movement (REM) sleep, the phase of rapid electrical activity in the brain that is most closely associated with dreaming, has been described as a "third state of brain activity" in addition to waking and the non-REM stages of sleep. So, too, sleep has practically as many functions as being awake does, involving distinct actions of the endocrinological, neurological, respiratory, muscular, and sensory systems. As befits a subject this complex, sleep does not have one history but many. Although the overall structure will take us from the early modern period (from roughly 1500 to 1700) up to today, the book has a braided rather than a strictly sequential or chronological organization.

If sleep has been hidden beneath the covers of history, my hope is that peeling back those covers might also tell us much about the waking world. History does not pause when people go to bed. Wars, natural disasters, poverty, economic systems, and technologies of all sorts affect the way we sleep, and all in turn are affected profoundly by the ever-present need to organize life around ensuring sleep. The philosopher Thomas Hobbes even pointed to the need to protect citizens from the common defenselessness of sleep as one of the reasons why we need government in the first place. (Without basic protections, our sleep, like the rest of our lives, might be nasty, brutish, and short.) History is made by human actors, all of whom—consciously or not—organize their waking activities in relation to the need to shut down. So in addition to sleep being shaped by history, there is virtually no aspect of history that is not influenced by this silent pressure that mounts for each historical actor throughout the day.

For much of human history, sleep had profound spiritual meanings, many of which have been snuffed out as sleep was tamed in the modern world. For all of our current obsessiveness with sleep, our society seems to have radically restricted its meanings to the realm of medicine, hygiene, economics, and psychology: we need sleep—and we need to do it the right way—to be healthy, productive, and well-adjusted. Recovering sleep's hidden history might be one way of restoring some of its lost grandeur. Sleep's future, even more than its past, is also hidden; but by welcoming sleep into the arena of history, we might be able to change the rules that govern it—the rules that keep so many of us up at night.

PART I

The Invention of Normal Sleep

*I s'pose you are goin' a
whalin', so you'd better get
used to that sort of thing.*

—Herman Melville

CHAPTER ONE

Before Sleep Was Normal

What passes for "normal" sleep today is, by any historical standard, quite strange. Sleep now inspires unprecedented levels of medical concern, along with pervasive anxiety and countless attempts at micromanagement. Pills and sleep clinics are only part of this development, which also involves mattress companies, peddlers of self-help, big coffee chains, drowsy truckers, public health professionals, hyperstimulating electronic devices, napping consultants, high-speed travel and higher-speed communications, scientific researchers, military planners, risk assessment professionals, labor organizers, governmental regulators, space travel researchers, self-monitoring systems, smartphone sleep apps, sleep coaches, online sleep therapy programs, and even smart beds that analyze our patterns of movement, breath, and perspiration. All of these proliferating consumer choices, expert voices, and manipulators of sleep either produce sleep difficulties, claim to remedy them, or both. It seems that the more we try to fix our sleep, the more we put it under pressure, creating a vicious insomniac cycle.

Beyond this apparently chaotic set of phenomena lies an elusive but deeply ingrained set of social norms that governs much of what we think about sleep—and our efforts to enforce these norms have cost us untold sums of money, time, and psychological energy.

People living in the contemporary world do not all sleep in the same way, yet my guess is that most people reading this book share an idea of what standard-issue sleep is supposed to look like, even if the rules are honored in the breach: Sleep through the night, in one straight shot, for about seven or eight hours. Form a habit of preparing for sleep at roughly the same time every night, no matter what season, preceded by similar pre-bed rituals. Sleep in a bed in a sealed-off, noise-free space. Do it alone, or with, at most, one other consenting partner. Train your children to sleep on their own, and through the night, from an early age. If something goes wrong, consult a doctor, read a sleep-training book, or pop a pill. All of these elements of contemporary sleep wisdom are so firmly entrenched in our culture that it's hard to see that there might be other sensible ways to get the job done. And yet none of these rules is anything close to universally sanctioned across cultures or historical periods, and several of them would seem quite odd to people in times and places other than the twentieth- or twenty-first-century West. Even worse, many of these practices feel oddly mismatched to the social and technological worlds we inhabit, which make the idea of regular sleeping hours and routines seem next to impossible.

What's strangest is that although all of these features are taken as natural or normal ways to sleep, *not one* of them seems to have been in force at any time anywhere before around 1800 in Europe and North America. This is worth reiterating: virtually *nothing* about our standard model of sleep existed as we know it two centuries ago.

For starters, the notion of sleeping in a private bedroom, out of view of strangers or even most other family members, turns out to have shallow roots. Contrast the modern North American or European middle-class bedroom, which typically harbors just one or two children or two consenting adults, with scenes of sleep from other times and places.

In a recent volume called *Sleep Around the World*, anthropologists describe the sociable sleeping patterns of the cultures they study. Rules for sharing beds can be quite elaborate and even insistent. On his first night among the Asabano people in Papua New Guinea, for instance, Roger Lohmann was surprised when a man in the village apologized for not being able to sleep with him, because he had to sleep with his own wife. Lohmann arranged for a house to be built for himself with a private sleeping room in the back, but this seemed to trouble the villagers. As he stayed in the town, a number of men offered to sleep with him—and he allowed several of them to stay in his common room. Offering companionship in sleep, he learned, was a basic kind of hospitality, and in this cool mountainous region, in which homes lacked climate control, snuggling up was also a way to keep warm at night. Additionally, the Asabano believed that solitary sleepers were dangerously vulnerable to spiritual forces unleashed at night. In the homes of the Cook Islanders in the South Pacific, another anthropologist notes, bedrooms tend not to have doors, and entire families often sleep together. In Maori ancestral meeting-houses, extended family gatherings after the death of a relative end with the sacred act of communal sleeping; there are elaborate rules involving the positioning of elders, and women are prohibited from stepping over the legs of sleeping men.

Although many of these practices persist, they are on the retreat worldwide. In places that experienced colonial rule, missionaries and other European authorities actively tried to stamp out sleeping arrangements that they considered perverse, backward, or unhealthy throughout the nineteenth and twentieth centuries. Such efforts to "improve" the lives of the natives were part of the justification for often violent systems of control. But in those pockets of the non-Western world where communal sleeping persisted despite the efforts of colonialists, the introduction of electricity sometimes did the trick—as soon as some people could watch television, others wanted to find another place to sleep.

For most people in Europe, private sleeping quarters were a rather new phenomenon in the nineteenth century. Until the industrial era, only the aristocracy possessed sufficient wealth for such luxury. Historian Sasha Handley reveals that even the idea of a "bedroom," denoting a room primarily associated with sleep, is rather new. Throughout the eighteenth century in England, most homes had rooms with overlapping functions depending on the time of day; and well into the nineteenth century, it was common for travelers to share beds with strangers. In 1530, the Dutch scholar and theologian Erasmus wrote, "If you share a bed with a comrade, lie quietly; do not toss with your body, for this can lay yourself bare or inconvenience your companion by pulling away the blankets." And the great eighteenth-century diarist Samuel Pepys noted his preferences in choices of bedmates, ranking them by quality of conversation and their proper behavior in bed. He particularly enjoyed sharing a bed with merchant Thomas Hill, with whom he conversed "with great satisfaction" about music as well as "most things of a man's life."

Pockets of social sleep persisted into the nineteenth century: in colleges and boarding schools, in prisons, on slave plantations (as I will address in Chapter Four), in poorhouses and hospitals, on the battlefield, at sea, and in boardinghouses and lower-end hotels. But even these group sleeping arrangements were under assault. Some indication of the changing dynamics occurs early in Herman Melville's *Moby-Dick* (1851), when Ishmael—or the guy who wants us to call him Ishmael—holes up for a night at the Spouter Inn in New Bedford, Massachusetts, before setting sail. There he is told he must share a bed with a strange, tattooed Polynesian harpooner named Queequeg. "I s'pose you are goin' a whalin', so you'd better get used to that sort of thing," says the innkeeper. But Ishmael has his proprieties: "No man prefers to sleep two in a bed," he ruminates. "In fact, you would a good deal rather not sleep with your own brother." Yet he consents to bed down with Queequeg, after which he reports that he never slept better in his life. In fact, after two nights, the strange bedfellows are snuggling as close as newlyweds, referring to each other as married, and joking that Queequeg's tomahawk is their baby. In the mornings, they lounge and nap, "with Queequeg . . . affectionately throwing his brown tattooed legs over mine."

This famous passage is wonderful for many reasons, not least of which is its breaking down of cultural barriers through a startling invocation of same-sex interracial physical intimacy. But I cite Melville's treatment of this episode for comedic shock value as evidence that values on land had changed: by 1851, a rather unambitious man on a downward trajectory from the middle class could say that "no man prefers to sleep two in a bed." Sleeping with Queequeg isn't the oddity; as Handley points out, travel throughout the seventeenth and eighteenth centuries provided men and women of different ranks and social classes the opportunity to bed down together "in the pursuit of new forms of sociability." What's new in the history of sleep, as Ishmael sets off on his mid-nineteenth-century whaling voyage, is the fact that he has been brought up to think there is something wrong with this tradition. From this perspective, sleeping with Queequeg isn't what's strange; the oddity is Ishmael's initial aversion to it.

———

Even while early modern travelers frequently shared beds with strangers, voices of authority warned about the moral and physical risks of communal sleeping. Norbert Elias, one of the great sociologists of the twentieth century, wrote of sleep's slow historical movement from a sociable activity to one that became "more intimate and private." Across the seventeenth, eighteenth, and nineteenth centuries, he argued, "to share a bed with people outside the family circle, with strangers, is made more and more embarrassing." Embarrassing, and also dangerous. Some voices warned against the health risks of sociable sleeping as early as the seventeenth century. In 1682, the English merchant and commentator on health Thomas Tryon painted a vivid picture of the horrors that might befall readers who shared beds, or who passed on beds from generation to generation, in his wonderfully titled *A Treatise of Cleanness in Meats and Drinks, of the Preparation of Food, the Excellency of Good Airs, and the Benefits of Clean Sweet Beds, Also of the Generation of Bugs, and Their Cure: To Which Is Added, a Short Discourse of the Pain in the Teeth Shewing from What Cause It Does Chiefly Proceed, and Also How to Prevent It*. "Beds," Tryon wrote, "suck in and receive all sorts of pernicious Excrements that are breathed forth by the Sweating of various sorts of People, which have Leprous and Languishing Diseases, which lie and die on them: The Beds, I say, receive all the several Vapours and Spirits, and the same Beds are often continued for several Generations, without changing the Feathers, until the Ticks be rotten."

European slave traders, too, noticed that sleeping arrangements seemed to play a role in disease. In the large shared spaces of slave ships, dysentery and other maladies began to spread. Reports of the ill health effects were challenged by defenders of the slave trade, who argued that the circulation of free air at sea actually improved the health of Africans. The English Parliament, however, grew concerned: white sailors were dying at alarmingly high rates. Although, in terms of profits, the human cargo that the slave ships were transporting was more valuable to the ships' owners than the crew, it was the effect on the white sailors that raised enough alarm to cause a response. The Dolben Act of 1788 stipulated that the slave ships must contain less crowded sleeping quarters below decks for the (white) crew members. Some crew members, including at least one captain, nevertheless slept with the enslaved masses in order to prevent mutiny. As for the enslaved Africans, the sleeping quarters were abysmal. Former slave Olaudah Equiano reported that the apartments of ships in the Middle Passage were "so crowded that each had scarcely room to turn himself." The stench became "absolutely pestilential, with the shrieks of the terrified, and the groans of the ill and dying keeping others awake."

Efforts to stamp out sociable sleeping in Europe took on a sense of urgency in the thick of industrialization in the nineteenth century. These efforts were motivated by health-related as well as moral concerns. Large concentrations of people in cities led to tight sleeping quarters, and workers in factories and mines often slept in large boardinghouses, "lodging shops," or other communal arrangements. A particular fear was the lack of ventilation in shoddily constructed buildings where large numbers of people slept huddled together, breathing and rebreathing the same foul air. According to pioneering health reformer Edwin Chadwick—one of the most important public health champions of the nineteenth century—disease and immorality ran rampant in these crowded spaces. His widely publicized 1842 *Report on the Sanitary Conditions of the Labouring Population of Great Britain* reads almost like a catalog of dangerous and improper sleeping practices: two or three families sleeping together, workers coughing and snoring together in rooms without windows or chimneys, and everyone on beds without sheets. The result was a "dense accumulation of bodies" and noxious, suffocating smells. Chadwick quotes one miner who called the lodging rooms "not to be fit for a swine to live in." This man reported that as many as fifty miners would try to sleep in sixteen beds at one time. "The breathing at night when all were in bed was dreadful," he said. "The workmen received more harm from the sleeping-places than from the work." Other workers complained of the filth and lack of ventilation of the sleeping quarters; at a time when the chief theory of contagious disease involved fetid air, or "miasma," such reports were alarming to the authorities. Chadwick thought that such cramped conditions led to cholera, a theory that was later debunked by John Snow, who discovered that it was carried by contaminated water. But the miasmic theory put social sleeping on the defensive, especially among the poor. The threat of disease within workers' lodging houses was so rampant that by 1851 Parliament passed a Common Houses Lodging Act specifying the hygienic measures to be undertaken in dormitories. The need for basic privacy was included.

By the late nineteenth century, social sleeping in ordinary life was decidedly on the wane across mainstream European and North American society, as high-minded authorities actively tried to eliminate it wherever they found it. Chadwick had written about indecent practices in communal sleeping arrangements among the laboring poor; the general Victorian squeamishness about sex extended the campaign to all matters involving shared bedding. One Dr. Richardson, writing in 1880, proposed single beds for all adults, because "the system of having beds in which two persons can sleep is always, to some extent, unhealthy." The bedroom, he wrote, "should be a sanctuary of cleanliness and order, in which no injurious exhalation can remain for a moment, and no trace of uncleanliness offend a single sense." Although cholera was no longer understood to be airborne, unhealthy miasmic effusions continued to permeate the Victorian imagination; a journalist in 1884 argued that the advantage of single beds was that sleepers did "not inhale each other's 'breathed breath.'" And an American doctor estimated that up to 40 percent of deaths in America resulted from overexposure to foul air during sleep.

Jacob Riis's influential 1890 study of poverty in New York, *How the Other Half Lives*, chronicled the unhealthy conditions of poorly ventilated tenements with "a hundred and fifty 'lodgers' sleeping on filthy floors in two buildings," lodging houses with long rows of "bunks with yellow sheets and blankets as foul," and tramps sleeping in doorways. Massive group sleep was really only for the neglected or unwanted members of society, such as disabled people, who often lived quarantined in institutions, or beggars in workhouses. The American physician William Whitty Hall, for instance, wrote in 1863 of the baneful health effects for "imbecile children" sleeping together in public asylums, where they breathed "putrid" air and kept each other awake with their screams and moans. "A single sleeper," Hall said, "requires a chamber twelve feet square" that is clean and well-ventilated: "It seems little short of a murderous process for more than one person to sleep together in a chamber of ordinary size."

So an industrial society, which depended on large concentrations of people in cities to supply labor for industry, began making efforts to supply privacy and unfouled air for the workers at night. This was not only a matter of health; society needed a sense that the populace was more than a mass of interchangeable, writhing bodies. This self-image was often explicitly invoked to bolster the idea of the superiority of whites to other peoples. Hall, as part of his campaign to provide adequate space for solitary sleepers, evoked the image of the "Calcutta Black Hole" from 1756, a Calcutta jail in which 136 British prisoners of war had been held in abysmal conditions and forced to breathe each other's air at night: 123 of them had died. And one slave ship captain reported that the enforced communal sleeping of slaves—in which as many as ten captives were forced to retire at night chained together—was not a problem, since Africans preferred to "crowd together . . . by Choice" at night. Europeans were supposedly more worthy of being treated as individuals, and their superior temperaments required that each person have a room of his or her own.

Indeed, keeping private sleeping quarters was one way that Europeans liked to mark themselves as superior to "savages," who slept in groups. White European and North American laborers were supposed to be better, in essence, than the slaves on a ship, the prisoners in a foreign cell, or the natives lying on a communal mat. Hall wrote disparagingly of co-sleeping societies, comparing them to "the vilest, and the filthiest of the animal kingdom—wolves, hogs, and vermin" who "huddle together." In contrast, in civilized societies, "as men improve in their condition, there is a strong desire for greater domestic conveniences and comforts; the very first of these is 'more room;' and eventually, instead of several members of a family sleeping in the same bed, each child, as it grows up, has a separate apartment." Hall echoed a late eighteenth-century French travel writer, who hinted darkly of incest among Hottentots in southern Africa: "The savages sleep all promiscuously together, in the same hut; and are neither acquainted with difference of age, nor that invincible horror which separates beings connected by blood." And missionaries among the Asabano tried to combat what they perceived as immoral group sleeping in order to promote the ideal of Western-style nuclear families: in New Zealand, collectively owned communal sleeping houses gained potency as spaces of resistance to colonial rule. And so just as Europeans were encountering a range of communal sleeping practices in parts of the world over which they were taking control, health experts and industrialists were stamping out the group sleeping of European workers. If the natives slept in groups, then to be "English" or "European" or "white" meant to sleep apart. Elias didn't spell out these racial connotations, but as he wrote, a new sense of shame became attached to sleeping in public, or with strangers.

Yet at the same time a new perception arose that sleep among "civilized" white people was broken. Across the nineteenth century, medical and popular writers alike noted a rise in insomnia, which they often linked to the progress of "civilization." According to the 1872 book *Sleep and Its Derangements* by the influential early American neurologist William Alexander Hammond, "as nations advance in civilization and refinement, affections of the nervous system become more frequent, because progress in these directions is necessarily accompanied by an increase in the wear and tear of those organs through which perceptions are received and emotions excited." The implication was that while white people had advanced over the rest of the world through superior exertion of their intellectual organs, their sleep suffered. Sleep loss even became somewhat modish, a sign of what came to be known as "sensibility." In the novels of the eighteenth and nineteenth centuries, nothing was more indicative of a young hero or heroine's superior refinement and thoughtfulness than inability to sleep. White Europeans were, in a sense, like so many delicate versions of the princess and the pea: tossing and turning on their ever-so-slightly uneven downy mattresses while savages snored lustily, huddled in groups, on whatever rough surface they could find.

It is impossible to know whether insomnia was "really" on the rise among whites in nineteenth-century Europe and America, but certainly the spread of such theories speaks to a widespread sense that there was something wrong with sleep, that it wasn't satisfying or fulfilling. Could it be that the era's perception of poor sleep was in part a byproduct of the loss of sleep's social dimension? Dozens of physicians and health reformers weighed in on the subject of collective sleep loss on both sides of the Atlantic in the nineteenth century; they all addressed the problem of afflicted individuals tossing and turning in their private beds: just the kind of orderly, quarantined sleepers that colonial authorities and public health officials were trying to produce. Whether or not the loss of sociable sleep was to blame for disordered sleeping, it's arguable that when sleep began to be shut off from social life, walled away behind closed doors, it became less pleasurable, more pressurized, more fragile, and more subject to the vagaries of individual psychology. Perhaps Queequeg really did cure Ishmael of insomnia.

————

Like the private bedroom and the twin bed, the ideal of eight hours of unbroken sleep is a modern, Western concept that may be a recent invention.

The first scholar to put consolidated sleep—today's standard "one straight shot throughout the night"—under the microscope was historian Roger Ekirch. In his fascinating 2001 essay "Sleep We Have Lost: Pre-Industrial Slumber in the British Isles" (expanded in his 2005 book *At Day's Close: Night in Times Past*), Ekirch revealed that across a wide range of nationalities and social classes in early modern Europe and North America, the standard pattern for nighttime sleep was to do it in two shifts of "segmented sleep." These two sleeps—sometimes called first and second sleep, sometimes "dead sleep" and "morning sleep"—bridged an interval of "quiet wakefulness" that lasted an hour or more. (The interval itself was sometimes called "the watching.") Ekirch's subsequent work offered evidence that a segmented nighttime pattern persisted well into the twentieth century in many non-Western locales, including among indigenous cultures in Nigeria, Central America, and Brazil. During the period of nighttime wakefulness, Ekirch showed, different cultures elaborated rituals—of prayer, lovemaking, dream interpretation, or security checks—and while the rituals varied, the pattern itself was so pervasive as to suggest an evolutionary basis that somehow became disrupted in the modern West.

So why did this mode of sleeping fall by the wayside, in favor of the eight-hour, lie-down-and-die model that has become an unquestioned norm? According to Ekirch, the main culprit was the spread of powerful artificial lighting in the nineteenth century in Europe and North America, and later in other locales. As activities that were previously nearly impossible to conduct under cover of darkness became fashionable under an ever-widening penumbra of powerful light, Europeans and Americans gradually shifted their bedtimes later. And as the available space between first and second sleeps shrank, the pattern of two nocturnal sleeps—and the enchanted space between them—became untenable. So complete was the transition to consolidated sleep that an American newspaper advice column in 1911 counseled readers who couldn't sleep well to take their sleep in two shifts—as if this were a novel suggestion! Ekirch argues that the reason so many of us experience middle-of-the-night insomnia (the kind that comes after a few hours of sleep), is that ever since electric lights reordered our sense of time, we've disrupted our ancestral—perhaps our evolutionary—rhythms. And while Ekirch eventually came to view the reasons for the shift from segmented to consolidated sleep as more complicated than just exposure to light—including shifts in technology, changing cultural attitudes toward work and rest, and the economic pressure to manage time more efficiently under industrial capitalism—powerful artificial lighting, he wrote, still "exerted the broadest and most enduring impact upon sleep's consolidation."

Ekirch's thesis has taken surprising hold in some medical and scientific circles. In 1993, at about the same time that Ekirch was doing his historical research into the erosion of segmented sleep patterns by the advent of electric lighting, psychiatrist Thomas Wehr of the National Institutes of Health was conducting clinical experiments in which subjects were deprived of artificial lighting for several weeks. Wehr found that under these circumstances, the subjects began to gravitate toward a common pattern of waking up for approximately an hour after midnight. During this interval, the brains of Wehr's subjects showed higher levels of prolactin, a hormone that reduces stress and that is also released during orgasm. Struck by the congruence with his own historical findings, Ekirch contacted Wehr and the two exchanged notes. Perhaps this hormonal activity, they speculated, was the biological basis for the fertility rituals that were so common during the interval between first and second sleep and that seemed to have vanished in the modern world. (The sixteenth-century physician Thomas Cogan, for instance, advised that intercourse occur not "before sleepe, but after the meate is digested, a little before morning, and afterward to sleepe a while.") Sleep specialists in the United States and Europe have begun to take these findings seriously, reevaluating the common wisdom that healthy sleep means uninterrupted nocturnal slumber. Russell Foster, a professor of circadian neuroscience at Oxford University, saw a therapeutic value in this new view of what constitutes normal sleep: "Many people wake up at night and panic," he said in an interview. "I tell them that what they are experiencing is a throwback to the bi-modal sleep pattern."

So does that mean, as Ekirch's and Wehr's work suggested, that humans are evolutionarily adapted to sleep in two shifts at night?

Not all scholars agree. The historian Sasha Handley, for example, questioned whether Ekirch's sources were representative enough to indicate a universal model of sleep across millennia of human history. Recent scientific studies also present a very different evolutionary scenario. Studying sleep patterns in three contemporary hunter-gatherer societies in Tanzania, Namibia, and Bolivia that lacked electricity, a team of researchers led by Jerome Siegel of the University of California at Los Angeles found little evidence of segmented sleep at night, but some evidence of daytime napping, especially during the summer months. Surprisingly, the average sleep time among these societies was approximately six hours per night, but the lower number, compared to the eight hours recommended in contemporary Western medicine, had none of the adverse health effects—including obesity, diabetes, and mood disorders—that authorities so often link to sleep deprivation. Even more surprisingly, this supposedly ancient sleep pattern more closely resembles the contemporary Western predilection for consolidated sleep than the preindustrial segmented variety that Ekirch documented, except that six hours a night is usually deemed unhealthful and often blamed on overexposure to artificial light, computer screens, and the like. In a coauthored article, Siegel's group claimed that because the tribes they studied shared environments similar to those in which the human species evolved, their sleep patterns represented the truly natural way to sleep: they were the "core human sleep patterns . . . characteristic of pre-modern Homo Sapiens."

Yet this claim, too, may be too sweeping. Ekirch, in a response, allowed that segmented sleep may not have been the pattern for "all preindustrial peoples in the non-Western world," but he pointed to dozens of examples provided by anthropologists to show that it was a predominant one. In a commentary on the Siegel group's article, another group of prominent sleep researchers rejected the conclusions as an "over-interpretation" of data, arguing that without a control group, their study simply could not yield "normative values" for an evolutionary default pattern for human sleep. The Siegel group defended their conclusions and in a sense doubled down, suggesting that the evolutionary pattern they had discovered should make sleep clinicians question the notion that sleeping less than seven hours a night is detrimental to the health of adults. Meanwhile, several anthropologists who study sleep patterns weighed in with their own doubts about the Siegel team's conclusions. No culture, Kristen Knutson argued, is a "living fossil," and so extrapolating from current practices to a universal evolutionary basis for sleep is problematic. Matthew Wolf-Meyer went further, pointing out that the very societies that Siegel and his team studied were far from premodern hunter-gatherers: all three groups had centuries of experience in dealing with colonial administrations and state governments; one had a burgeoning tourist industry; another had members working for big logging companies; a third had extensive trade networks with other communities—and all of these historical factors likely had some effect on their patterns of sleeping and waking. The arguments are still spinning out as I write this summary.

So is it "natural" to sleep through the night, or instead to break sleep up into segments? The dispute between the Siegel camp and the others raises profound questions not only about what might be the natural way to sleep, but about whether any particular sleep pattern is more natural for *Homo sapiens* than others. The argument seems irresolvable, at least by me; but it does indicate the depth to which our society—including its academic researchers—feels dissatisfied with sleep: we are looking to the ancestral past as well as to medical experts for solutions. Because sleep is always governed by society's rules and environmental pressures as well as by physiological needs, though the search for one unchanging "natural" way to sleep seems unlikely to solve our current collective sleep frustrations. The efforts are noble, and they yield fascinating accounts of sleep's mutability; but as the experts present conflicting visions of the best, most naturally human way to sleep, they may only feed sleep anxiety rather than conquer it.

Perhaps we can view these conflicting visions of sleep's evolutionary forms the way we view different consumer products, picking the one that suits our particular sleep quandary the best. Each of the positions staked out in this academic battle might be psychologically comforting to contemporary troubled sleepers in search of some historical or evolutionary perspective on their troubled passage through the night and their drowsiness during the day. The Ekirch position suggests that if you can't stay asleep through the night, you're not an insomniac, but simply more in touch with ancestral rhythms than your culture wants you to be. The Siegel position says, in a sense, that we should stop worrying about sleep loss, since, for all our distractions, we don't need as much sleep as the experts tell us we do. And those who argue that there is no single way to sleep naturally or correctly give us license to be more forgiving of our own sleep patterns, to stop thinking that there is a "right" way that we're failing to achieve.

———

As difficult, or even as impossible, as it might be to determine a single evolutionary basis for sleep patterns, one can still point to several features of nineteenth- through twenty-first-century life that exerted novel pressures on how people slept and that continue to shape sleep to the present day. Perhaps the most commented upon development is the spread of lighting and electricity. Historians, anthropologists, and medical researchers alike have all reinforced the idea that electricity and all the gadgets that eat it up have made healthy sleep a casualty. Sleep hygienists regularly advise avoiding electronic screens around bedtime; workers who suffer from "shift work sleep disorder" are often treated with controlled lighting to mimic natural rhythms of sunlight and darkness; and many sleep researchers counsel that exposure to natural daylight is the best way to avoid jet lag and other disturbances to the sleep cycle. At least as far back as Thomas Edison's invention of the incandescent light bulb, ubiquitous electricity has created a challenging sleep environment that can hardly be construed as similar to the conditions of our evolutionary ancestors—no matter how many hours people sleep or what patterns that sleep takes. (Edison himself famously thought that sleep was a waste of time.)

But what drove the need to colonize the night with light? Did the switches go on because people wanted to stay up later, or did people stay up later because the switches went on? As with many questions in social history, cause and effect can easily be made to switch places. And the answer depends on whose perspective we are looking at: patrons of brightly lit nighttime operas and late-shift factory operatives clearly had different responses to artificial lighting, even if the sleep patterns of both groups were affected. Yet it seems clear that without the needs of industry, there would have been no great technological shift in the history of lighting, and likely no corresponding shift in the patterning of sleep at night.

The age of artificial lighting was, after all, the age of industry, which had a vested interest in manipulating the sleep patterns of workers. In 1867, Karl Marx wrote in *Das Kapital* that industrial capitalism "oversteps not only the moral, but even the merely physical maximum bounds of the working day. . . . It reduces the sound sleep needed for the restoration, reparation, refreshment of the bodily powers to just so many hours of torpor as the revival of an organism, absolutely exhausted, renders essential." But as capitalists sought new ways to push bodies to their limit, they hit upon the stumbling block of darkness, or at least dimness. Certainly, artificial light had been used to illuminate pockets of the night since humans figured out how to produce fire, and some workers had always had to stay up while others slept: night watchmen, bread bakers, brewers, glassmakers, iron smelters, privy cleaners (or "night scavengers," as they were sometimes called), servants who cleaned up after feasts, prostitutes, and other medieval and early-modern night owls often found nighttime the best time to work, or were forced by circumstance to do so. But the industrial revolution created possibilities for round-the-clock work on a scale that went beyond anything that had come before; and the weak light shed by candles and oil lanterns was no match for the cavernous interior spaces of the factories. From the late eighteenth century through the early twentieth, industrial growth both triggered a revolution in light and was escalated by it—beginning with gas lighting and culminating with the development of the incandescent electric light bulb. A fundamental shift took place, from taming flames to harnessing chemical processes in order to increase both the intensity and the durability of a single light source.

The new light, it seemed, allowed industrialists to manipulate the sleep-wake cycles of workers—a practice that reached its peak with the development of continuous-process industries like petroleum and steel-making. (These industries were especially conducive to round-the-clock production because the materials involved are continuously in motion and subject to chemical changes that have no clear endpoint.) A survey in 1927 showed that 40 percent of all workers making rubber, sugar, iron, and steel worked the night shift. Particularly challenging to sleep schedules was the dreaded "long turn" in early twentieth-century steel mills—a day when an individual worker switched over from twelve-hour days to twelve-hour nights. But it wasn't just workers who were affected. The same industrial economy that pushed factory hands to churn out a staggering array of goods under a strong, cheap source of light also drove the market for lighting itself. Throughout the seventeenth century, before the eras of cheap gas and electric light, it was mainly only aristocrats who had been able to spend the night in sociable revelry and dissipation; by the end of the nineteenth century, staying up late to do what one wanted seemed an ideal within reach of many—a sort of unspoken democratic right. Cheap, powerful lighting also helped to increase demand for new products popping out of the factories—magazines and books, then phonographic records and radios, and so on: for all of these, artificial light was needed, so that consumers had enough usable leisure hours in which to enjoy them. The genie was unleashed: soon streets were flooded with powerful unnatural light beams; theater stages were emblazed into the small hours; and the interiors of middle-class homes could be nearly as bright as day in the middle of the night. Light came full circle: it enabled the work that produced the goods to be consumed under the same beams that had been used to make them.

What did all of this do to sleep patterns? First, it put them on a strict and often punishing schedule, then it disrupted those schedules, which in turn fed demands for increasing regularity. Early in the process of industrialization, observers could imagine that simple fortitude and moral forbearance would allow workers to adapt cheerily to the new sense of time brought on by industrial work rhythms and an eroding distinction between day and night. The early American writer Sarah Savage, in her 1814 novella *The Factory Girl*, tells the story of an orphaned young woman who goes to work in the textile mills, where she is called to the factory floor each morning at the same early hour. Through prayer and clean living she easily adapts to the strict regimentation of her time, even telling her kindly aunt, "I will wait no longer for the factory bell to [wake] me up." Her own sunny Christian morality serves as a sort of internal alarm clock. But by the next century, chronic fatigue—or what today might be called shift-work sleep disorder—was a standard feature of accounts of life on the factory floor.

For his 1919 exposé, *Steel: The Diary of a Furnace Worker*, the Yale graduate Charles Rumford Walker posed as an ordinary workingman in the steel mills. He wrote that after the night shift, "I wash up, go home, eat, and go to bed. . . . Anything that happens in your home or city that week is blotted out, as if it occurred upon a distant continent; for every hour of the twenty-four is accountable, in sleep, work, or food, for seven days; unless a man prefers, as he often does, to cheat his sleep-time and . . . take a drink with a friend." Similarly, Thomas Bell's 1941 novel, *Out of This Furnace*, about turn-of-the-century immigrant steel workers, had this to say about the long turn's effect on the protagonist: "The second twelve hours were like nothing else in life. Exhaustion slowly numbed his body, mercifully fogged his mind; he ceased to be a human being. . . . At three o'clock in the morning of a long turn a man could die without knowing it."

Even in less extreme scenarios, the sense of rhythms shifted in a world lit up at night. Industry hours shaped much of the sense of time outside the factory walls: factory whistles blew; train schedules were coordinated with deliveries to and from the factories; shops opened and closed in sync with workers' schedules; regular times were set for school and entertainment. All of these activities fell into patterns that were directly or indirectly tied to the new industrial economy: they were relatively invariant across seasons, governed by clocks rather than by the rising and falling of the sun or the change in seasons, and timed to take advantage of prevailing labor schedules. Clocks had been around for centuries, and they had long been used to synchronize social activities in athletic contests, law courts, and gambling dens, but never before the industrial revolution did they have such broad regulatory force. Time itself became a chief product of the industrial age, and when clock time did not correspond to natural rhythms, artificial lighting could help enforce it.

Despite, or perhaps because of, the factory system's role in creating havoc with sleep schedules, the idea of a standard model for healthful sleep—eight unbroken hours—took hold. The factory system clearly made its own special demands on times for working and resting with little regard for human health, but both employers and workers played a role in creating new expectations for the timing of sleep. Some nineteenth-century industrialists sponsored research into the physiology of rest in order to promote efficiency and safety on the factory floor. The exhausted factory workers themselves reinforced the emerging standard model when they agitated for labor reforms that would address their irregular and punishing schedules. The rallying cry chanted in labor halls and union meetings beginning in the late 1800s was "Eight hours for work, eight hours for rest, eight hours for what you will." Eight hours, not four and four with one in the middle for interpreting dreams or making love, or six at night and two after lunch.

———

Nevertheless, many societies around the world continue to practice napping during the workday (although some are actively trying to suppress it in the name of efficiency, as I will explain in Chapter Seven). Less well-known than the prevalence of napping is that in many times and places, human sleeping patterns have varied greatly according to the season—with some of the most extreme variations approaching hibernation in the winter. The sixteenth-century English physician Thomas Cogan wrote that "concerning the quantity or time, how long we should sleepe, it cannot bee certainely defined a like for all men, and for all seasons. But it must be measured by health and sicknesse, by age, by time of the yeare, by emptinesse or fulnesse of the body. . . . In winter, longer sleepe is requisite than in Sommer." Cogan, whose popular book on hygiene was consulted for at least half a century after it was first printed in 1584, based this idea on early modern theories of sleep that focused on the importance of heat regulation: sleeping longer in the winter was a way to retain more of the body's natural heat. But even without a doctor's advice, many people in cold climates stayed in bed longer in the winter out of necessity. With reduced food supplies and limited sources for heat other than animal skins or other coverings, they simply had to conserve energy.

Some economically isolated societies preserved this kind of seasonal variation well into the modern age. Historian Graham Robb wrote that in remote regions of the French Pyrenees throughout the late nineteenth century, a year consisted of "two seasons . . . the season of labour when even the longest days were too short, and the season of inactivity when time slowed to a crawl and seemed in danger of stopping." As late as 1880, one observer said that residents of the Eastern Pyrenees were "as idel [sic] as marmots" during the cold months. Entire mountain regions would essentially shut down in late autumn, with some villages essentially "entombing" themselves through the early spring. One geographer wrote in 1909 that "the inhabitants re-emerge in spring, disheveled and anaemic." Even some lower-lying regions, with more temperate weather, showed signs of prolonged torpor. An official report in 1844 described what happened to Burgundian day laborers after the harvest season had ended: "After making the necessary repairs to their tools, these vigorous men will now spend their days in bed, packing their bodies tightly together in order to stay warm and to eat less food. They weaken themselves deliberately." And in 1908, the French chronicler of rural life Jules Renard wrote that "in winter, [peasants] pass their lives asleep, corked up like snails." Robb concluded that "human hibernation was a physical and economic necessity. Lowering the metabolic rate prevented hunger from exhausting supplies."

The economically dominant British, whose industrial might was powered in part by regular work schedules across the seasons, tended to look down their noses at such backward habits. A 1900 report in the *British Medical Journal* mentioned that "a practice closely akin to hibernation," known as *lotska*, "is said to be general among Russian peasants in the Pskov Government, where food is scanty to a degree almost equivalent to chronic famine." Since there was not enough food to last the year, peasants spent "one half of it in sleep." At first snowfall, the entire family would lie down by the stove, and everyone would wake up once a day to drink some water and eat a piece of hard bread, a six-month supply of which had been baked in the autumn. Afterward, everyone went to sleep again. Family members took turns on a vigil "to watch and keep the fire alight." Six months later, they would all go out, like human groundhogs, to check and see whether the grass was growing. The writer of the report found "economic advantages" to this kind of hibernation, but in general he speaks with a condescending faux-envy, betraying his sense of British superiority: "We, doomed to dwell here where men sit and hear each other groan, can scarce imagine what it must be for six whole months out of the twelve to be in the state of Nirvana longed for by Eastern sages, free from the stress of life, from the need to labour, from the multitudinous burdens, anxieties, and vexations of existence." Certainly this account reveals as much about the writer's own fantasies of non-Western life as it does about the actual sleeping patterns of Russian peasants; yet at its core, his observations comport with more sober accounts of extreme seasonal variations.

Such variations persisted into the twentieth century in northern regions with relatively few economic and social ties to the more temperate (and more industrialized) regions to their south. Consider the case of native peoples in the northernmost regions of North America. In his 1948 account of his sojourn among the Ihalmiut of northern Saskatchewan, the Canadian writer Farley Mowat chronicled the lives of people facing a forbidding environment that brought plentiful supplies of protein and fat in late summer and autumn, but next to nothing in the winter. In such conditions, they needed to adjust themselves to "the rhythm of the elements," which included holding long sleepless vigils during the caribou-hunting season of the fall. During this time, "huge fires burned all day and all night and blocks of white deer fat began to mount up in the tents," wrote Mowat. In the following season, when temperatures could dip to fifty below zero, came long periods of dormancy, when the only source of heat was the "fat . . . being burned—within their bodies." People would "eat a little and then go to sleep." But the few waking hours were not merely times of deprivation, for although "the almost continuous darkness and cold could well drive men mad," the Ihalmiut people composed and sang songs for great "song-feasts" before retiring to their igloos. Periods of prolonged torpor in today's world might be considered signs of depression or seasonal affective disorder; but in these other times and places, they were simply part of the established order of things—a way that the body responded as a natural system to environmental cues. Changing sleep patterns were part of a cyclically occurring ebb and flow of supply and demand: sleep occurred in inverse proportion to supplies of food and heat.

Although some onlookers to such scenarios have referred to wintertime periods of extended dormancy as acts of "hibernation," the term—sleep scientists tell us—doesn't quite fit. Humans lack the ability of other mammals, such as bears and squirrels, to experience the prolonged periods of suspended animation that occur in true hibernation, which are physiologically quite different from sleep. During hibernation, the need for nourishment is minimized and blood flow to the brain drastically reduced. (Researchers are trying to understand why such oxygen depletion, or cerebral ischemia, is fatal to humans but not to our cousins.) And yet seasonal variations manifestly do exist across cultures, pointing to the wide flexibility of sleep patterns necessary for survival during much of human history. Workers in Arctic and Antarctic regions, for instance, exhibit profoundly different sleep cycles in winter than in summer, and for good reason.

Compare this ecological attunement of the sleeping body to its changing natural environment with the advice given by sleep experts from the nineteenth century to the present. "Let there be an appointed time [for sleep]," wrote William Whitty Hall in the mid-nineteenth century, "not to be changed for any common reason." A century later, Nathaniel Kleitman, the University of Chicago physicist who is generally considered the father of modern sleep research, also argued for the importance of "following a definite routine with respect to daytime and evening activity and the time of going to bed." Kleitman's follower William Dement, who taught the first course on sleep science in an American medical school and wrote the most authoritative sleep hygiene text of the late twentieth century, followed the idea of an unchanging routine even further. "Managing your sleep is a lot like managing your money or your weight," he wrote in *The Promise of Sleep*. One needs to study one's sleep patterns to find out "how much sleep you need on the average in each 24-hour period." And a 2015 *New Yorker* article surveying the science of sleep loss offers the conclusion that "sleep variability"—going to bed without a strict routine—is one of the surest routes toward insomnia. While this may seem like sound advice—certainly many sleep experts have echoed it—it is remarkable that Dement and most of his followers make no allowance for change of season in determining "how much sleep you need." The "hibernating" peasants or the caribou-hunting Inuit would have seen such regular patterning of sleep as disastrous to their well-being.

———

Modern advice about regularizing sleep stems from an understanding of the body's rhythms, which are seen as being independent of, but interactive with, external forces. Nathaniel Kleitman launched his career in the late 1930s by studying the natural circadian rhythms of human sleep, that is, the daily cycle inherent in the body's physiological processes, untouched by the rhythms of the sun rising and falling or the needs of society. Along with his graduate student Bruce Richardson, Kleitman holed himself up in Kentucky's Mammoth Cave and studied what happened to his sleeping and waking patterns in the absence of fluctuations of light, temperature, and social obligations. Their goal was to see if they could acclimate themselves to a six-day week made up of twenty-eight-hour days.

While Kleitman himself was unable to adapt, his younger colleague readily did so, which led Kleitman to conclude that the diurnal sleep-wake rhythm of humans was not a steady clock, but an intricate system that could be reset to different environmental and psychological cues. As anthropologist Matthew Wolf-Meyer pointed out, however, Kleitman specifically forbade napping in his experiment: even this pioneering sleep researcher had assumed that consolidated sleep was somehow "natural." In addition, his insistence that "true" human sleep rhythms could be understood in isolation from changes in temperature and levels of light reflected a sense that one could study sleep best by isolating it from its natural habitat. In a sense, his project was like trying to study the breathing systems of fish out of water.

Kleitman's main claim to scientific fame was his later discovery, with Eugene Aserinsky in 1953, of the REM sleep cycle and its association with dreaming. But this earlier research about sleep rhythms tells us a great deal about one major thrust of sleep research in the twentieth century: Kleitman's work was funded by corporate and military sponsors who wanted to see how adaptable humans were to the rhythms of imposed schedules, and they wanted advice about how to create productive employees and soldiers. Kleitman, to his credit, pushed back against some of the more exploitative practices, including frequent radical changes in workers' shifts. Yet he still treated sleep patterns as something that should be manipulated and rationalized in a machine-like way. His advice about invariant sleep routines was conveyed in his important 1939 work, *Sleep and Wakefulness*, and was recirculated in a 1942 article in *American Business*.

Other scientific research gives the lie to the notion that humans are wired to sleep the same way every night. The field of chronobiology, which studies the effects of time on living organisms, supplies intriguing clues about the flexibility of the human sleep system, which depends on multiple factors: genetically encoded circadian rhythms tied to the brain's chemical surges, length of time spent awake, availability and type of light, force of habit (known as *entrainment*), and so on. In an early 1960s experiment that helped launch the field, the German physician and biologist Jürgen Aschoff took Kleitman's Mammoth Cave experiment several steps further. Many scientists at that point believed that one could never create a "time-free" environment for the human body, because internal rhythms were somehow dependent on the earth's rotation. In response, Aschoff and his colleague, physicist Rütger Wever, built a carefully controlled sleep bunker, which consisted of two apartments within a hillside that shielded against everything that could indicate the passage of time to research subjects: it lacked windows, it was completely soundproof, it maintained a consistent internal temperature, and it could even block fluctuations in the earth's electromagnetic fields. (The bunker did have electric lighting, which the subjects were free to turn on and off.) The subjects of their experiment entered their apartments through a corridor separated by two thick doors, which could be opened only one at a time. In order to replenish their supplies, they placed shopping lists in this corridor—along with urine samples, so that researchers could examine their metabolic and hormonal output. In some experiments, subjects were alone in the apartments; in others, groups lived in the same apartment so that the researchers could examine how the body clocks of different individuals affected one another.

Most subjects retained a basic pattern of sleeping approximately one-third of the time. But after a few weeks, strange things began to happen. The majority of subjects retained something close to a twenty-four-hour pattern; but a significant minority—close to a third—began to carve up their time in forty-hour segments, while a smaller number experienced days that were significantly shorter than twenty-four hours. Even stranger, these new elongated or truncated "days" were at odds with the basic rhythms of other body functions: changes in body temperature and hormonal flow occurred in twenty-four to twenty-five hour cycles, indicating that the internal timing system of humans works on multiple levels, and that not all systems are intrinsically timed to work together. The bunker-dwellers' reported sense of subjective time provided further evidence of "internal desynchronization." When those who had a warped sense of the length of a day were asked to estimate the passage of time, they were not far off for intervals of short duration (a minute). But when they were asked to estimate the passage of an hour, their responses were in sync with the stretching or contracting of time indicated by their new sleep-wake cycles.

These internal timing systems, subsequent researchers have found, are governed by a small group of neurons above the optic chiasm called the suprachiasmatic nucleus (SCN). But given that the internal sleep clock is so wildly variable, as well as independent from the timing of other body functions, this multiplicity of timing systems must have some evolutionary basis. Contemporary chronobiologists theorize that internal desynchronization has evolved out of the body's need to remain flexible to changes in the external environment. If all of the body's clocks were set to one rhythm, one could never adapt to changes in season, to sleepless vigils on the trail of caribou, or to any other deviations from a regular pattern of sleep and waking. The search for one ideal, natural, evolutionary, prehistoric, immutable, universal pattern of sleep seems to be contradicted not only by the diversity of sleep across the globe, but by the interconnectedness of the body's own mysterious inner processes.

———

So what explains the supposed wisdom, often peddled by the medical establishment, that sleep should proceed more or less uniformly, from night to night, with the regularity of a household budget (okay, not my household budget), preceded by strict routines and mapped according to a schedule? It's easy to notice that in these schemes, the human body is treated like a machine, either well-oiled or not; sleep routines, like factory-made goods, are a product of the industrial age. (The human body, wrote the nineteenth-century neurologist Hammond, is a "complex machine," differing only from other machines in that "it possesses the power of self-repair"—by which he meant sleep.) As we have seen, from the nineteenth century onward, human rhythms became estranged from natural ones; artificial light pushed back the night and mechanical clocks synchronized travel, commerce, and work with little reference to the rising and falling of the sun, the falling of snow, or the changing of leaves. Sleep seemed sufficiently strange and difficult in this new industrial environment that it warranted intensive study, often funded by the industrialists themselves.

In addition to the mechanical control of time and the electrical taming of night, another relatively unexplored aspect of the way we have controlled our sleep environments over the past two hundred years has been the development of modern climate control and big agribusiness. In societies with abundant energy reserves and a worldwide food distribution system, we consider it natural to sleep independently of changes in seasons and differing lengths of day and night. That's not because regularized sleep schedules are healthy, or because our bodies are built to switch on and off in that way, but because we're simply trained to sleep in places where it doesn't matter much what time of year it is, how long the day is or how short the night, how cold or hot the season, and how plentiful the nourishment.

Although the Siegel team's conclusions about supposedly pre-modern sleep patterns in hunter-gatherer societies are controversial, one aspect of their research was not disputed: they found that the timing of sleep was more dependent on changes in temperature than on changes in light. Across the three widely dispersed subject groups they observed, arousal occurred not at sunrise, but at the time when the temperature stopped dipping and began to rise. And in these relatively temperate zones, only fifteen or twenty degrees removed from the equator, sleep duration was one or two hours longer in the winter than in the summer; in Berlin, by contrast, where both the temperature and the length of daylight decrease far more dramatically in winter, the difference between winter and summer sleep averaged only eighteen minutes. The presence of climate control and Western expectations for regular sleep routines apparently accounts for the difference.

In wealthy industrialized societies, work and eating can go on in the same way regardless of temperature, availability of natural light, or harvest. And so does sleep. The privacy of modern sleep is not simply a withdrawal from other people into the sanctuary of a quiet bedroom; it's also a withdrawal from nature. "Hibernating" peasants appeared exotic and backward in the nineteenth century: how much more so does a Tanzanian hunter-gatherer or Inuit caribou hunter appear to someone living in Maine who can eat Chilean corn grown in January, dial up the thermostat, seal out the noise of wolves or hooting owls, and drive off to work at eight the next morning, the same as in May? After all, such people are told by the medical establishment to fall asleep and wake up at the same time every day. And if the routine doesn't work, it's easier—and cheaper—to pop a pill than to try to harmonize the body with natural rhythms.

———

Fast-forward from the distant past, through the industrial age, to the present and into the future of sleep—and back to the past. (The future, to quote the science-fiction writer William Gibson, is already here, it's just not distributed evenly. Ditto for the past, as in my use of the word "ditto.") One of the more popular movements reflecting unease with contemporary life is the Paleo movement, a so-called "caveman-inspired lifestyle" that peddles hygienic advice based on supposedly evolutionary health principles. The centerpiece of this movement is the Paleo diet, which has spawned magazines, cookbooks, diet books, cooking apps, and cookware—and has attracted a range of celebrity adherents who attest to its wonders. The main article of Paleo faith is that humans are evolutionarily poorly adapted to the modern diet, with its heavy reliance on grains, dairy products, and processed sugar, and should revert to grass-fed meat cooked over flames, nuts and fruits, and other staples of the hunter-gatherer menu. As the movement expanded, however, it began to cover other aspects of health that are supposedly threatened by the diseases of civilization: exercise (favoring CrossFit-style regimens that don't depend on machines); natural cosmetics and cleaning supplies; attachment parenting; and avoidance of overreliance on electronics.

Sleep, too, has an important role in the Paleo lifestyle. In his 2008 book *The Primal Blueprint*, the founder of the movement—a former world-class marathon runner named Mark Sisson—writes that "for billions of years, the evolution of nearly all life forms on earth has been driven by the consistent rising and setting of the sun." He (incorrectly) claims that "sleeping and eating patterns as well as the precise timing of important hormone secretions, brain wave patterns, and cellular repair and regeneration [are] based on a 24-hour cycle." In his picture of primal sleep, nighttime was often disrupted by the intrusion of dangerous predators or the need to care for the young, and cave-dwellers retired frequently for naps to make up for these nocturnal disturbances. These ancestral rhythms, according to Sisson, have been profoundly disrupted by "excessive artificial light and digital stimulation after sunset, irregular bed and wake times, jet lag, graveyard shift work, and alarm clocks," with negative effects on health and happiness.

John Durant, in his book *The Paleo Manifesto*, takes this evolutionary criticism of modern rhythms even further. Updating early modern medical theorists like Cogan, who believed that sleep was a matter of the body regulating its own internal heat, Durant argues that modern humans have suppressed the body's ability to thermoregulate itself by relying on climate control, aspirin, and avoidance of seasonal extremes to keep the body at an unvarying temperature. Drawing on the historical literature on sleep, he blames the industrial age for keeping people indoors and severing humans' relationship with the sun. This fundamental shift made old, evolutionary patterns of sleep, extending back to the hunter-gatherer phase of human existence, untenable. Segmented sleep, with common naps, was replaced by the eight-hour consolidated version, and less rigidly controlled sleep environments (harder surfaces, fluctuating temperature and seasonal variation, myriad noises from the natural environment) could no longer be tolerated. The soft-bodied, sunlight-hating, computer-loving, coffee-drinking, carb-bingeing, pill-popping, climate-controlling humans of modern times have become fussy about soft mattresses, intolerant of other people and noise, and obsessed with packaging their sleep into one neurotic bundle. The difference between modern and caveman sleep, in other words, is like the difference between working in Dilbert's cubicle and roaming the savannah for the chance of a fresh kill.

More than most health and fitness fads, the Paleo movement takes history, evolutionary biology, and anthropology seriously; I was impressed to discover that these nonacademic "professional cavemen" had consulted many of the same sources about the science and culture of sleep as I had from my university perch. Like Ekirch and Siegel, Durant offers a vision of a default evolutionary sleep pattern for humans; unlike those scholars, though, he is part of a commercial enterprise that promises to reform modern society by selling products that are supposed to help humans escape the modern world's unnatural ways.

In the Paleo literature, "natural" sleep is presented, paradoxically, as something to be achieved through quintessentially modern, Western means: strict diets and daily plans, trips to the gym, and the right products. Paleo sleep, for all its nostalgia, needs to be rigidly scheduled—Sisson tells us that we must "follow consistent bed and wake times." And Paleo manuals rather shamelessly hawk such modern products as self-help books, exercise classes, training manuals, beauty products, T-shirts, action figures, cookbooks, cooking utensils, workout gear, and even amber-tinted glasses, which Paleo adherents wear in the evening, claiming they help them sleep better because they block out the blue light of computer screens. Sisson's book includes a link to a website where you can purchase sleep aids—like an eye mask to use when you can't achieve total primal darkness in your corrupted modern bedroom. And Durant recommends purchasing software packages to monitor the intensity of your screens, so that they don't emit too much blue light late in the evening; light boxes to simulate sunrise in your bedroom; and special alarm clocks that can measure your sleep cycles and wake you up at an optimal time in your sleep cycle. Sleeping like a caveman sounds more like a trip to a shopping mall for cyborgs.

One additional aspect of caveman sleep that the Paleo movement has not really addressed—the prolonged torpor associated with cold winters in extreme latitudes—is making a comeback in an unlikely place—if you can call outer space a place. Researchers at the National Aeronautics and Space Administration (NASA) and other interplanetary types have long sought a way to reduce the payload on spaceships and extend the period during which humans could safely travel while minimizing their need for supplies. The idea of induced hibernation—or, more precisely, prolonged torpor—has thus generated a great deal of research. But as we have seen, the human sleep-wake cycle is not like that of hibernating bears and squirrels. Our inability to hibernate has made it difficult to adapt to the food shortages and extreme cold weather of the polar regions of the planet: despite the adaptability of human circadian rhythms to changing environmental cues, prolonged states of suspended animation have never been possible. Now space agencies, scientific and medical researchers, and pharmaceutical and bioengineering firms are trying to push beyond what seemed like a species-based limitation to see if they can bring about the safe suspension of human consciousness.

The idea of hibernating one's way into the future has had a serious hold on the popular imagination for centuries. Ever since the 1771 publication of Louis-Sébastien Mercier's fantasy *Memoirs of the Year Two Thousand Five Hundred*, putting humans to sleep for long periods as a way to enable them to zoom into a new world has been a staple of fantasists and sci-fi writers. Washington Irving's "Rip Van Winkle," H. G. Wells's *When the Sleeper Awakes*, Edward Bellamy's *Looking Backward*, and Woody Allen's *Sleeper* are some of the better-known examples. The hit film *Interstellar* gave new impetus to the idea, with astronauts fleeing a climate-change-ravaged earth by strapping themselves into sleeping pods for a long voyage outward. Little is made in any of these works about the medical challenges of inducing, let alone maintaining, such a state: in *Interstellar*, the astronauts emerge a little groggy and disoriented, but really none the worse for wear.

But maybe crossing the evolutionary threshold and learning to hibernate can save humanity, or at least give us more reliable satellite networks for our smartphones. NASA and the European Space Agency (ESA) are understandably concerned with finding ways for humans to adapt to environmental conditions for which the course of evolution never prepared us. And they want to do it inexpensively. According to the ESA's website, the agency's Future Technology Advisory Panel has identified "TORPOR & HIBERNATION as a possibly game-changing technology for human spaceflight." The website adds: "It is conceivable that lowering the metabolic rate of Astronauts would not only lead to reduced consumption of air, water and food supplies, but it might also lead to a lower susceptibility to radiation damage." Drawing on medical research that has used hypothermia (lowered body temperature) to induce prolonged sleep-like states as a therapy for certain kinds of brain damage, the advisory panel is seeking to enable humans to enter extended states of suspended animation in order to make deep penetration into space.

David Dinges, a noted sleep researcher at the University of Pennsylvania, has examined the effects on circadian rhythms and cognitive functioning during prolonged space flight. In an ESA-funded project, MARS 500, in which astronauts inhabited a faux spaceship for 520 days, Dinges found that the crewmembers unknowingly and steadily decreased their activities and entered a state of what the researchers called "behavioral torpor." There are dangers associated with such states—but where some see risk, others see potential. NASA has also funded projects studying the health implications and cost-saving possibilities of prolonged space-flight torpor, including the design of *Interstellar*-like sleeping pods for insensate astronauts. One such project, developed by a company in my home town of Atlanta called Space Works, Inc., involved designing a template for an environment that would induce prolonged torpor in astronauts, who would be fed intravenously for up to six months on a manned mission to Mars.

Little progress has been made. Undeterred, however, researchers persist in the quest to make the human sleep-wake cycle more flexible than history and anthropology show us it already is. Kelly Drew, a hibernation researcher at the University of Alaska at Fairbanks, initially received US Army funding to study how prolonged states of torpor might benefit soldiers who have lost blood on the battlefield. In the wake of the terrorist attacks of 9/11, however, military funding went in other directions, and so she turned her attention to space, ultimately receiving a grant from the ESA to study . . . ground squirrels. How, she wanted to know, could squirrels' brains avoid damage when blood flow is reduced during hibernation? The trick, she found, was the interactions between a neuromodulator called adenosine and its receptor adenosine A1, which allow a squirrel's body and brain to cool to ambient temperature and then, as it rewarms, to regenerate synapses that might be lost during long periods of inactivity. "There are drugs that stimulate this in ground squirrels," she told me—and she is working to find out how to bring them safely to human trial.

So perhaps what we have seen in the past two hundred years is a small blip in the long history of sleep. Sleep, for most of human history, was social; it was generally distributed in several chunks throughout the day and night; and its duration and patterning varied greatly depending on the season, natural lighting, the availability of resources, and other environmental cues. Only since the industrial revolution has sleep become privatized, packaged into one standard time slot, and removed from nature's great rhythmic cycles of temperature and light. As these space-age explorations—and, on a different wavelength, such fads as the Paleo movement—portend, we might be entering an era that takes the variability of sleep even further, using new means to wrest control of our sleep patterns. In such a scenario, the unyielding routine of an eight-hour straight shot in a private, noise-free, climate-controlled bedroom will seem as quaint an artifact of the past as the hibernation of peasants in winter does now.

On a deeper level, the industrial age of sleep is only prelude to sleep's unevenly distributed futures. The will to tinker, to *engineer* sleep according to the dictates of industry, commerce, travel, and communication, will likely only grow more intense in the digital age, the space age, the cyborg age, or other emerging futures. Only, instead of a one-size-fits-all product—that mystical "natural" sleep that Nathaniel Kleitman sought in the depths of Mammoth Cave, or that historians and scientists alike seek in the records of the past—science, medicine, technology, and culture seem to be offering us new ways to package sleep in whatever forms we or our employers find most profitable. The age of normal sleep may be drawing to a close, and new technologies for optimizing the human body may be ushering in an age of customized or individually optimized sleep.

We'll explore some of the developments challenging the reign of "normal" sleep in the last chapter. But let's not get ahead of ourselves. There's still a lot of history to cover.

CHAPTER TWO

A Different Drummer

What happened to sleep in the industrialized world also happened, with particular intensity, to Henry David Thoreau. But unlike most nineteenth-century sleepers, Thoreau was, while awake, an astonishingly sensitive observer and recorder of changes to his environment both large and small and the human place within it. Along with such writers as Marcel Proust and Virginia Woolf, Thoreau is one of the great *noticers* in the history of world literature, one who could sense in such phenomena as ripples on the surface of water after a bug skates across it, or changes in the behavior of his countrymen after the railroad line comes through town, significant alterations of our physical, emotional, spiritual, and social landscapes. Whenever he mentions sleep and waking—and he does this with surprising frequency in his great work *Walden*—one can feel the earth turning and history moving. *Walden*, along with Thoreau's own personal story of battling the forces that were creating modern sleep, tells us as much as any book about the origins of sleep troubles in our times.

In *Walden*, Thoreau turned a private complaint into an act of personal liberation and a source of great insight, and that insight resonates today more powerfully than ever. The work is recognized as a masterpiece of environmental writing, one that continues to be of interest to casual readers, scholars, nature-lovers, and even

environmental scientists and climatologists. It is also a classic memoir, a story of heroic American individualism and nonconformity, of
absolute commitment to higher principles and of refusal to accept
society's demands for convenience's sake. What has been missed is
that the book provides an unusually vivid picture of an emerging
modern world in which the human sleep-wake cycle has been fundamentally damaged: people have forgotten both how to sleep and
how to be fully awake.

Throughout this famous work, Thoreau portrays his fellow
countrymen as being deranged by novel pressures and expectations
concerning sleep, to the point that the rhythms of their bodies are
completely out of sync with the rhythms of the natural world. The
residents of the world he left behind exhibit a panoply of sleep disturbances: chronic exhaustion, sleepwalking, frequent sleep interruptions, caffeine addiction, and an inability either to unwind or
to remain alert. The society's obsessive demands for high-speed
commerce, travel, and communication was running workers and
consumers alike into the ground. The restructuring of time was
wreaking havoc on the body's most elemental rhythms: "To be
awake is to be alive," Thoreau wrote, and yet he had "never yet met
a man who was quite awake."

That lack of wakefulness, or really a blurring of sleeping and
waking states, was not just a matter of individual well-being for
Thoreau. If you follow the sleep-waking thread in his work, you get
a remarkable account of how the most intimate, private behaviors
linked nineteenth-century sleepers to a world well beyond their
bedrooms: to industry, commerce, environmental damage, war, and
even slavery. Sleeping and waking, after all, are the totality of life:
reading Thoreau with this in mind flashes a brilliant light on how
our own sleep-wake cycles are affected by the great historical forces
that still shape our world today.

What Thoreau did about his own troubled sleep was to move to
a cabin that he built on the northeast shore of Walden Pond. In the
book, he lists many reasons for going: he wanted to live deliberately,
to front only the essential facts of existence, to suck the marrow
out of life, to live sturdily and Spartan-like, to know what is mean

and what is sublime, to conduct some private transactions with the woods. But apparently none of these activities could be undertaken if one was "overcome with drowsiness." Thoreau wanted to know what it was like to be truly awake, to be alive to the world. To do this, he had to remember how to sleep.

Walden was first published in 1854, and it chronicles the two years, two months, and two days that Thoreau spent in his cabin by the pond nearly a decade earlier. (In order to reflect the rhythm of the seasons, the book presents this sojourn as one year.) Yet it is not simply a historical record: it speaks with uncanny urgency to the present moment, because the problems he diagnosed have only grown deeper over the generations. Commercialism, materialism, infatuation with technology and speed—at the time called "the annihilation of time and space"—via a communications network fueled by new technologies (telegraphs, cheap printing technologies, railroads, and a postal network), all fueled a sense that too much of nineteenth-century life was being lived in an unnatural pursuit of acquisition and on a schedule that had nothing to do with the body's own rhythms. In prose that veers from acerbic satire to meditative rapture, *Walden* speaks powerfully to the origins of many of our contemporary sleep troubles, and it presents a more capacious way of thinking about the human sleep-wake cycle than the supposedly expert advice with which we are so frequently bombarded today.

Before we look more closely at Thoreau's ideas about sleeping and waking, though, it's useful to know how he arrived at them. Like many aspiring writers and nonconformists, the young Thoreau kept strange hours. Partly this was a matter of preference: he loved moonlit walks through the woods, the shine of still water reflecting the starry sky, the serene sounds of whippoorwills and owls, the sight of fireflies, the subdued tones of the landscape. But biology shouldn't be ruled out: his body's incapacity to shut down when it was supposed to would likely be called a sleep disorder today.

The trouble started when he was small: his mother would often find Henry up late, staring out the window. He began to worry that he had a hereditary condition; as he wrote in his famous book, he suspected that his "lethargy" was connected to a "family complaint":

his uncle, for instance, "goes to sleep shaving himself." Matters worsened when Thoreau experienced health problems and emotional troubles. He contracted tuberculosis in college and relapsed on several occasions, with coughing fits that kept him up late. During one of his periods of good health, his brother, John (also tubercular), died in his arms after contracting tetanus from a shaving cut. In the wake of this tragedy, Henry worked a series of jobs—teaching, tutoring, helping to run his family's pencil-making factory—but he found trying to abide by a strict schedule of waking up on time every morning impossibly taxing. Fine particles from the factory's graphite mill aggravated his coughing attacks, which worsened his sleep, and he was beset by worries about his future, fearing failure as a writer. He felt himself running down. As he wrote in his journal: "I am a diseased bundle of nerves standing between time and eternity like a withered leaf." He was wracked by insomnia and chronic fatigue, an infirmity so profound that it became almost impossible for him to read or write.

Concord, Massachusetts, was undergoing a startling transformation during Thoreau's boyhood in the 1820s and 1830s. At the turn of the nineteenth century, this storied site of one of the first Revolutionary War battles was a small hub for farmers and tradesmen, with only about two hundred households. But as new roads were laid connecting the town to Boston and other commercial centers, and new technologies took hold, the way of life began to change. By the time Thoreau left to live in the woods in 1845, there were still farmers and cabinetmakers, but also now water- and steam-powered mills that enabled new industries to spring up, including a lead pipe factory, a steam-driven smithy, two gristmills, two sawmills, a cotton mill, and six warehouses. The factories were nowhere near the scale of the textile mills in nearby Lowell, but the industrial economy slowly began to change certain basic features of town life. Patterns of work and rest were less tethered to seasonal changes or the weather. The clattering of machinery and the increased bustle of trade created new kinds of sounds. Other rhythmical and regular sounds, like birdcall, receded as the canopy of forest decreased and was eventually almost completely cleared. Strangers came and

went, doing new kinds of business and bringing new cultural practices, new patterns of conversation, even new religions. By the time
Thoreau was in his twenties, passengers could arrive by train on
the new railroads. The railroads also allowed for more efficient and
widespread sale of factory-made goods. As these changes quickened
the pace of life and increased the level of noise, they challenged old
sleep patterns. New expectations emerged to conform one's life to a
rigid schedule, and there was a new sense that one had to live one's
life in a hurry.

Nineteenth-century sleep was beginning to change. We saw evidence in the previous chapter that people in some traditional rural
communities used to sleep longer in the winter than in the summer, storing up calories, conserving body heat, and responding to
a diminished need for labor. But with factory bells ringing at the
same time every morning to call workers to the factory floor as the
machines were powered up, sleeping in was no longer a possibility for many nineteenth-century Concordians. Midday naps became
less frequent and came to be seen as a sign of indolence. Adding
to the pressure to develop regular sleep schedules was the increasing number of parents who worked outside of the home and the
development of compulsory education for children. Rising wealth
from the industrial economy allowed middle-class homes to become
larger, with the once-unthinkable prospect of separate bedrooms for
children starting to take hold. Slowly, sleep was becoming a private
and regulated activity: something one was ashamed of doing in public, at odd hours, or entangled with bodies other than a spouse's.

Changes such as those don't happen all at once—they come
haltingly, at different rates, and in different sequences in different
places. In Concord, the Thoreau family was experiencing many of
the changes that were transforming the broader economy of the
Western world. When Henry was young, his father, John Thoreau,
moved the family around greater Boston as he followed a series of
odd jobs: painting signs, selling groceries, and peddling ardent spirits. But in 1823, six years after his youngest son was born, he moved
the family back to Concord in order to take over a pencil factory
that his brother-in-law, Charles Dunbar, had founded with a partner

but had proven too erratic to maintain. It was a modest start for an aspiring industrialist. The factory never made the family rich, but it secured them a measure of comfort and stability. Henry would contribute to the family business as an inventor, engineer, and manager intermittently throughout his young adulthood; factories were a fact of life that structured his expectations about work, commerce, and daily rhythms. When he wrote in *Walden* that he wished people could be "awakened by . . . Genius" rather than by "factory bells" and other "mechanical aids," he was drawing on personal experience that reflected a broad economic and social shift.

The precise schedule of work in the Thoreau pencil factory is unknown, but it's safe to assume that it was not as labor-intensive and exhausting as the work at the famous Lowell Mills and other nearby factories. Newspaper reports were already exposing the dangers and health risks of thirteen- and fourteen-hour shifts, particularly for the mills' female factory workers, who complained of chronic lack of sleep. "The labor of the southern female slave is neither so hard," read one article, "or so wearing upon the constitution as the burdens imposed upon the factory operative of the north." But the comparatively light industry of pencil-making still required discipline, steadiness, and regular hours of labor. Interestingly, one of the reasons that Thoreau's father took over the factory from the cofounder, Henry's uncle, was that Charles apparently had a severe sleep disorder. In addition to falling asleep while shaving, he was on several occasions found knocked out cold during odd hours at the kitchen table. Regular hours, early rising: these were virtues preached in sermons, advice and etiquette books, and—increasingly—in medical texts. Although they powered the new industrial economy, several of the Thoreaus had trouble adhering to them.

Other aspects of sleep and waking were little changed in the Concord of Thoreau's youth. Coal didn't become commercially available there until the 1830s, and so on cold nights the family warmed their beds with warming pans. (Later, in college at Harvard, Thoreau was given a cannonball to warm in his dorm room's fireplace; it was then transferred to an iron skillet where it would radiate heat through the night.) Gas light was mainly available for the rich, and while Thoreau was living at home his family still used candles. In this dim light, there was relatively little inducement to stay up late. Railroads—and the accelerated pace of life that came with them—didn't reach Concord until 1844, a year before he departed for Walden. And family members still often shared sleeping space to a degree that would be unimaginable a few generations later.

As a youth Henry shared a trundle bed with his brother John: his parents rolled it out from under their own four-poster bed on casters every night. John was long-limbed, angular, and a sound sleeper. Their bed was a simple, Spartan affair, padded only with blankets rather than a straw or feather mattress. Parents did not typically make much fuss about bedtimes, as there was little inducement to stay up late in the dim light. They were generally advised not to give children beds that were too comfortable, lest they become used to them and thereby spoiled for other sleeping arrangements when they traveled. Despite its hardness, the real warmth and comfort that John and Henry's bed provided was the intimate contact of the two boys' bodies, with the psychological security of the parents sleeping in the same room. That stiff bed must have seemed a refuge from a chaotic nighttime world, for the Thoreaus began to take in boarders when Henry was about ten. Short-term business visitors needed somewhere to stay, so many families opened their doors, charging for rooms by the week. Typically, boarders shared bedrooms, sometimes even beds, and ate in common meal areas. Not unlike today's Airbnb, such arrangements allowed families of modest means to make some extra money, which they used to keep up larger and better-appointed houses than they would have otherwise been able to afford. Thoreau's sister, complaining about the atmosphere at home in her diary, said the noise and hubbub were enough to make one want to live on an uninhabited island, oddly prefiguring her brother's trek off to solitude at Walden Pond. Indeed, Thoreau himself wrote of his desire to sleep alone: "I think I had rather keep a batchelor's hall in hell than go to board in heaven. . . . The boarder has no home." Such imposed group sleeping seemed to impel a desire to sleep alone, a not insignificant component of Thoreau's famous individualism.

In addition to trying to shut out the noise from boarders, Henry, two years younger than John, was forced to find a comfortable position as his bigger brother shifted in the night. Unsurprisingly, he was often restless in bed. One time when he was a young child, his mother, bringing a candle into the room, found him awake in the middle of the night staring out at the stars. "Why, Henry dear, don't you go to sleep?" she asked him. He may have had trouble sleeping, but the wakefulness itself evoked a memory of tranquility. "Mother," he replied, "I have been looking through the stars to see if I could see God behind them." (Insomnia as a cause of transcendental moonshine has been infrequently diagnosed.)

And so despite the morning peal of factory bells, the clatter of carts and machines, and the economic changes that were affecting his family's schedule, Henry grew up in a world where people slept pretty much the same way their ancestors had, which was pretty much the same way people still sleep today in many traditional communities around the world. Despite the challenges of sleeping in the clamorous Thoreau boardinghouse, the night for him was enchanted, and sleeping was a social activity undertaken in close contact with other bodies. He both gravitated toward that security of contact during sleep and found himself longing for isolation, a way to slip out of the social world and fall into himself.

Private sleeping—one child to a bed, or, at most, two consenting adults, and one bed in each room (or, at most, two for children sharing a room)—has become a hallmark of Western bourgeois life (as will be explored in depth in Chapter Five). But sleeping was a social activity in the Thoreau household, as it still is in much of the world. The brothers' bond was thicker than that experienced by many siblings in middle-class homes today, and one likely factor is their close bodily contact through the night. When John and Henry reached adolescence and early adulthood, they continued their almost conjoined nighttime relationship. On outdoor adventures, they camped out together under the open stars, sharing a buffalo-hide blanket in a tent of their own making. They briefly opened a school together. They even fell in love with the same woman, each proposing to her and each in turn getting rejected. The two brothers were both tubercular, perhaps having contracted the disease in the close board-inghouse atmosphere of their childhood home, and their bouts of coughing likely woke each other up.

A final, and tragic, intimacy came when John died of tetanus in 1842; afterward, Henry, twenty-five years old at the time, developed sympathetic symptoms of lockjaw and went into an emotional tail-spin. While he was living at Walden Pond, three years after John's death, he wrote his first book, *A Week on the Concord and Merrimack Rivers*, about a trip he had taken with John in 1839, dedicating it to "my Muse, my Brother." "Whenever we awoke in the night, still eking out our dreams with half-awakened thoughts," he wrote, "it was not till after an interval, when the wind breathed harder than usual, flapping the curtains of the tent, and causing its cords to vibrate, that we remembered that we lay on the bank of the Mer-rimack, and not in our chamber at home." With their heads on the bare earth, they listened to the river "whirling and sucking, and laps-ing downward, kissing the shore as it went," and to the wind rustling the oaks and hazels "like an inconsiderate person up at midnight, moving about, and putting things to rights." But then, as the wind died away, "we like it fell asleep again." From his shared nocturnal experience with John, he learned that the night might be his com-panion, full of sounds and clues and meanings.

What started as nearly a fused identity in the Thoreau broth-ers' childhood nights remained an emotional bond unmatched by any other in either brother's life. But since Thoreau's time, such a nighttime bond has become almost unthinkable. By the late nine-teenth century, as middle-class houses grew larger, more and more families chose to put children in separate bedrooms. Thoreau him-self came to be a solitary sleeper, although at Walden his sleep was still a kind of intimate communion with his surrounding world, not a retreat from it. Some might have considered his stay at Walden Pond a lonely endeavor, but, as he wrote, solitude was an excellent companion. He had the sounds of the woods to wake to, owls and tree frogs at night. And though he was alone, the night was good for reverie about his lost sleeping companion. On the lift-top green writing table in his cabin by the pond, he memorialized the nights shared with his brother: "Perhaps at midnight one was awakened by a cricket shrilly singing on his shoulder, or by a hunting spider in his eye, and was lulled asleep again by some streamlet purling its way along at the bottom of a wooded and rocky ravine. . . . It was pleasant to lie with our heads so low in the grass, and hear what a tinkling ever-busy laboratory it was." On these trips with John, even disturbed or broken sleep seemed natural—a responsiveness to crickets and creatures burrowing in the grass rather than some kind of disorder. To be a writer, he imagined in this early work, was to be so attuned to the rhythms of the natural world that one would practically hibernate in winter: "The poet is he that hath fat enough, like bears and marmots, to suck his claws all winter. He hibernates in this world, and feeds on his own marrow." Even when the two brothers took refuge in a boardinghouse, Thoreau felt free to follow his own poetic hours: long after everyone else retired, he frequently stayed up by an open window listening to the river.

Despite these interludes of sleeping in nature, before Thoreau set out for Walden he had to learn how to make his sleeping and waking patterns conform to the demands of society. As a young man, he had ambitions, and his family had ambitions for him. First among these was to go to Harvard College, which he did in 1833. He was not a top student, but he showed flashes of brilliance, and among those brilliant episodes was a graduation-day speech he gave on the subject of "The Commercial Spirit of Modern Times." He spoke of telegraph lines and railroads crisscrossing the continent and quickening the pace of life. "Man thinks faster and freer than ever before," he proclaimed. "He, moreover, moves faster and freer. He is more restless, because he is more independent than ever." At this point in his life, he spoke of such developments with raw excitement, perhaps because he saw them mainly in the abstract. But he also had plans; he wanted to get somewhere fast.

His body, however, wouldn't cooperate with the tempo of the times. His first bout of tuberculosis had forced a withdrawal from Harvard in the spring of his sophomore year. Tuberculosis was, in fact, a check on the fast-paced life indicated in Henry's speech. Contagion spread in close quarters among factory workers, which accounts for the epidemic spread of a disease that was the leading killer in Massachusetts and that took the lives of many in Thoreau's family, including his grandfather's, his father's, his sister's, and ultimately his own. And it spread as well in such cramped and poorly ventilated spaces as college dormitories and boardinghouses. Tuberculosis, or consumption, as it was called, was considered a "disease of civilization," spurring many sufferers to seek restoration in nature. Because the cause was unknown, it inspired a kind of paranoia about improper management of the body, which led many sufferers to subject the minute details of diet, exercise, and sleeping and waking to new scrutiny.

Thoreau's tuberculosis was bad enough that several relatives advised him to quit school; nonetheless, he returned to finish, taking the common medical advice that frequent outdoor trips would improve his health. Trips to the country and the woods with friends planted the idea of a different way of life that might be more healthful and satisfying. But after he graduated, with the disease likely in a period of remission, he moved back with his family in Concord and set about making himself useful. He did several stints as a schoolteacher, including one in a school that he ran with his brother—but they had to close it down when John's health declined. As a fallback, he continued to work in the family pencil factory. One rarely thinks about Thoreau in this way, but he had significant talent as an industrial engineer: he invented a machine to grind graphite in such a way that, when mixed with German clay (a mixture he also developed), the lead would adhere better to the grooves in the pencil wood, without snapping. The result was the finest line of pencils America had yet produced, which became preferred by artists, teachers, architects, surveyors, and engineers. Dust from the graphite mill exacerbated his respiratory problems, and his chronic fatigue made the schedule of tending to the factory ultimately too grueling for him. Fortunately, he had attracted the attention of an established figure in the literary firmament—Ralph Waldo Emerson—who in 1841 invited Thoreau to live in his family's well-appointed home in exchange for doing odd jobs around the house and in the garden. The great writer enjoyed Thoreau's fascinating conversation.

Thoreau was beginning to explore his long-held ambition of becoming a writer, but John's death in his arms, in 1842, nearly sent him over the edge. First he suffered sympathetic symptoms of lock-jaw, refusing food and conversation for weeks, staring at the ceiling, not reading or writing, and of course sleeping poorly. Gradually he grew out of his melancholia and began to read seriously in Emerson's library (which had volumes from all over the world—from ancient Greek philosophy to Hindu mystical tracts). In time he recovered his health somewhat and returned to taking long walks and, in winter, skating on Concord's ponds. He was writing seriously for the first time, and Emerson thought he should go to New York to make some publishing contacts. To that end, he secured for Thoreau a position tutoring his brother's children in Staten Island.

It was a disaster, on all counts. Thoreau didn't get along well with his main pupil, William Emerson's oldest son. He couldn't abide by the strict routines: breakfast at 6:30, lunch at noon, dinner at 5. He failed to impress any editors in New York enough to gain regular magazine work. Like many an idealistic aspiring writer, he was dismayed by the artificial way of life and frenetic pace of the city. Unsurprisingly, his health and mental state again began to falter. When he received news that a close college friend had died, he developed insomnia so severe that reading and writing became almost impossible. "I must confess," he wrote in his journal, "there is nothing so strange to me as my own body. I love any other piece of nature, almost better." For someone who, despite bouts of illness, had always been considered vigorous, for whom long walks in the woods were one of life's great pleasures, this was a calamitous realization.

Thoreau retreated to Concord to work in the pencil factory. But he also began planning a personal liberation from modern life and its pressures: the pressure to work on someone else's schedule; the pressure to earn, spend, and consume; the pressure to accept social convention; the pressure to make something of oneself. And, not insignificantly, the pressure to wake up when others demanded, to ignore both his internal timekeeper and the pulsating rhythms of the natural world in favor of the dull, regular rhythms of the clock and the factory.

Emerson had recently bought a plot of land along Walden Pond, and he agreed to let his promising young friend try out an experiment in literary self-discovery there. And so after purchasing boards and nails and borrowing an axe, Thoreau built his little cabin in the woods. In his time many people turned to drugs—opium, bromides, caffeine (cocaine would come a few decades later)—to pull their bodies into rhythm. Some of the most extreme cases of fatigue, insomnia, and other varieties of unruly sleep even wound up in insane asylums, where (as we will see in the next chapter) sleep was regulated more thoroughly than perhaps in any other nineteenth-century location. Today we have more precise chemical means of manipulating our rhythms; we have greater expertise in monitoring the problems, and more specialized medical clinics and technologies for observing and correcting disordered sleep. But in shrugging off this impending future—our present—Thoreau gave himself over to the erratic rhythms of his own body to see where they would lead him.

———

Once Thoreau stopped fighting his sleep patterns, he entered a period of astonishing creativity and lucidity. In a way, his abnormal sleep-wake cycle enabled him to produce some of the most powerful poetic prose ever to emanate from an American writer. On July 4, 1845, he moved into his cabin, where he declared his own independence not just from his society, but in a way from time itself. He left behind his clock, but he brought along a wagon full of furniture, some of which he had made himself: three chairs, a three-legged table, a writing desk, and a thin hardwood bed—he had carved its maple legs and stretched out its rattan cane bottom. The rattan slats came from palm trees, likely imported from China by a Concord importer. So in his little retreat, snug in bed, he was supported in part by the global trade, which was powered by new industrial wealth. Ironically, in stepping aside from the modern world and its commercial values, he slept on an artifact of that world.

The cabin itself was not exactly in the wilderness, or even in a frontier outpost. His neighbors included geese and wildflowers, but there were also a few vagrants squatting nearby. His neighbors included several poor Irish families and free blacks—at least one of them had escaped from slavery. The cabin was less than two miles from town, which he visited regularly to get "homeopathic" doses of civilization: the sights and sounds of workers going about their business, carts rattling, villagers reading the newspaper aloud or gossiping at the post office. Even back at his cabin, he was not completely isolated from the outside world. Workers passed through his retreat, most notably in the winter, when they came to cut sheets of ice from the pond to bring to market. And he had frequent visitors, friends and family members who sat in his three wooden chairs and engaged him in long, boundaryless conversations. Sometimes his mother brought him pies. On one famous occasion, he found himself back in town involuntarily, when he was hauled off to the Concord jail for refusing to pay his taxes, which went to support the Mexican War, an American land-grab that he and many others saw as upholding the interests of slaveholders.

But no reminder of the modern world's proximity was more potent than the trains that passed less than half a mile from his cabin. The Boston-to-Fitchburg line had been extended as far as Concord just a year before Thoreau began his experiment of living by the pond. The very boards used to make his cabin were purchased from an Irish railroad worker who had left his cabin for work further up the line. The train, shrieking through the valley, occasioned some of Thoreau's most impassioned writing. He felt he was witnessing the birth of a new god, a mechanical beast that stomped through the hills, throwing him out of bed with its violent reverberations: "I hear the iron horse make the hills echo with snort like thunder, shaking the earth with his feet, and breathing fire and smoke from his nostrils. . . . All day the fire-steed flies over the country, stopping only that his master may rest, and I am awakened by his tramp and defiant snort."

That mechanical beast, which traveled "without rest or slumber" and awakened people at odd hours, signaled the coming of a new economic order that depended on a new structuring of time. Railroads, which served the new factories by speeding up the delivery of raw materials and then rushed the finished products to distant markets, played an important role in the changing conceptions of time that were taking place in the nineteenth century.

A great problem facing the new railway companies was how to make sure everyone knew when the trains would be arriving and departing. Certainly, measuring time was nothing new: from sundials, hourglasses, and devices that dripped water in regular intervals, mechanical means of timekeeping had existed since antiquity. Even wheeled clocks—wound by hand or water-driven—were a fairly ancient technology, probably dating back to thirteenth-century monasteries, where daily schedules were subject to strict regimentation long before anyone ever worked in a factory. But the development of an industrial way of life brought timekeeping into new prominence, especially as it pertained to regularizing labor. And setting those clocks precisely was an especially difficult and pressing problem in an era of high-speed travel. For centuries, timepieces had been calibrated to the rising and falling of the sun, which meant that as you moved thirty or forty miles to the east or west, your clock would need to be reset. But if a train heading from Boston to Fitchburg was supposed to arrive at Concord heading west at 7:19, whose 7:19 would prevail?

At first, railroads set their clocks by the location of the railway's headquarters, but synchronizing workers and passengers in far-flung places to this standard proved nearly impossible. National standardized time zones would be developed in the 1910s, but well before that, railway companies took the lead in establishing regional standards for setting the clocks. All sorts of ingenious means were used to promote temporal conformity, from the dropping of balls in town squares (a ritual that is still with us on New Year's Eve celebrations) to the practice among telegraph companies of selling subscriptions to hourly readings of the correct time to businesses and private homes. As the historian Michael O'Malley put it, in this way, time itself became a commodity, "a thing identifiable, quantifiable, packagable, and saleable."

The overwhelming feeling one gets when reading *Walden* is one of repose. Time pulses through every chapter, but its rhythms are patterned mainly by the rising and falling of the sun and the change in seasons. And yet when the trains hurtle through its pages, they shake Thoreau out of his meditative state, jolting him into a different kind of jagged alertness—one more attuned to the rhythms of the industrialized social world that he had ostensibly left behind. Part of Thoreau's project of living by the pond and writing *Walden* was to understand more fully what such shocks to the system were doing to him and to his society. He thought a good deal about the effects of the trains on his fellow citizens' sense of time. Some of the effects were positive: "The startings and arrivals of the cars are now the epochs in the village day," he wrote. He noticed a new punctuality: the need to arrive at the station precisely on time created a kind of temporal discipline that had never before been necessary. The trains, he noted, "go and come with such regularity and precision, and their whistle can be heard so far, that the farmers set their clocks by them, and thus one well-conducted institution regulates a whole country. Have not men improved somewhat in punctuality since the railroad was invented?"

But railroad time also created a frantic panorama of people scrambling to adjust, stringing their minds and bodies tight under the new pressures of clock time. Even as railway companies promoted standardized time, for riders, the ability of the speeding train to collapse physical space led to a profoundly disorienting experience. It was as if time were melting, giving passengers a sense of becoming unmoored, of exhilarating hurtling. Thoreau's contemporary Nathaniel Hawthorne captured the experience in his 1851 novel *The House of the Seven Gables*, as two elderly passengers ride a train for the first time: "Everything was unfixed from its age-long rest, and moving at whirlwind speed in a direction opposite to their own." The old man, Clifford, is moved to exclaim: "I have never been awake before!"

In *Walden*, Thoreau points to another frightening dimension of the railroad's effect on daily rhythms of sleep and waking. In a famous passage that begins as a pun about railroad "sleepers" (the wooden ties that support the rails), he crescendos to an indictment of a technology-mad society that cares little for the collateral damage its machines leave in their wake:

We do not ride on the railroad; it rides upon us. Did you ever think what those sleepers are that underlie the railroad? Each one is a man, an Irishman, or a Yankee man. The rails are laid on them, and they are covered with sand, and the cars run smoothly over them. They are sound sleepers, I assure you. And every few years a new lot is laid down and run over; so that if some have the pleasure of riding on a rail, others have the misfortune to be ridden upon. And when they run over a man that is walking in his sleep, a supernumerary sleeper in the wrong position, and wake him up, they suddenly stop the cars, and make a hue and cry about it, as if this were an exception.

The "sound sleepers" living under the rails are men, presumably workers who build the railroad only to find that "the rails are laid on them." The implication may seem simply that some can afford to ride the rails while others must build them, but Thoreau is clear that this is not simply a critique of labor exploitation. His "us" is broadly inclusive: "We do not ride on the railroad; it rides upon us." When the train runs over an unfortunate sleepwalker, it is news. But in fact, no one is "quite awake" in his contemporary world, as he explained earlier, and the violence of the railroad extends to everyone: there are no exceptions.

As with so much of Thoreau's writing, these passages work both as a wildly imaginative metaphor and also as a careful, literal description. On the one hand, the railway and its "sleepers" are a metaphor for the modern condition of mechanized, routine labor: a life, as he put it, in which "men have become tools of their tools." But at another level, Thoreau is arguing quite literally that the modern age of machinery is creating severe risks. As the train comes whipping through the woods, it wakes all who slumber within earshot; the result is sleep deprivation, a deranged sense of time, and ultimately a nation of sleepwalking citizens. One might wander across the tracks only to be crushed. Thoreau is sounding a warning note that would reverberate across governmental reports, industry exposés, and medical advice books all the way up to our time.

Half a century after Thoreau wrote *Walden*, a spate of railway accidents led the US Congress to investigate railway worker fatigue. Union activist Henry Fuller testified, "It seems almost beyond belief that a man who has been a railroad man for years will absolutely sit down on the track and go to sleep, when he knows that another train is liable to come along and kill him, but they will do it. . . . When a man goes without sleep a certain length of time, he is not responsible for what he does." The problem extended well beyond railroad work. Sleep deprivation, wrote psychologist Stanley Coren in his popular 1976 book *Sleep Thieves*, is "a danger to the general public because of the probability that a sleepy individual might cause a catastrophic accident." Sleep deprivation has been blamed for such high-profile industrial and transportation accidents as the Chernobyl nuclear meltdown, the Exxon Valdez oil spill, and the *Challenger* space shuttle disaster, as well as less spectacular but more systemic problems such as loss of worker productivity, impaired memory, and increased health and emotional problems. In other words, we have been walking across Thoreau's tracks in a daze now for over a century and a half.

––––––

In Thoreau's time, as ours, people increasingly responded to the hazards of the new tempo of work and rest by fueling themselves with caffeine, primarily in the form of coffee. The Thoreau household was strikingly coffee-averse, as his mother reportedly eliminated coffee from the household budget in order to pay for piano lessons for Thoreau's sister, Sophia. When Henry was courting Ellen Sewall—the young woman who had formed an attachment to him as well as to his brother John—one of his tokens of affection was a letter about the perils of coffee. (Whether this lecture to her confirms the speculation that he never really had any interest in courting women is beyond the scope of this investigation.) Throughout his career, Thoreau exhibited a love-hate—mostly hate—relationship with coffee. "Like many of my contemporaries," he wrote, "I had rarely for many years used animal food, or tea, or coffee, etc.; not so much because of any ill effects which I had traced to them, as because they were not agreeable to my imagination." And "Think of dashing the hopes of a morning with a cup of warm coffee, or of an evening with a dish of tea!" Yet occasionally he did succumb to the allure of caffeine. He wrote of a muscular, simple-yet-wise Canadian woodchopper who passed by his cabin in the woods for conversation and who carried with him a supply of "coffee in a stone bottle which dangled by a string from his belt; and sometimes he offered me a drink." The effects of caffeine on this vital man seem not to have diminished his natural hardiness, for when Thoreau asked him if he was "sometimes tired at night, after working all day," he cursed quaintly: "Gorrappit, I never was tired in my life." One gathers from this exchange that the offer of coffee from the stone bottle was accepted; yet later Thoreau wrote of the feelings of self-loathing that followed consuming such stimulants: "Ah, how low I fall when I am tempted by them!"

We tend to think of obsession with coffee as a new phenomenon, one that sprang up with the emergence of chains like Starbucks with shops on practically every corner of city streets and in every suburban strip mall. But coffee has a long history, which had reached a jittery high point in Thoreau's time. The first people who used coffee appear to have been the Oromo people of territory now incorporated into Ethiopia, who ground it together with animal fat as a staple of their diet. The Sufis of today's Yemen were the first to use it in beverage form to help them stay alert, particularly during their evening devotionals. From there it spread through the Arab world, where it was celebrated as a mentally stimulating yet sobering drink—an appropriate beverage in a part of the world that renounced alcohol and developed much of modern mathematics. Via trade routes through Turkey in the seventeenth century, coffee eventually reached Europe, and by the turn of the next century a European coffee mania was taking hold.

Coffee was celebrated as a wonder drug that promoted a range of physical and mental benefits: it could cure colic and dropsy, aid in digestion, fortify the liver, regulate the appetite, and serve both as a sleep aid and a wakefulness extender. By 1700 there were three thousand coffeehouses in London alone; it is no accident that some of the greatest works of eighteenth-century Enlightenment philosophy and literature were composed in these centers of intellectual and political activity. Fueled by this new stimulating drug, the men of the Enlightenment (women typically weren't allowed in the coffee-houses) helped fashion a new style of thinking, a new political ethos, and new forms of artistic expression, all of which were marked by hyperrationality, attentiveness to evidence, and sociability. As literary scholar Roger Schmidt argues, the public orientation of eighteenth-century intellectual life would have been nearly unthinkable earlier, when public houses serving wine and beer rather than caffeinated beverages were the dominant gathering places.

New cultural forms arose from this chemically and socially stimulating environment. One of them was journalism: Richard Steele, editor of *The Tattler*, categorized news according to which coffee-house it was gathered in, and he gave the paper's address as the coffeehouse of the Grecian. Long novels became popular: reading works by Henry Fielding and Samuel Richardson required heroic feats of extended consciousness fueled by coffee. At around the same time, Johann Sebastian Bach composed "Wachet Auf," or "Sleepers Awake," as well as "The Coffee Cantata," just as coffee was threatening to displace beer as the most popular beverage in Germany. And, according to Schmidt, the rise of coffee in Europe came with a cultural devaluation of sleep. Alexander Pope's "The Rape of the Lock," for instance, uses drowsiness as a metaphor for cultural collapse and celebrates coffee for keeping the senses alert.

There is, of course, a darker side to the history of this stimulant. Like sugar, cotton, and rubber, coffee was a staple of colonialism and New World slavery. By 1788, San Domingo (today's Haiti) supplied nearly half of the world's coffee; the coffee beans that gave Voltaire, Rousseau, and Diderot the energy to write their treatises on intellectual and political liberties were harvested by slaves laboring under some of the most brutal conditions imaginable. "I do not know if coffee and sugar are essential to the happiness of Europe," wrote a French traveler who was horrified by the conditions he saw in the Caribbean, "but I know well that these two products have accounted for the unhappiness of two great regions of the world:

America has been depopulated so as to have land on which to plant them; Africa has been depopulated so as to have the people to cultivate them." Thoreau's mentor, Emerson, commented acerbically on these networks of violence and commodification in an 1844 antislavery speech. "The sugar they raised was excellent," he wrote of West Indian planters; "nobody tasted blood in it. The coffee was fragrant; the tobacco was incense; the brandy made nations happy; the cotton clothed the world. What! all raised by these men, and no wages? Excellent! What a convenience!"

Although Thoreau was a more committed antislavery activist than Emerson, his rejection of coffee was primarily a matter of his hatred of wasteful expense and his notions about health. By the nineteenth century, health reformers and writers realized that many of the earlier claims about coffee's salubrious properties had been overblown, and new concerns arose. Commentators were complaining that too much coffee ate away at the stomach's lining, disturbed sleep, and caused irritability and a host of other mental ailments.

One of the most famous coffee-drinkers of the nineteenth century, French novelist Honoré de Balzac, reportedly drank anywhere from twenty to fifty cups of coffee per day. He claimed that enormous amounts of "finely pulverized, dense coffee," which he swallowed without adding water, on an empty stomach, inspired his work. He acknowledged that the health risks were severe, as the habit "brutalizes the stomach linings." But he believed the intellectual payoff was worth it: with caffeine, "sparks shoot all the way to the brain," and "from that moment on, everything becomes agitated": "Ideas quick-march into motion like battalions of a grand army to its legendary fighting ground, and the battle rages. Memories charge in, bright flags on high; the cavalry of metaphor deploys with a magnificent gallop; the artillery of logic rushes up with clattering wagons and cartridges; on imagination's orders, sharpshooters sight and fire; forms and shapes and characters rear up; the paper is spread with ink." This extreme intake allowed him to write for fourteen to sixteen hours a day, yielding seventeen volumes of his masterpiece *La Comédie Humaine* within a six-year period. Balzac's work is, in a sense, the opposite of his contemporary Thoreau's: its urban settings swarm with people on the move, on the make, in a hurry. Thoreau's praise of slowness, idling, and release from the social weave would make a coffee fiend like Balzac bounce off the walls. "Of all ebriosity," Thoreau wrote in one of his anti-coffee bromides, "who does not prefer to be intoxicated by the air he breathes?" The answer would be Balzac, who is rumored to have died from his massive caffeine intake. (For the curious, you can now take a test online to see how much coffee will kill you. In my case, apparently 128.5 shots of espresso in a day would do the trick.)

Thoreau was not just concerned about the health effects or the unnatural patterns of thought that coffee produced. To drink coffee was to create a craving that could only enslave the drinker in a cycle of spending and consuming. His encounter with the Irish immigrant farmer John Field one rainy afternoon sums up his protest against this cycle. Field, who worked himself to exhaustion each day by "bogging" his neighbor's field in order to support his family, is—according to Thoreau—enslaved not by poverty or prejudice, but by his reliance on artificial stimulation. Thoreau tells him,

I did not use tea, nor coffee, nor butter, nor milk, nor fresh meat, and so did not have to work to get them; again, as I did not work hard, I did not have to eat hard, and it cost me but a trifle for my food; but as he began with tea, and coffee, and butter, and milk, and beef, he had to work to pay for them, and when he had worked hard, he had to eat hard to repair the waste of his system . . . and yet he had rated it as a gain in coming to America, that here you could get tea, and coffee, and meat every day. But the only true America is that country where you are at liberty to pursue such a mode of life as may enable you to do without these, and where the state does not endeavor to compel you to sustain the slavery and war and other superfluous expenses which directly or indirectly result from the use of such things.

Thoreau doesn't come off particularly well in this exchange: he is self-righteous, hectoring, and remarkably dismissive of a hard-working man who simply wants some comforts in his life (and at least a little racist to boot: when his arguments fail to take hold, he sniffs that "the culture of an Irishman is an enterprise to be undertaken with a sort of moral bog hoe"). John Field's wife certainly doesn't take the harangue well. As soon as the rain stops, this mother of "several children" discreetly cuts off the lecture offered by this peculiar highfalutin idler and urges her husband back to work: "You'd better go now, John."

And yet there is something quite remarkable about Thoreau's compact analysis of the relationships among consumerism, commodities, labor, violence, coercion, and the body's energy. Field had come to America because here you could "get tea, and coffee, and meat every day." But he finds himself trapped in a system—a "false" America—that "compels" him to want these things as a way of sustaining slavery and war. "Slavery" meant both chattel slavery and the indentured servitude (like Field's) that made such products available on the cheap, as well as a psychological dependence bordering on a physical addiction for those very substances. Thoreau believed that a vicious cycle of craving and "waste" had set in: without the products that the body toiled to secure, the laborer would not have the needed energy reserves to do the labor necessary to support the system.

Coffee made the system go. But it wasn't just a matter of keeping manual laborers sufficiently fueled. Neural jolts became pleasurable in and of themselves, and a craving for them permeated the culture. Life in the "restless, nervous, bustling, trivial nineteenth century" was punctuated by micro-sleeps and compulsive, caffeinated awakenings. Earlier I quoted Thoreau's rumination that began with "Hardly a man takes a half-hour's nap after dinner, but when he wakes he holds up his head and asks, 'What's the news?' as if the rest of mankind had stood his sentinels." He continues: "Some give directions to be waked every half-hour, doubtless for no other purpose; and then, to pay for it, they tell what they have dreamed. After a night's sleep the news is as indispensable as the breakfast. 'Pray tell me anything new that has happened to a man anywhere on this globe,'—and he reads it over his coffee and rolls, that a man has had his eyes gouged out this morning on the Wachito River; never dreaming the while that he lives in the dark unfathomed mammoth cave of this world, and has but the rudiment of an eye himself."

It is with a shock of recognition that one reads these lines in the twenty-first century. The obsessive question "What's the news?" about anything that happened anywhere on the globe, the inability to sleep soundly for fear of missing out on some piece of trivial gossip—this seems like a direct precursor to the midnight hand compulsively tapping on the digital headlines, stock prices, and social media updates. Thoreau ingeniously, perhaps presciently, links this state of mind to the chemical cravings of a nation of neurotically overstimulated insomniacs, who have been turned into nonstop consuming machines.

In Thoreau's time, reporters for the ubiquitous commercial newspapers—fueled no doubt by heavy doses of caffeine—were indeed able to create a sense of instantaneous information flow, especially in urban areas. Telegraph transmission meant that news could be gathered from distant sources in a matter of seconds; cheap paper-making techniques and improved distribution routes (canals, railroads, and postal systems) meant that the printed product could reach millions within hours. The rush to provide news as fast as possible fueled a competitive market that was barely less intense than today's, and a news junkie like the one portrayed in *Walden* might well have experienced a novel kind of sleep deprivation. In the communications revolution of the mid- to late nineteenth century no less than the one we are living through today, it became a journalistic commonplace that the wired world was inhospitable to human sleep. One nineteenth-century Chicago lawyer, for instance, wrote that "the practical annihilation of time and space by . . . telegraphs and railroads" was largely responsible for the rapid spread of "sleeplessness" among the populace.

It wasn't just newspaper readers and telegraph users whose rhythms were thrown off in this new media environment. New York City diarist George Templeton Strong told of being awakened in his Gramercy Park home at 11:30 one night by "a herd of highly excited newsboys" crying a story about the arrival of a missing ship. The newsboys themselves were near the bottom of the economic ladder, doing a new kind of work that demanded irregular hours. Known as "street Arabs," they were typically semi-vagrant children who were also engaged in begging, harassment, and faking of headlines. And they often could be found sleeping on the streets, typically in groups for protection and companionship. As Jacob Riis put it, "like rabbits in their burrows, the little ragamuffins sleep with at least one eye open, and every sense alert to the approach of danger." But much of this night work was invisible to affluent city dwellers. Historian Peter Baldwin explains that "a city resident who began the day by reading the newspaper, eating breakfast, and visiting the privy could easily forget that this morning routine was made possible by the night labor of many men."

Thoreau's critique of modern life is aimed mainly at the middle-class newspaper reader who has been hoodwinked into thinking he needs the infotainment peddled so assiduously by the commercial press; the disturbed sleep rhythms he chronicles are more those of the consumer than of the low-level worker who has no choice but to stay up, like the newsboys. But at moments, he reflects an awareness that sleep, like other valuable resources, is unevenly distributed. Lying alone in his little cabin by the pond, he wrote of workers being awakened by "factory bells" and other "mechanical aids" to get themselves to their appointed places in the economic order, after trying to catch sleep in boardinghouses even less quiet and conducive to sleep than the one in which he grew up. The female factory operatives in the famous mills at Lowell were reportedly wakened by bells calling them to work at five every morning, and they often worked by lamplight into the evening hours. "Consider the girls in the factory,—never alone, hardly in their dreams," Thoreau wrote. "It would be better if there were but one inhabitant to a square mile, as where I live."

———

The extraordinary accomplishment of *Walden* is not simply its diagnosis of social problems, including those involving time, speed, consumerism, labor, and technology (all of which affected sleep). The book is primarily remembered as one of the first great pieces of nature-writing, one that continues to resonate with the environmental concerns of our time. No American writer, said the scholar Lawrence Buell, "comes closer than [Thoreau] to standing for nature in both the scholarly and the popular mind." Thoreau's prose is at its most electric when he is describing walks in the woods or by the pond, especially when he makes minute observations of the natural world, such as in his account of the thrilling battles of ants, who disembowel each other even as the author lifts the leaf on which they are fighting and carries it into his cabin for closer inspection. His gift for noticing details arose from a lifelong practice of simply watching and recording. *Walden*'s language can soar on wings of metaphor (far better metaphors than the one I just used), but rigorous empiricism is at its base. Thoreau had read deeply in ancient classics, but he also closely followed the work of modern naturalists, from Alexander von Humboldt to Charles Darwin.

Like those great scientists, Thoreau kept exacting records of what he saw in nature. His daily notebooks formed the basis for his literary output, and in a twist that Thoreau would have appreciated, contemporary scientists have begun to use them as primary evidence of the changes that have taken place on our planet in the industrial and postindustrial age. When Richard Primack, a conservation biologist at Boston University, wanted to find evidence of climate change in his own backyard, he turned to the journals that Thoreau kept while he was living by Walden Pond from 1845 to 1847, and for eleven years thereafter. There, he found meticulous recorded tables documenting the flowering times of more than three hundred plant species, which he and his team compared to those same plants' springtime openings a century and a half later. They found that spring was actually arriving weeks earlier, direct evidence that climate change had come to Walden Pond. Primack considered adding Thoreau as coauthor to the first scientific papers he published on the topic: "Thoreau was a climate change scientist whose research was more than a century ahead of its time."

Part of what makes Thoreau's writings of such great interest to contemporary climate researchers is precisely what interests me in relation to what has changed about human sleep. The industrial forces that Thoreau decried have been responsible for a dangerous shift in the rhythms of the seasons over the past two centuries; those same forces have also disrupted the seasons within. There are many different layers of time in *Walden*, some social (factory bells, train whistles, news criers) and others natural (whippoorwills, seasons, body rhythms). But the most elemental way that we mark and submit to the passage of time is in our movement from sleeping to waking and back again. The timing of the human body, as chronobiologists have taken pains to show, bears a very complex relationship to these external cues: like all living beings, we are fashioned to live in sync with daily and seasonal changes, but we also can be "entrained" to ignore them, at least to an extent.

From Thoreau's journals, we see a steady fascination with the daily and seasonal patterns of different life forms. Starting with humans, at age twenty-three: "How we eat, drink, sleep, and use our desultory hours . . . determines our authority and capacity for the time to come." At age thirty-three, birds: "I hear, just as the night sets in, faint notes from time to time from some sparrow falling asleep,—a vesper hymn,—and later, in the woods, the chuckling, rattling sound of some unseen bird on the near trees. The nighthawk booms wide awake." Insects and worms at thirty-five: "What is the earliest sign of spring? The motion of worms and insects? The flow of sap in trees and the swelling of buds? Do not the insects awake with the flow of the sap?" Early on Thoreau notes that he seems out of sync with himself: "My soul and body have tottered along together of late, tripping and hindering one another like unpracticed Siamese twins." But in his mature phase, at Walden, he notices, without rancor, a lack of correspondence between his own inward rhythms and the rhythms of other life forms: "Methinks my seasons revolve more slowly than those of nature; I am differently timed. I am contented." A sense of peaceful repose comes over him during a rainstorm: "I feel as if I could go to sleep under a hedge.

The landscape wears a subdued tone, quite soothing to the feelings; no glaring colors." All of which rises, eventually, to a hard-won observation: "Health is a sound relation to nature."

This peaceful submission to nature takes on added pathos when we remember Thoreau's lifelong sleep troubles, troubles that seemed nearly to unhinge him as a young man living and working in a succession of environments that only made matters worse: boardinghouse, factory, dormitory, school, town, city. While his compatriots in the northeastern United States were spending increasing amounts of time in such unnatural environments, losing a sense of the seasons and the pace of day and night, Thoreau preached that health lay outside—or rather in a synchronization of the body's interior with the rhythmical cues of the environment. Environmental historian Donald Worster wrote that Thoreau had a "visceral sense of belonging to the Earth and its organisms"; critic Christopher Sellers specified that that belonging involved submitting his body to the natural rhythms of the sun, both on a daily and a seasonal basis. "Drink of each season's influence as a vial, a true panacea," Thoreau wrote. "The vials of summer never made a man sick, but those which he stored in his cellar." Sleeping under a hedge in a gentle rain seems a far better salve than the bromides and opiates that were being used during his time to treat those with similar problems. His opinion on such things is in accord with his overall sense of health as a matter of being attuned to nature—his recognition that the human body was a part of the environment, rather than something separate from it. When we bombard sleep with pills, rules, and routines, when we subject it to scrutiny, measure it with machines, convert it into statistics, consider it fuel for productivity at work or a hedge against catastrophic risk, we mark our own alienation from the natural world and turn our sleeping and waking alike into mechanical operations rather than natural processes.

In writing *Walden*, Thoreau also drew on his fascination with the ways in which living things interacted with time. He was most effusive about mornings: "The morning, which is the most memorable season of the day, is the awakening hour. Then there is least somnolence in us; and for an hour, at least, some part of us awakes which slumbers all the rest of the day and night. . . . Morning is when I am awake and there is a dawn in me." But how should he awaken? The lack of a clock in his cabin gives a clue:

> Little is to be expected of that day, if it can be called a day, to which we are not awakened by our Genius, but by the mechanical nudging of some servitor, are not awakened by our own newly acquired force and aspirations from within, accompanied by the undulations of celestial music, instead of factory bells, and a fragrance filling the air—to a higher life than we fell asleep from. We must learn to reawaken and keep ourselves awake, not by mechanical aids, but by an infinite expectation of the dawn, which does not forsake us in our soundest sleep.

Here Thoreau is at once empirically astute (we are more awake when we are attentive to what are now called circadian rhythms than we are when we sleep and wake by the clock) and intensely spiritual (this attentiveness leads to a "higher life than we fell asleep from"). His fascination with natural rhythms stems in part from his interest in the work of chronobiology's predecessors, including Carolus Linnaeus, who first systematically studied the opening and closing times of various plants to find the mechanism that he called the "flower clock." And the mystical overlay comes in part from his long reading in Eastern sacred texts. In 1843, two years before he set out for Walden Pond, he translated a selection from the Hindu sacred text *The Laws of Menu* for the Transcendentalist journal *The Dial*. Included in his selections was this rapturous aphorism:

> Not solicitous for the means of gratification, chaste as a student, sleeping on the bare earth, in the haunts of pious hermits, without one selfish affection, dwelling at the roots of trees; for the purpose of uniting his soul with the divine spirit.

In *A Week on the Concord and Merrimack Rivers*, the book Thoreau wrote during his time at Walden about the earlier trip he had taken with his late brother, he paid homage to this spiritual zone of midday slumber: "While lying thus on our oars by the side of the stream, in the heat of the day . . . our thoughts reverted to Arabia, Persia, and Hindostan, the lands of contemplation and dwelling places of the ruminant nations." But nighttime also held moments of spiritual transcendence: its glorious, enchanted qualities are to be found on occasion in *Walden*, as when he stumbles back from the village through the woods in complete darkness late at night. Feeling for his own footprints with his feet, touching the bark of familiar trees, he experiences a kind of dreamlike synesthesia or estrangement of the senses: "Sometimes, after coming home thus late in a dark and muggy night, when my feet felt the path which my eyes could not see, dreaming and absent-minded all the way, until I was aroused by having to raise my hand to lift the latch, I have not been able to recall a single step of my walk, and I have thought that perhaps my body would find its way home if its master should forsake it, as the hand finds its way to the mouth without assistance."

Despite these rapturous nocturnal perambulations, there is still a sense of melancholy, even fear, in some of Thoreau's writing about the night. "I believe that men are generally still a little afraid of the dark, though the witches are all hung, and Christianity and candles have been introduced," he wrote. One senses that the fear might be Thoreau's own. He confesses at one point that the solitude at night leads to "a slight insanity in my mood." This response is sometimes triggered by the strange sounds of owls and other animals, which remind him of "ghouls and idiots and insane howlings." He admits to a deeper aloneness in these passages about solitude at night than elsewhere in the book. The thin bed in his cabin, after all, was big enough only for one. Unlike so many modern sleepers who are sealed off in their noise-free, climate-controlled chambers, he may have experienced his body blending into nature at night; but like so many of us then and now, he slept—ever since John had died—alone.

———

After two years, Thoreau left Walden Pond because, as he said, he had other lives to live. He never wanted to reject the restless, nervous, bustling, trivial nineteenth century completely, just to stand apart from it and watch it from a slight distance. He came out into the world a bit more as a writer; he cut a figure as a lecturer on the lyceum circuit, published more essays and poems, as well as two books (more were published after he died), and became more outspoken on social issues, especially slavery. Thoreau was known not just as a naturalist, but as a great proponent of civil disobedience against society's crimes against one's conscience. His biggest moment in the limelight came when he daringly lectured in support of the rebel John Brown after Brown was apprehended in October 1859. Far from being the maniac that his sleepwalking countrymen— whom Thoreau characterized as "sluggish by constitution and by habit"—presumed him to be, the heroic Brown was actuated by the highest principles. The thought of Brown suffering in jail awaiting execution, and the thought of the slaves who remained imprisoned in their living hell, reactivated Thoreau's insomnia. Under the current circumstances, with the country heaving violently toward war, insomnia was the true mark of a humane soul: "We aspire to be something more than stupid and timid chattels," Thoreau wrote, and "if there is anyone who gets his usual allowance of sleep," he wanted nothing to do with them. In the night, he put his sleepless angry pencil to use: "I put a piece of paper and a pencil under my pillow, and when I could not sleep I wrote in the dark."

Brown was executed, and those who loved liberty and abhorred war, as Thoreau did, were losing hope. He himself had only a short time to live. His health had been failing again, with a strange illness sapping all the vigor from his legs. His father died from tuberculosis in early 1860, and Thoreau tried unsuccessfully to take over the family pencil business, but tuberculosis was catching up with him, too. From Brown he tried to take a lesson in dying. He had written in *Walden* that he had never met a man who was truly awake; in his "Plea for Captain John Brown," he wrote, "It seems as if no man had ever died in America before; for in order to die you must first have lived." In the midst of his prolonged bouts of sleeplessness, he told a friend he wished his bed were like a shell, that he might curl up in it. In his last days, the doctors offered him opiates to alleviate his pain, but he refused to take them. Thoreau had learned what it was to be awake, to sleep, and to live in a natural relation to the universe; now he wanted to know what it felt like to die.

PART II

Taming Sleep

*More slaves are whipped
for oversleeping than for
any other fault.*

—Frederick Douglass

CHAPTER THREE

Lady Macbeth's Doctor;
or, Sleepwalkers and Lunatics

Over the centuries, sleep and sleeplessness slowly began to lose their lofty spiritual implications—those insane hootings and howlings, as well as the intimations of a higher will—that are still alive in Thoreau's writing. Instead, disordered sleep came to be treated as a purely mechanical phenomenon. How we came to this state, of trying to tame sleep medically, rather than letting it run its wild and mysterious course, is a tangled story involving drugs, doctors, ministers, institutions—and visionary sleepwalkers. In a famous dramatic scene that encapsulates much of this history, a doctor in Shakespeare's *Macbeth* witnesses Lady Macbeth's strange behaviors in the night—including sleepwalking and speaking in monologues that drip in blood imagery ("Out, damned spot!")—and concludes that "more needs she the divine than the physician." Subsequent generations of doctors would not hesitate to take such matters into their own hands.

For Thoreau, no pill could "keep us well, serene, contented" as effectively as "our great-grandmother Nature's universal, vegetable, botanic medicines." The sustained, full-body alertness that came with sleeping and waking in tune with natural rhythms—both inside and outside his body—and rejecting chemical disruptions of those rhythms, gave his writing a tactile, sensual responsiveness that more artificially induced states would likely have inhibited; his work retains some of the spiritual grandeur long associated with sleep. But Americans in the nineteenth century, as in our own times, increasingly emphasized "fixing" unusual sleep patterns, either through subjecting them to the surveillance and discipline of professionals, by means of medication, or both. In our overmedicated age, perhaps we have lost some of the creative and spiritual potential of troubled sleep. That loss, strange as it may seem, began with the fate of nineteenth-century sleepwalkers—particularly young female somnambulists—who became the great test case for the powers of medicine to supplant those of religion in the effort to tame sleep.

———

Treating problematic sleep medically was not exactly new in the nineteenth century. There is a long history of medicinal remedies for sleep, particularly insomnia, stretching back for centuries, even millennia. Coral, anise, onions, garlic, lettuce, rose flowers, valerian, saffron, iris, almond oil, wine, bitter almonds, and wild pomegranate roots were all in circulation as sleep aids through the early modern period in Europe and North America, as was castoreum (a secretion from a gland near the anus of a beaver). Even such exotic techniques as applying the lungs of a freshly killed sheep to either side of the head inspired local enthusiasm.

None of these techniques, though, seemed more effective than various concoctions derived from the poppy plant. There is some evidence that opium was used for medical purposes, including perhaps as a sleep aid, as far back as prehistoric times. But it was the Renaissance that saw the drug's true emergence as a global commodity—one that could be packaged in all sorts of ways. The sixteenth-century French physician André du Laurens, for instance, found that the best way to use it as a sleep aid was to allow blood-sucking leeches to bore holes behind the patient's ears, and then place a grain of opium in each hole. Italian physician Marcelo Ficino presented a more inviting scene. He advised eating lettuce after the evening meal, then drinking pure wine, rubbing an ointment made of the oil of violets or camphor on the temples, listening to pleasant songs, and then downing a potion made of lettuce seeds, balsam, saffron, sugar, and—you guessed it, poppy seeds—before lying down in a bed covered with the leaves of fresh, cool plants.

The leeches, cool leaves, violet oil, and soothing songs began to fall by the wayside in subsequent centuries, as those innocent little poppy seeds came to fuel a massive global drug trade that reached its height in late eighteenth-century Europe, when the British East India Company established a virtual monopoly on opium. In 1758, the botanist Carolus Linnaeus decisively classified opium as a "sleep-inducing" agent; for the next century and more, strung-out, exhausted Europeans and Americans and their doctors turned to it in the form of pills, smokable resin, snuffable powder, injectable or potable liquid, or really in whatever form they could get it: morphine, laudanum, codeine, and later, heroin. It killed pain, it relieved the bowels, it produced unparalleled feelings of tranquility and peace, and it could give you sleep. (It could also, of course, produce deadly addictions.)

———

Loosely accompanying the medical treatments of disordered sleep over the millennia were theories about its physical process and function. The reigning theory, which held sway in Europe from the time of ancient Greece through the early nineteenth century, was that sleep was mainly a matter of digestion. Historians of sleep research remark at the extraordinary staying power of Aristotle's *De somno et vigilia (On Sleep and Waking)*, which maintained that the function of sleep was to turn food into blood, which it did via the process of evaporation. When the warm vapors of digested food reached the brain, the head became heavy, causing the eyelids to close and the head to nod. The mixture of "spirit" and blood in the brain was then forced down the veins to the heart, causing a "seizure" of the heart that inhibited the rest of the body from experiencing sensation. Accordingly, sleep usually came after meals, and waking occurred when digestion was complete. Many of the substances used to treat sleep loss—from crisp lettuce leaves to nutmeg, dandelion, and onions, were thought to dissipate excess heat in the stomach and therefore reduce the warm vapors rising to the brain, or to slow down the restless vibration of the nerves by cooling them.

Aristotle also believed that sleep constituted a retreat from the particular qualities that made humans *human*—those higher elements of consciousness that we can only truly access while awake. The soul, he believed, had three parts: the human, the animal, and the vegetable. The highest, the human, was the seat of the "rational powers of intellect"; the animal, or sensitive soul, was the source of powers of movement, emotion, and senses; and the lowest, the vegetable, "included the functions basic to all living things: nutrition, growth, and reproduction." Sleep involved the shutting down of the two higher portions of the soul. Sleepers were, in a sense, vegetables—on par with all other living things, but lower than waking humans and even beasts.

Medical theories of sleep twisted and turned across the centuries, but through the sixteenth and seventeenth centuries in Europe, most of them centrally involved digestion and the circulation of the body's four "humors"—blood, black bile, yellow bile, and phlegm. By the late seventeenth century, physicians had begun to explore the role of blood flow to the brain, but that flow itself was typically understood as induced by the digestive process. Fresh air was also fundamental, as susceptibility to putrid miasmic waves bearing disease was thought to be heightened during sleep. Yet while you could tinker medically with digestion, with the flow of bile, and with ventilation of rooms, ultimately these forces had to be brought back into the service of the immaterial soul: the reason to sleep well was not so much to be healthy, wealthy, and wise, as a later age would have it; rather, it was to be spiritually on balance, to serve god fully. According to historian Sasha Handley, for many early modern households, learning to sleep correctly was "a core feature of what it meant to be a devoted Christian." Conversely, sleep disorders were signs of spiritual disfavor, or of active attacks by the devil.

———

Accordingly, the first profession to subject sleep to more or less systematic surveillance, with the aim of regularizing it, was the ministerial one. In seventeenth- and eighteenth-century New England—that is, in the centuries before young Thoreau staggered toward Walden—Puritan ministers asserted the need to exert some degree of control over where and when their congregants slept, because the devil was always lurking—especially when he could take one away from worshipping God. And so before the medical control of sleep, there was religious control; before the invention of normal and disordered sleep, sleep was a matter of sin and salvation.

The New Testament story of Eutychus in the Book of Acts pointed to the mortal dangers of losing control of sleep. Eutychus is described as an unfortunate "certain young man" who was sitting in a loft while the apostle Paul preached well into the night. When Eutychus nods off and succumbs to sleep, he falls from his lofty perch and is "taken up dead," only to be restored to life by some mysterious agency in the next verse. "And Paul went down and fell on him, and embracing [him] said, 'Trouble not yourselves, for life is in him.'" Puritan ministers in eighteenth-century Britain and in the American colonies were much taken with the story. To them, it represented the inherent depravity of man, the need for constant vigilance over one's spiritual faith, and, above all, the vital importance of heeding the word not only of God, but of the ministers themselves.

In 1684, Increase Mather, the influential minister of the North Church of Boston (later to become president of Harvard College), used the Eutychus story to warn his congregants of the constant snares that Satan was setting for them and the punishments that God could hand out for succumbing. Sleeping in church was akin to breaking the third commandment—taking the Lord's name in vain—because "by sleeping at Sermons, [you] practically say, that the Word of the Lord is contemptible." Eutychus, Mather explained, at least had decent excuses for falling asleep during worship: Paul's sermon lasted for hours, and the incident took place late at night, when "men are more naturally inclined to sleep." (This was so, Mather explained, because early Christians had to meet clandestinely, in order to escape the notice of the non-Christian authorities.) Even so, God saw fit to smite him dead for his transgression—if only to raise him again. Think, then, how awful might be the fate of the good Christians of Boston, who had no such excuse for dropping off during a service. "If thou dost find thy self inclined to sleep under the hearing of the Word," he intoned, "think how Satan is busie about thee."

And yet drop off they clearly did. Mather even mentions "some woful Creatures" who "have been so wicked as to profess they have gone to hear Sermons on purpose, that so they might sleep, finding themselves at such times much disposed that way." Sleeping in church was a favorite topic for ministers of many denominations in the seventeenth and eighteenth centuries, with examples of similar sermons on record for a wide range of them, from Bavarian Catholics to Swiss and Scottish Reformed. But the theme had pride of place in New England Puritan sermons. "Is it possible! What! *Sleep*, when you have a Blessed SAVIOUR at *Prayer* in your company?" begins the 1719 sermon "Vigilius, Or, The Awakener," by Cotton Mather, son of Increase. He reminded congregants that the unsleeping Satan had the upper hand: ever at the ready "with his *Energy* to make us *Drowsy*, when we should *Awake*, and be *still* with *GOD*," he had "*Hidden Ways* of dozing us; *Hidden Ways* of coming at us." Mather's distant cousin, the Connecticut minister Azariah Mather, delivered a sermon called "Wo to Sleepy Sinners," in which he compared the preacher's task to that of someone trying to rouse a perpetually drowsy friend. The ultimate task of the religious leader, he wrote, was "the Convincing and Awakening of poor sleepy Souls"; otherwise, "Sinners, there's no sleeping in Hell whither you are going."

For the Mathers, the regulation of sleep was not simply a matter of individual will, but a communal imperative. Increase Mather warned that if yawns and snores began to spread across the congregation, then God might decide to "take his Word away from them." Cotton Mather frequently referred to Christians as "watchmen," and in "Vigilius" he told his followers not only to "Shake off" their own "Sinful Sleep, if you find yourselves at any time growing sleepy in your *Devotions*." No, because we are our brothers' keepers, and because maintaining a proper state of alertness was the task of the entire community of true believers, a timely pinch or nudge of a nodding pew-mate is sometimes required: "We must not be afraid of *offending* our Neighbour with the Ill Manners of disturbing his *Repose*. No, be afraid of offending the Glorious GOD, by neglecting your Duty to your Neighbour. The Neighbour must either take your Jog very *Thankfully*, or else put off the Christian, and express a shameful Impiety; a shameful Ingratitude; a disposition to *Evil-doing*."

No one who makes a living by holding the attention of an audience, whether minister, lecturer, actor, politician, or magician, likes to see people dozing off when he or she starts to speak. (In the battle for the 2016 Republican presidential nomination, Donald Trump mocked Jeb Bush in a fake commercial touting him as a cure for insomnia, showing that the same principle has lasted since Increase Mather's time.) But why were these religious authorities so obsessed with regulating the sleep of their congregants? The early eighteenth century was a challenging period for colonial New England religious leaders: Cotton Mather, a third-generation minister, had struggled to exercise the kind of influence over his community that his ancestors had held. Generations of warfare with surrounding native tribes had tried the faith of parishioners in their leaders; and splinter groups and outright blasphemers began to challenge the rule of ministers who had once held almost unchallenged authority in their communities. According to historian Craig Koslofsky, exhaustion was sometimes taken as a sign that congregants had been up to no good, since the rival groups, fearful of detection, often held their meetings at night—an activity that left them physically and spiritually spent the next day.

Cotton Mather certainly seems to have worried about this sort of thing; in particular, he condemned the "riots" that could attend nocturnal threshing parties, and admonished local farmers to "let the *night of your pleasure* be turned into *fear*." Worse than riotous parties could happen at night: Indian raids, attacks of wild beasts, and even the cavorting of witches. The most famous such challenge culminated in the Salem witch trials of the 1690s, in which Cotton Mather offered evidence of the demonic possession of two young

Salem girls who had been spotted engaging in suspicious activities in the night. He was ambivalent about the eventual executions that followed the trials; but the grim necessity of policing the night in this way was surely a factor in his warnings about controlling sleep.

With all of these forces from within and without pulling apart the once cohesive religious communities, a jolt of energy was needed to stop Christian heads from nodding and keep butts in the pews, as it were. Contemporary neuroscientists understand that the brain needs regular shots of a neuropeptide called *orexin* to maintain a prolonged state of arousal; many drugs that promote wakefulness increase the flow of orexin, and now some that promote sleep suppress it. Puritan ministers turned to fear, rather than pills, to keep congregants awake, but this was only one tactic; others found more novel ways to keep the orexin flowing. The religious revival movements of the generations following Cotton Mather were known as the Great Awakening, and they featured hyperkinetic, possibly over-caffeinated ministers waving their arms, breaking out into sweats, and inspiring followers to speak in tongues. The ultimate result was often a visible frenzy. "The world is in a deep sleep," the famous revivalist George Whitfield said in 1739, "and nothing but a loud voice can waken it." A former slave who was in attendance at one of Whitfield's sermons admiringly described Whitfield as "sweat[ing] so much as I ever did while in slavery. . . . I had never before seen divines exert themselves in this manner." Whitfield's follower John Wesley (with his brother Charles a founder of Methodism) wrote of oversleeping as a kind of gateway drug to all manner of social ills: "It sows the seeds of foolish and hurtful Desires. It dangerously inflames our natural appetites. It breeds and continually increases Sloth, so often objected to the English nation. It opens the way and prepares the soul for every other kind of Intemperance. . . . It totally unfits us for *enduring hardship as good Soldiers of Jesus Christ:* and consequently for *fighting the good fight of faith, and laying hold on eternal life."*

For all of these spiritual dangers of sleeping in the wrong way, at the wrong time, for the wrong duration, these ministers never lost sight of the fact that sleep was also a matter of the flesh. Cotton Mather was a towering intellectual figure who pioneered not only in theology but also in natural sciences and medicine. He is famous in the history of medicine for writing the first medical treatise published in the Americas and for performing the first smallpox vaccine (a technique he learned from his enslaved African-born servant Onesimus). Mather's sermons often took natural phenomena—including the phenomena of the body—as indications of God's mysterious will. He viewed insomnia as a medical malady, but he also believed that God might visit this affliction as punishment upon parishioners who became drowsy during worship. ("What if an Holy GOD should punish your Drowsiness with Diseases wherein Sleep shall be withheld from you?") In his 1724 book *The Angel of Bethesda*, he mixed medical and ministerial modes. On the one hand, he appealed to his "SAVIOUR," asking that he might "cause me to *Awake unto Righteousness*." On the other, he tinkered like an unlicensed pharmacist with cures for nightmares and insomnia (which he referred to as "Waking *Coma*"). If "gentle Purges" and forced vomiting didn't work, then other remedies might: "a Bath made of *Rain Water*," perhaps, or "a Bath of Anodyne-Herbs, as *Lettice, Poppy, Water-Lillies, Camomil-flowers*, for the *Feet*, yea, and for the *Head* also." Or "the Head Shaved, and a Napkin dipped in a Mixture of *Water* and *Vinegar* and a little *Spirit of Wine*." And if that didn't work, he suggested "*opiates* (and *Opium* itself) moderately given," or "oil of Roses, mixed with some Rose Water." Speaking as both physician and minister, he imagined his role as helping those who were weak in physical and spiritual health maintain proper vigilance over their bodies and souls.

Which brings us back to Lady Macbeth's doctor. Confronted with disordered sleep, he had thrown up his hands and left the matter to the divines. But by Thoreau's time, Lady Macbeth would likely meet a different fate. Much more than insomnia or any of the array of other sleep disorders and difficulties that so preoccupy us today, somnambulism, or sleepwalking, was the first medical sleep problem of the modern age: a phenomenon that required study, empirical observation, and medical correction—and one that inspired widespread social consternation. Across the eighteenth and nineteenth centuries, physicians began to investigate the role of the brain in producing or disrupting sleep. Drawing on new neuro-logical theories, medical men who were far less modest than Lady Macbeth's doctor eventually stole sleep from the control of religious authorities.

————

One night in 1811, and for many nights thereafter, a young woman named Rachel Baker rose from her bed in Marcellus, New York, and—apparently in a sleeping state—announced that she was going to die and proceeded to pour out a sermon of religious dread and impending doom. Baker came from a Presbyterian family that was caught up in the fervor of the Great Awakening's revival movement centered in Onondaga County, the heart of the so-called "Burned-Over District" (so named because its inhabitants had all been con-verted, leaving no "fuel" left over for the fire of faith to ignite). According to a local minister, she formed strong religious senti-ments early in life, and from the age of nine, "the thoughts of God and eternity would make her tremble." During her waking hours, she was meek and proper; before bed, she offered her nightly devo-tions with decorous expressions of love and gratitude for her maker. There was nothing particularly striking about her waking self: in the words of her minister, she was "far from possessing very quick perceptions, a penetrating discernment, or lively sensations." But in the middle of the night she took on personality traits that veered between the disturbing and the miraculous. The episodes began with her "sighing and groaning, as if in excessive pain, which caused great alarm to the family." She then began to talk in a disordered way, "like one somewhat deranged. . . . [S]he would be one min-ute begging for mercy like one in extreme anguish; another minute warning her mates, telling them not to do as she had done, but to take warning by her; she was going down to hell!"

By the time she was nineteen, Baker was attracting curious onlookers, who gathered around her bedside to hear her "evening exercises," which began with prayer, then exhortation, and a clos-ing prayer. One of the thirty or forty neighbors who showed up described her as a "plump, hale country lass, . . . rather above the middle size," with a "tranquil" face that showed no sign of "mental vivacity or vigor." Yet apparently in the midst of sleep, she gazed at her visitors with an "unsteady, wild and capricious" eye distorted by "sickly dilation of the pupil." She prayed for the church, the minister, and sinners alike, asking "that God would give them a sense of their danger, and enable them to apply to the Saviour, who is willing to save all them that come unto him, even the chief of sinners." She seemed to refer obliquely to her own sleeping state by exhorting the sinners to stay awake: "She would beg them not to give sleep to their eyes, nor slumber to their eye-lids, till they had made their peace with God." Her public sleep-talking went on in this way for two months, after which it reached a dramatic apex: "Soon after she went to bed, she was seized with horror and trembling; she gave a loud shriek, and awoke greatly terrified with a sense of her deplorable condition. . . . She said that one of the infernal fiends was grasping her, and would drag her down to the bottomless pit! A fathomless abyss! A dread eternity in full view!" Baker's family rushed to comfort her, assuring her that her sins were all forgiven, and she announced that henceforth she would only praise and bless the holy name of God. The horrifying vision seemed to create a spiritual breakthrough for her, and throngs of as many as three hundred people began to visit her nightly. She did not disappoint.

In these nocturnal visitations, after half an hour of prayer, Baker's chest began to heave, she grated her teeth, her breathing became irregular, and her moans filled her visitors with dread. One night, her eye met that of a visiting church elder, and she told him of "the shuddering terrors of eternal damnation"; her warnings of mortal danger caused visitors to "shudder and shiver in sublimity." But then her sleeping incarnation composed itself, and she delivered an address full of learned reference to scriptures in a commanding voice. At the end of her sermons, she would shake violently, as if casting off an unseen tormentor, and then collapse on her bed, "colourless as the dead." Despite such terrifying performances, many visitors were struck by her lucidity and composure. Astonishingly, despite the fact that in her waking state she "[did] not appear to be possessed of a clear mind in the scriptures, a retentive memory, nor a good judgment," her sleeping sermons exhibited a minute understanding of "the great doctrines of grace" that testified to "eminent attainments in Christian knowledge."

Baker's deranged sleep—if that's what it was—was interpreted entirely as a spiritual matter, as such altered states of consciousness had been understood for centuries or even millennia. Scattered reports of sleepwalking and sleeptalking go back to ancient times, and they were often associated with religious visions that might be manifest in fits, trances, and convulsions. All of these phenomena were thought to emanate from an alternating consciousness that was caught between the earthly and the sublime, the angelic and the demonic, an ascent up to heaven and a slide into hell. It was after one of his visions that the apostle Paul had said, "It is no longer I who live, but Christ who lives in me"; upon seeing lights and hearing voices, he wondered "whether [I was] in the body or out of the body." Ministers in colonial New England had feared this sort of experience, especially when it took place at night, and even more so when women and girls were the ones arising from their beds in this disordered and untimely way to explore the supernatural world. The Salem witch trials were only the most famous instance of women getting up to no good under such circumstances. Ecstatic experiences and trances received the approval of authorities only when they took place in the proper time and place: otherwise, they might be evidence of witchcraft, spirit possession, rebelliousness, or even prostitution.

In the eighteenth century in Europe and North America, mainstream religious authorities began to challenge the spiritual interpretation of such unruly sleep, often drawing on the rationalistic worldview of philosophers and scientists, who viewed it as evidence of mental instability rather than religious inspiration or demonic possession. The clash of scientific and theological interpretations of sleepwalking and associated altered states became a matter of public concern shortly after a group of French Huguenots, who had been expelled from France when Protestantism was outlawed there, arrived in London in the early eighteenth century. These so-called "French prophets" all reported common mystical experiences: the young women in their group frequently fell faint or swooned and began to "Prophesie and Preach in their Sleep," generally without any memory of the event when they awoke. Opponents of the immigrants and their unsettling religious behaviors refused to acknowledge the validity of these spiritual states. Instead of religion, they saw "enthusiasm," a term that connoted mental imbalance and false religious impressions, and was often used to tar opponents as being both dangerously radical and mad. As much as a century later, leaders of the revival movements, in part because they gave credence to the ecstatic, sometimes somnambulistic, voices of women and others of low status (such as Rachel Baker), were often referred to dismissively as "French prophets" and charged with promoting social unrest. By encouraging those who lived on the margins of society to proclaim their spiritual visions in public, the revivalists elicited the scorn of the more established religious leaders of the late eighteenth and early nineteenth centuries, who considered such uncensored outpourings to be dangerous, even possibly dangerous enough to promote the spread of insanity. Old-line Congregationalist minister Charles Chauncy found such enthusiasm to result from "bad temperament of the blood and spirits." Because of "the Weakness of their Nerves, and from hence their greater Liableness to be surpris'd, and overcome with Fear," women—in his view—were more prone to be thrown into "these *Agitations* and *Terrors*" than were men.

Nonetheless, sleepwalkers continued to enthrall onlookers on both sides of the Atlantic. Even strict rationalists admitted that such behaviors existed, and that often, they came bundled with extraordinary powers. Wrote physician John Bell in 1788, "People struck with Somnambulism, given up to a sound sleep, walk, talk, write and perform many other actions as if they were awake; nay, even sometimes with more discernment and exactitude." There were other notable examples: A late eighteenth-century Swiss teenager could reportedly eat, drink, and dress himself while sleeping without aid of light, even composing a complex piece of music in that state. A divinity student in Bordeaux composed sermons and musical works more elegant than those he was capable of producing while awake. A poet who published his sleep-writing attracted favorable notice in Britain.

Not surprisingly, sleepwalking was often understood as an eruption of special mental powers associated with genius, an explanation that some in the medical community accepted. But it could also
indicate disease of the brain. Preeminent American physician Benjamin Rush (a signer of the Declaration of Independence) treated
sleepwalking as a rather straightforward medical problem that could
be cured by bleeding, gentle purges, low diet, exercise, and perhaps a "draught of porter, a glass of wine, or a dose of opium." He
explained that sleepwalkers have nervous systems that are "so free, as
that vibrations can descend from the internal parts of the brain, the
peculiar residence of ideas, into them." He viewed somnambulism as
"a higher grade" of dreaming, or "a transient paroxysm of madness":
"Like madness," he wrote, "it is accompanied with muscular action,
with incoherent, or coherent conduct, and with that complete oblivion of both, which takes place in the worst grade of madness." It is
a state in which complex activities can be undertaken—"the scholar
resuming his studies, the poet his pen, and the artisan his labours . . .
with their usual industry, taste and correctness." Novelist Charles
Brockden Brown took this idea of sleepwalking-as-madness to
its logical conclusion, picturing in his gripping 1799 novel *Edgar
Huntly; or, Memoirs of a Sleepwalker* a man who commits murders in
his sleep. He is captured and taken to a lunatic asylum—a fate that
predicted the case of a notorious American killer in 1833 who was
the first to claim the sleepwalking defense in court.

Older, nonscientific interpretations of sleepwalking (and sleep
generally) persisted through the nineteenth century, although they
weren't always tied to the frameworks of organized religion. Reports
of the experience of sleepwalkers frequently included supernatural
abilities. A Rhode Island woman was said to be able to leave her
body during sleep: when she "travel[ed]" to New York in this manner, she described the pictures on the wall of her physician's house
in the city and suffered seasickness on a steamboat ride across the
Long Island Sound. A German woman reported visiting the moon.
A Scottish sleepwalker spontaneously learned tenets of astronomy
and geography. A young man in Gloucester, Massachusetts, published a long account of a mystical experience that he claimed he

had only been able to write while holding a pen in his teeth during sleep. And another young woman, from Rachel Baker's upstate New York, claimed that during her sleep she had visited the borders of a lake where she encountered "continual weeping and lamentation": she almost fell in. Her vision of a deranged man lunging after her from out of the lake of fire, unable to reach her only because of the chains holding him back, is horrifying. But she was then treated to a view of Christ with angels cavorting about him before being returned to her sleeping body. For all of the remarkable features of Baker's case, it was not particularly original, but it did clearly fall under the heading of religious trance, rather than medical problem.

Medical interest in Baker's case eventually followed the hubbub over her performances. In 1813, she went to New York City to stay with her aunt, and there, away from the revivalist culture of her frontier community in Marcellus, she came into contact with medical men who had absorbed some of the most advanced teachings from Europe. Unlike Lady Macbeth's doctor, these early nineteenth-century doctors were not always willing to cede authority over such fantastical behavior to the "divines"; they had little interest in the immaterial soul, and instead offered explanations of the behavior that were based on the idea that the body, including the brain, was a machine that ran on regular principles. It was these doctors who were, in a small way, responsible for turning sleep and its derangements into a medical problem rather than a spiritual threat (or opportunity, depending on your perspective).

Most of the seemingly supernatural events that these men subjected to their scientific gaze befell women. As historian of medicine Kristen Keerma Friedman has noted, women had few opportunities to voice their views in public, and sleepwalking sermons and other visionary utterances gave them a chance to speak. Medicine was an exclusively male province, and so it made sense that as doctors became involved, they would use such episodes to demonstrate their mastery over the bodies of the young women, who, after all, were challenging societal roles when they acted as if they were claiming spiritual authority, even if it was only when they were sleeping. As

Friedman points out, Rachel Baker herself alluded to this dynamic in some of her nightly orations: when one skeptical onlooker asked why an illiterate woman should presume to preach on religion, she retorted, "It is a strange thing, and it is a mystery to many. . . . Truly, I have not had the advantage of education; I am but a poor, ignorant child; but what I speak my God seemeth to reveal to me."

Samuel Latham Mitchill, a professor at the College of Physicians and Surgeons and editor of the first medical journal published in the United States, was eager to examine Baker when he heard reports of her visit to his city. Mitchill was an extraordinarily accomplished man: he was an early exponent of Antoine Lavoisier's chemistry and sometimes wrote in verse on complex scientific matters. In addition to his medical practice, he held a law degree; studied geography, zoology, botany, and cartography; founded the New York Lyceum of Natural History, which later became the New York Academy of Sciences; and was elected to the New York State Assembly in 1789. While praising Baker's message, he worried that there might be "some cunning, or some concealment," lurking "under feminine disguise." Nonetheless, he came away convinced that the occurrences were so complex and regular that "more faith is required to suppose it a consummate and practical piece of deceit, than to consider it the result of devotional somnium" (the term given for spiritual visions received during sleep). Without venturing too far into causation, he speculated that her behavior had something to do with disturbed digestion—an explanation for all manner of sleep disturbances going back to Aristotle.

Others suggested different theories. Charles Mais, the stenographer who recorded Baker's performances, speculated that the onset of her somnambulism was triggered by the beginnings of puberty, "a period when the female frame acquires additional sensibilities, and undergoes a peculiar revolution." (Erasmus Darwin, the famous eighteenth-century physician who was the grandfather of Charles Darwin, had earlier popularized the notion that somnambulism in females could be triggered by menstruation.) But John Douglass, another medical man and former health commissioner of New York City, wasn't ready to throw out the idea of the workings of the spirit.

In his introduction to a booklet called *Devotional Somnium*, which collected accounts of Baker's behaviors by his friend Mitchill and the minister David Rathbone, he announced that "the case is indeed interesting to the physician, philosopher, and divine." Unable to determine whether medical or theological explanations would win the day, he threw up his hands: "Will it not confound the theory of those who think that the soul is matter highly organized? And the kindred opinion that the soul sleeps?" After this flurry of notoriety in New York, Baker returned home in 1815, where her health soon deteriorated. She died not long thereafter, at the age of twenty-eight, of unknown causes. Two decades later, the contest between medical and spiritual interpretations of this peculiar disturbance of sleep would be over.

———

In the spring of 1833, Jane C. Rider, a well-liked servant to a reputable family in Springfield, Massachusetts, began to act very oddly in the night. This nineteen-year-old daughter of "a respectable mechanic" first experienced intense, intermittent headaches, especially on the left side of her cranium. She slept more than usual, and she reported feeling highly sensitive to light. Eventually, she began to rise from her bed while still asleep. On some occasions, the *Springfield Republican* reported, she seemed to perform a somnambulistic parody of her normal work routine: "She has got up and set the table for breakfast, with as much regularity as she does when awake, selecting the right articles, and placing them upon the table exactly as they should be." But more often, something was slightly askew: "She frequently goes to the drawers where her clothes are kept, changes the position of the articles, or takes them out, and in some cases has placed some of them where she could not find them when awake." Some of her behaviors bordered on the marvelous. One night, an eyewitness reported, she threaded a needle twice, sewed a piece of fabric to make a bag for boiling squash, then searched the house for a squash and, not finding one, threw in a piece of meat and placed the bag in a pot of water over the fire. All of this she accomplished with her eyes closed, and "in a place where there was not sufficient light" to see what she was doing. Other actions seemed at first more mundane: often, she just sat up in bed talking to herself, reciting poetry, praying, or singing. Even here, though, something strange was going on, for when she awoke, Jane C. Rider generally could not repeat the same tunes or lines—most of which she seemed to have learned in early childhood.

As with the case of Rachel Baker's upstate New York town, the Springfield of Jane C. Rider was experiencing a wave of religious revivals. In the weeks before Rider's case was reported in the local papers, the *Republican* ran an account of a "sleeping preacher," an adolescent girl from New Haven, Connecticut, who would arise in her sleep to preach the gospel. When word spread about this miracle, locals flocked to her home, and "the fervor of her praying brought forth a kind of simultaneous panting from all around her." Rider's employers sought a medical cure rather than a demonstration of spiritual prowess, and so they summoned Lemuel Belden, a local doctor with an interest in mental functioning. A graduate of Yale College and a firm believer that all mental phenomena could be explained by physiological rather than spiritual processes, Belden sought both to banish her troubling symptoms—which must have been increasingly vexing to her employers—and to explain her case to the wider public.

He originally diagnosed her with *chorea*, a term broadly used to describe disordered movements, spasms, and tics. Yet upon observing her nighttime behaviors more closely, Belden became convinced that the disordered sleep he was observing emanated from a malfunctioning or malformed brain. He noted that she slept more often than most people and that she was intensely sensitive to the light. In her sleepwalking, she started by dressing herself, going to the kitchen, and preparing breakfast, with her eyes closed and the lights off, not noticing anyone around her. Her sudden attacks, or paroxysms, became more frequent as he observed her over the summer; she would move things about her room and be unable to find them in the morning; she sewed a ring on a curtain. And yet she remained almost entirely insensitive to her surroundings, which Belden took as the chief indication that she was asleep.

Belden was interested in the fashionable science of phrenology, whose adherents believed that the shape of the head revealed underlying aspects of character and mental capacity. In his phrenological examination of Rider's skull, he noted a particularly tender spot on the left side of her head, near what phrenologists referred to as "the organ of marvelousness." Sometimes she complained of pain near that spot ("It ought to be cut open, it ought to be cut open"), and occasionally she would take on "the appearance of a person in a violent fit of hysterics." In accordance with the still prevalent digestive theories of sleep, Belden treated her with emetics to induce vomiting, which he thought might relieve pressure on her brain from a too intense flow of blood following digestion. This experiment yielded some improvement in her condition, but no cure.

And yet the paroxysms unleashed fantastical abilities: tests of her vision, for instance, revealed that she could read the motto on the seal of a letter in the dark. She began to have fits in the daytime, and one attack lasted forty-eight hours. When word of these episodes got out, locals started flocking to see her. "During this time," Belden wrote, "she read a great variety of cards written and presented to her by different individuals, told the time by watches, and wrote short sentences," despite having handkerchiefs over her eyes. She also sang frequently, despite never having learned how to sing and never singing during waking; and she recited passages of poetry that she had not seen since childhood. Like a magician who doesn't want to give away a trick, Belden described in some detail how he took precautions to ensure that her eyes weren't open—he would wad up a cloth and seal it to her eye cavities, or use thick blindfolds. But she could always read the cards and even write responses, dotting the i's in the correct places, and making corrections whenever she left out a letter. However, there were some errors; for instance, she once mistook her father for a little boy in her village.

Belden was described by a later biographer as a modest and diligent physician "who made no bustle in his business, and no display in the community in which he resided." Yet one is struck by the stagey appearance of all of this: a doctor presenting a celebrated patient performing miraculous feats of skill and perception in her sleep before a crowd of gaping onlookers, who apparently never came away disappointed. It is hard to tell where medical curiosity shaded into showmanship. Did Rider pull one over on Belden, or was Belden in on it? Making matters more complicated, contemporary sleep researchers do find many of the reported symptoms to be consistent with certain types of "arousal disorders." I asked Carlos Schenck, one of the leading medical researchers of somnambulism and related disturbances, to comment on Rider's reported behaviors, and he was struck by the migraine-like symptoms—intense headaches, sensitivity to light—that she reported experiencing before her episodes; these, he explained, were often precursors to somnambulism. Given that medical knowledge at the time rarely linked these phenomena, Schenck was inclined to give some credence to what may seem an incredible case history. Rider almost certainly sleepwalked, and, for whatever reason, she also performed a version of that experience for the public that accorded with fantastical accounts of other female somnambulists: writing while blindfolded, exhibiting otherwise buried poetic talents, and the like.

What happened next in Rider's career, though, leaves little doubt that somewhere behind the staginess of the displays was a genuine experience of bizarre sleeping patterns that caused considerable suffering. Belden decided to contact his old examiner at Yale, Samuel Woodward, who was one of the most eminent physicians in New England and was now the superintendent of the State Lunatic Asylum at Worcester. In November 1833, against her wishes, Rider was committed to Woodward's care at the asylum. ("She complained," wrote Belden later, "that she was locked up in the Hospital, and did not wish to stay, and that she would not have come here if she had expected to be locked up.") Yet her doctors felt that it was crucial to remove her from the strain induced by a "constant succession of visitors" and provide her with the "seclusion which seemed essential to her cure." The two doctors, the renowned mentor and his former pupil, set about trying to understand, or at least to tame, Rider's wild sleep.

The facility at Worcester was itself something of a marvel. With its grand pillared edifice looming imposingly on a hillside on the outskirts of this industrial city in Massachusetts, it was the first state-run asylum in the country erected on "modern principles." It had opened only ten months earlier. At first this seems an odd choice for a patient like Rider. By the time she was admitted, there were approximately 164 inmates at the asylum, more than half of whom had been sent from jails, almshouses, and houses of correction. Many of them were violent, and 8 of the first 40 had been convicted of murder. In fact, as historian Gerald Grob showed in his study of the hospital, jail keepers were often motivated to send insane convicts to the asylum not to protect them from ordinary criminals, but to protect the ordinary criminals from the "furiously mad."

Yet the asylum at Worcester also stood as a beacon for a new kind of humane treatment of the mad. The first superintendents of such state-run institutions, including Woodward, justified massive public expenditures, as well as their own powers to rescind the liberties of mentally afflicted citizens, by pointing to the extraordinary cure rates resulting from their system of treatment, which consisted of careful attention to the medical and social conditions of those deemed insane. The "moral treatment," as it was known, was said to cure the great majority of cases of insanity, even the most violent among them. Some estimates (later disproved) put the cure rate at over 90 percent, and in the more successful asylums over half the admitted patients were discharged as cured within a year. The asylum was really a citadel of faith in the new creed that medicine, rather than religion, could address problems of the mind, even problems as fantastical as young women who rose in their sleep to preach, prophesy, recite poetry, cook, or thread needles.

Into this unlikely environment walked—perhaps while sleeping—the young Jane C. Rider. One can speculate on the reasons for her involuntary admission. First is that as a serving girl she was becoming increasingly inconvenient to her employers. Why should they continue to support her when her sleeping self undid all the work that her waking self was charged with performing? And what about all the gawkers showing up to witness the strange theater performed by their domestic? The asylum offered a humane way for the family to get the troublesome servant off their hands, and at public expense. Asylum treatment was far better for the family's image than abandoning her to the streets or an almshouse. Second, Belden himself saw an opportunity to expand his solitary observations within the emerging science of psychiatry. (The name had not yet been invented, but most historians date the origins of the psychiatric profession to the emergence of what was then usually called "asylum medicine.") Belden also likely relished the chance to bolster his professional ties to the eminent superintendent of the asylum. For Woodward, who had only recently been installed as superintendent of this highly touted new institution, solving the already notorious Rider case would be another feather in his cap. And surely it was a relief to be offered such a fascinating specimen who was neither a furious maniac nor a convicted murderer.

Casting off centuries of religious interpretation of sleepwalking as mere superstition, Belden and Woodward—apprentice and master—had complete faith that Rider's case depended, as Woodward wrote, "on physical disease," and that it would "gradually disappear, if a judicious course be pursued." Praising the initial investigations of his younger trainee, Woodward wrote that his and Belden's views on the causes and treatment "perfectly coincide[d]." But despite the united front they presented in the final write-up of the case, Belden and Woodward seem to have been operating under different theories. Belden was inclined to believe from the outset that the seat of Rider's troubles was her digestive tract. Before she was admitted to the asylum, he started her on a course of emetics; while this did not cure her, he and Woodward experimented with her diet throughout her stay in Worcester. For his part, Woodward decided early on that Rider's case could be explained by the principles of phrenology. The soreness in Rider's head, Woodward believed, indicated that one of the brain's regions, or "faculties," was overexcited or distended, causing not only pain but also enhanced sensory perceptions during her trances. Both men, though, agreed that there was nothing mystical about Rider's experience. When she read those cards with her eyes closed, and a thick blindfold tied over her eyes, "she actually *saw*." A tiny amount of light must have penetrated the bindings, which was enough for her retina, with its "increased sensitivity," to record a sense impression; and "a high degree of excitement in the brain itself" enabled "the mind to perceive even a confused image of the object."

But how to "cure" such a case? As with so much early nineteenth-century medicine, the answer was essentially to try everything until something worked. Before coming to the asylum, Rider had been taking laudanum and ether before bed to help ward off the fits, and, as Belden wrote in an article for the *Boston Medical and Surgical Journal*, "this she was permitted to continue" until it was established that the drugs were ineffective. In order to "subdue that irritability of the brain which formed the bases of the disease," she was bled copiously, and then had her feet put in a warm bath with mustard flour. Her head was shaved and blisters raised on her scalp; she was given a laxative and told to exercise; and her diet was strictly monitored. But the paroxysms continued, and she was treated to a series of drugs whose names read like the catalog of a pharmaceutical museum: a nitro-muriatic bath, tincture of stramonium, guaicum, carbonate of iron with extract of conium, emetic of ipecac, sulphate of zinc, calomel, opium, sanguinaria, the liquor potassae arsenitis, purssiate of iron, sulphate of quinine, and nitrite of silver. There is no detailed record of how Rider responded to these interventions, but Belden does tell us that "some medicines . . . were almost invariably followed by a paroxysm." One can indeed imagine that a helping of opium followed by the powerful sedative conium might very well bring on something resembling a somnambulistic fit. During one of these paroxysms, Rider cried out, "My head, my head, do cut it open!" Whether this desperate cry could have been better explained by the presence of a migraine, by some phrenological imbalance, or by the massive intake of drugs is an open question.

Given Rider's clear desire to be cured and to leave the institution, the fact that her trances never completely vanished makes it almost certain that she was no faker, even if she had previously acted out and amplified her symptoms back in Springfield. The doctors congratulated themselves on the progress they made with her: after a few months in the asylum, wrote Woodward, "she has never appeared so cheerful, and in so good spirits." She even demonstrated that she could return to her proper station in life, as a servant: "In the absence of one of our attendants . . . she has done more or less work in the halls every day." There is a creepy geniality to some of Woodward's notes about his researches at this point, which one senses the patient bore rather stoically, with a smile plastered to her face. "During the last paroxysm I applied leeches to her head. She waked during the paroxysm, not a little surprised at her new *head ornaments*." Rider wrote a few letters to Belden expressing her thanks to her doctors and her assurance that her condition was coming increasingly under control. She hoped soon to be released—"not that I am discontented in the least, for I am not. The time has passed very quick and pleasantly. I take a ride almost every day—that I like very much, and think it does me good." Woodward, of course, had read this letter before it was sent and added his own postscript to it. Rider knew what her doctors wanted to hear and told it to them. It was this, as much as any improvement in her condition, that appears to have occasioned her release one month after writing the letter. Even Woodward admitted that she still had the occasional sleepwalking fit.

The fact that Rider never entirely stopped sleepwalking throughout this ordeal should convince us of the reality of her condition, no matter how theatrical it at first appeared. And yet at the end of her time at the asylum, her doctors had no real explanation for her condition, other than a vague confirmation of their initial hypotheses. The episodes seemed to be brought on by "the free use of fruit," particularly green currants—which Woodward suspected she was smuggling into the asylum despite his strict orders. Echoing Rachel Baker's doctors, Woodward and Belden considered the possibility that an irregular menstrual flow may also have been a precipitating cause, but, perhaps out of a sense of decorum, they said little about their investigations into this matter in their published report.

Yet at the core, a fundamental mystery remained. As Belden concluded: "If it be asked how a physical cause, acting either directly or indirectly on the brain, can . . . endow the brain with the power of perceiving relations to which it had before been insensible, I can only answer, I do not know. . . . We here reach a gulf which human intelligence cannot pass." Woodward was particularly flummoxed by the extraordinary snatches of memory that Rider's sleeping self could access. This symptom seemed evidence not only of certain overexcited faculties of the brain, but of the fact that "all knowledge once impressed on the mind, remains indelibly fixed there, and only requires a strong stimulus to call it forth." He strained at a grand summation of her medical state that verged back on the fantastical: he speculated that Rider's condition augured "a future state of existence" in which "all the knowledge which we gain in this world will, by the increased energy of mind, be restored to the recollection and be at the command of the will." (Or perhaps he was just predicting Google searches.)

As for Rider herself, she slipped back into obscurity after her release from the asylum. A magazine piece revisiting her case twelve years later reported that she had been "cured" by Woodward and Belden's treatment, and that since then there had been "no return" of the affliction. Rider had served her doctors well. When they publicized her case in pamphlet form, the story created a terrific advertisement for their own new institution: it could make a furious lunatic sane, it could turn a fantastically disordered sleeper back into an ordinary serving girl. Her own voice—sometimes submissive, sometimes anguished—emerged in poignant fragments throughout the account, as she begged the doctors to release her, or, in more desperate moments, to cut open her head. Through such moments we glimpse what it felt like to have one's unruly sleep turned from a visionary portal into a medical problem.

———

Despite Woodward's grand metaphysical proclamations about future states of mind, he and his generation of medical men never gave up on the power of modern medicine to cure the most unusual of mental and physical maladies. Sleepwalkers did not constitute a large portion of the patients who passed through his asylum, or through other asylums run by the same principles of the moral treatment, but correcting problematic sleep remained a major concern of early psychiatry. Asylums were, as the great sociologist Erving Goffman put it, "total institutions"—enclosed spaces like ships and prisons (and, one might add, slave plantations)—in which a group of individuals led their lives cut off from society, and which had to be formally administered 24/7. Such spaces, wrote Goffman, break down a general rule of modern society: that individuals "sleep, play, and work in different places." There were individual bedrooms in insane asylums—Goffman's chief example of a total institution—but sleep was hardly private there. Bedroom doors typically had a window facing the corridor, and patients knew they were subject to being watched by the medical staff at all hours. As such, asylums like the one in which Jane Rider found herself served to enforce society's rules, including the one demanding that sleep must be done in an orderly way, straight through the night, in private: those who could not manage this fundamental expectation of civilization had to have their sleep tamed.

The first superintendent of the New York State Lunatic Asylum, Amariah Brigham, reported that *"the want of sleep"* was by far the most frequent cause of insanity. "If they sleep well," he continued, "they will not go insane." Accordingly, controlling the sleep routines of patients became an almost obsessive preoccupation of his asylum staff, who rose every morning before 4:30 and 5:30, woke the patients, and made sure they were washed and appropriately dressed. Unruly patients, those who could not stay in bed at the appropriate hours or who disturbed others at night, were placed in a device called the "Utica crib," a slatted and completely enclosed structure from which they could not escape. Use of the crib spread to other asylums, but even when it was not used, patients who would not get out of bed on time were sometimes put on public view all day as a punishment; one former patient recounted in an exposé of her treatment in Illinois that those who overslept were often beaten. (This was a claim also frequently made by former slaves, as we will see in the next chapter; perhaps it was one reason that disaffected former patients often referred to the asylum as a novel kind of slavery.) And, of course, there were the drugs: opium to subdue the patients, and a host of stimulants to rev them up when they overslept.

Religious authorities had once policed troubled sleep for its potential to disturb the community of worshippers, but asylum authorities had more secular concerns. Much of their worry arose from the fear that patients might harm others or commit suicide; a critic of the Worcester asylum that held Jane C. Rider blamed Samuel Woodward for the deaths of suicidal patients who had been allowed to sleep alone, without being watched or restrained at night. Particularly disturbed patients' rooms had latticework that allowed medical staff to hear slight sounds easily; if patients weren't in cribs, their rooms often had only a mattress on the floor, so that they could not use furniture to hurt themselves; and night watchmen patrolled the wards regularly, with close attention to those on suicide watch. Rider's case may have been unusual, but it really represents only one particularly flamboyant story in this history of taming sleep institutionally.

We now have other means of taming. Over the next two centuries, the asylum doctors were displaced by an ever-proliferating array of experts and specialists who hovered over disordered sleepers: first neurologists, then physiologists, psychiatrists, pediatricians, pulmonologists—even dentists, who now treat such problems as nocturnal tooth grinding (bruxism) and pulmonary obstructions caused by overextension of the jaw. Over seventy sleep disorders are now recognized in the *International Classification of Sleep Disorders*, ranging from the garden variety ("idiopathic insomnia," "obstructive sleep apnea") to the fabulous ("exploding head syndrome") to the terrifying ("fatal familial insomnia"). Forty million Americans annually are diagnosed with at least one of these. Unruly sleepers are no longer checked into asylums, but they are put under equally intense surveillance in modern sleep clinics—albeit for briefer periods, and with freedom to come and go. More than 2,500 accredited treatment centers were in existence by 2013—double the number from five years earlier, and five times as many as five years before that. You can find them in universities, strip malls, hotels, and on the side of the highway.

Sleepwalking is not much of a going concern at these clinics, although specialty clinics for arousal disorders, such as somnambulism and REM behavior disorder, have their place. Insomnia used to rule the roost as the most frequent diagnosis in modern clinics; now sleep apnea is by far the most common. (Critics claim this is driven by the profitability of continuous positive airway pressure machines, or CPAPs; pills for insomnia can be dispensed quickly and cheaply by a general practitioner in a routine office visit.) Utica cribs have long exited the stage, as have opium, leeches, emetic purges, and bleeding. But now we have electroencephalographic (EEG) read-outs of the different phases of sleep and their interruptions, and late-working lab technicians who hover over them. Threatening to render these sites of medicalized sleep obsolete are a host of new technologies that you can use at home to self-diagnose: headbands, chest straps, wristbands, and mattress pads that monitor precisely how long and deeply you rest, how often you get up, how often your heart beats and how many times you breathe each minute; smart-phone apps that interpret your raw numbers and give you recom-mendations for changing your routines; even Wi-Fi-connected beds that assemble all of this data and produce reports about your pos-sible sleep pathologies. The pervasiveness of this technology only reinforces the sense that disturbed sleep is the new normal. And as my colleague and co-teacher David Rye cracked, they might be pro-ducing new forms of sleep-related obsessive compulsive disorder.

Despite being converted into reams of hyperrational data, the strangeness of sleep persists. For one thing, our contemporary drugs bring with them new curiosities: Ambien, as has been widely reported, apparently creates Jane C. Rider–like side-effects in some users, who tuck themselves into bed and find themselves hours later behind the wheel of a car they've driven for miles in their sleep, or in front of a refrigerator, whose nastiest contents they have con-sumed in complete oblivion. People afflicted with REM behavior disorder act out their dreams in often horrifying ways, sometimes inflicting violence on themselves or loved ones.

And yet the strangest person in the village is no longer the one who preaches in her sleep or recites poems or cooks bags of squash in the middle of the night. The real curiosity, in our sleep-obsessed and sleep-damaged world, is the person who says she sleeps soundly and tranquilly every night. The rest of us live in Jane C. Rider's world.

CHAPTER FOUR

Sleeping Slaves, Waking Masters

In other times and places, sleep was indisputably rougher than it is for privileged Europeans and North Americans today. Except in the poorest communities, our postindustrial society has vanquished vermin, the threat of nighttime fires, extreme heat and cold, hunger, and other ills that could make sleep truly dangerous in earlier centuries. Professional police forces have been patrolling the night since the mid-nineteenth century; and although powerful artificial lighting—first gas, then electric—has been blamed for disrupting natural sleep patterns, in another sense it provides unprecedented nighttime security by scaring off criminals and helping the police do their job. As opposed to the fear and raw discomfort that were obstacles to steady sleep in earlier times and less wealthy regions, the battles that many readers of this book are likely to fight with sleep are more psychological and managerial than existential. According to the prominent British sleep researcher and sleep-panic skeptic Jim Horne, regardless of whether Europeans and North Americans sleep less today than people in other times and places, "sleep debt"—the cumulative effect of not getting enough sleep—"is the contemporary complaint of those of us who are well fed, well housed, and in full employment."

Yet while many economically advantaged people fight psychological demons and pop pills in secure and comfortable beds, plenty of people the world over still lack basic protection against the terrors of the night. "Normal" sleep is off limits to those whose sleep is disrupted by hunger, illness, war, natural disaster, or the need to hold down multiple jobs or work unreasonable hours. There is a long backdrop to this unequal distribution of sleep. The sleep norms that have been expected since the nineteenth century (sleeping in private, consolidating one's sleep at night, routinizing sleep behaviors, training children to reproduce these norms, and medicalizing exceptions) really applied only to some of the population.

The literature of poverty from the nineteenth century onward is also the literature of injured sleep: Edwin Chadwick's reports of the living conditions of the urban poor in London in the 1840s and Jacob Riis's accounts of squalid New York tenements in 1890 both present worlds in which restful sleep seems a structural impossibility. The American proletarian novelist Edward Newhouse put this scenario in the foreground of *You Can't Sleep Here*, his aptly titled 1934 novel about a newspaper editor who goes to live among New York's homeless poor. Across the Atlantic, George Orwell decided to cross over the line himself and experience such conditions firsthand. *Down and Out in Paris and London*, his classic 1933 memoir of menial labor and tramping during the height of the Great Depression, demonstrates that poverty is most acutely felt at night. Fighting off cold, vermin, dangers from other tramps, and the systematic abuse of the police, he shows that to be poor is to be acutely sleep-deprived, and that to sleep while poor is often to risk one's well-being or even life. Much of the book reads like a catalog of every imaginable way not to get a good night's sleep. In lodging houses, the pillows are hard and the sheets reek of sweat; you might be awakened by pickpockets, snorers, vomiting drunks, or fellow lodgers waking up to smoke, swear, or relieve their diseased bladders. On the streets, you might get robbed by thieves or beaten by police, and you have to contend not only with rough surfaces and natural elements but also with the noise of trams and light pollution from electrical signs. Being poor, he shows, means being unable to rest.

Across much of the world, such struggles persist. "Without a doubt, sleep is the biggest issue for homeless people," writes San Diego–based blogger and self-proclaimed "chronic homeless man" Kevin Barbieux, aka "The Homeless Guy." (Barbieux updates his blog either using a donated laptop or the computers at his local library, which, like many such facilities, has increasingly become a sleep sanctuary for homeless people.) In shelters, he writes,

> you will be in a room with anywhere from 25 to 150 other home-less people, and not all of them will be ready to go to sleep. They will be talking, laughing or yelling, getting into fights (verbal and physical) making noises, the mentally ill will be trying to wind down from their constant hallucinations. . . . If you like the cold, you'll sleep well, if not, you could have problems. . . . After a couple hours, most everyone has settled in to sleep, and you'll get some sleep. But then you'll be awakened, sometimes rudely, at 5 a.m. at most shelters. 5 a.m. every single morning.

The poetically haunting Indian documentary film *Cities of Sleep*, which chronicles the lives of homeless men attempting to secure safe sleeping places in Delhi, ekes out a street-level philosophy from such struggles. "If you want to seize control over someone," says one of the men, "never let them sleep."

"Normal" sleep, then—sleep undertaken in private, in an unin-terrupted stretch of seven or eight hours at night, and practiced according to a relatively unvarying routine each night—is a privi-lege that is simply unavailable to much of the world's population. The rules surrounding normal sleep may be constricting, and yet those constrictions seem like silken fetters in comparison to the sleep-worlds of those for whom the rules don't, can't, apply. To get a sense of the exclusiveness of "normal" sleep, we might look at the lives of those who were most actively pushed outside its walls during the time of its creation. Just as Thoreau was trying to liberate him-self from the expectation to sleep and wake on schedule in a world run by clocks, trains, and factory bells, an entire population to the south was struggling in a much more basic way to gain control over the rhythms of their bodies.

Offering a frightening view of what sleep looked like on the other side of normal is the story of how sleep was managed, controlled, and systematically manipulated on slave plantations. If slaves helped build the modern world, they were never afforded sufficient rest from the toils involved. Nor were they afforded the privacy that, according to the sociologist Norbert Elias, was becoming a hallmark of Western bourgeois sleep. And once excluded from normal sleep, they were punished for failures to maintain alertness and productivity, and branded as constitutionally lazy for any sign of exhaustion. Their supposedly different sleep patterns—those that marked them as belonging to an "inferior" race—were actually taken as a justification for race-based slavery by medical authorities and slavery propagandists (two overlapping categories). Out of this context, the popular racist idea of the "lazy black" person was born. The rough sleep environments that produced sleep disparities remain prevalent for many of the descendants of slavery today, as does the stigma that was associated with sleeping and waking differently. Sleep can be a respite from prejudice, inequality, and injustice; but, in a cruel twist, controlling sleep is a weapon that one group might use to impose its will on another, and interpreting the sleep of others can be a way to justify that control.

———

As early as 1684, English merchant and social reformer Thomas Tryon identified disturbed sleep as one of the damages wrought by slavery in the New World. (This is the same man who wrote of the health hazards of shared and unclean beds.) In *Friendly Advice to the Gentlemen-Planters of the East and West Indies*—a book urging the reform, if not the repeal, of British slavery in the colonies—he saw wretched sleeping conditions as an ordeal shedding light on the entire system of slavery. Writing in the voice of a slave, he condemned "inconsiderate masters" who heeded "neither the voice of *Nature* nor *reason*, but with Cruelty compel us to Labour beyond our strength, and allow us no competent time of *Rest* or *Refreshment*, in so much that often-times we are forc'd to work so long at the *Wind-Mills*, until we become so *Weary, Dull, Faint, Heavy*, and *Sleepy*, that we are as it were deprived of our natural Senses." He chronicled how slaves working at the copper pots sometimes became so "overcome with weariness and want of proper Rest" that they would "fall into the fierce boyling Syrups." The contrast between the chronic exhaustion of the slaves and the comfortable ease of the plantation rulers' lives was clear. Tryon's enslaved alter-ego says, "We rise early, and lie down late, and labour beyond our strength, whilst our luxurious Masters stretch themselves on their soft Beds and Couches." Despite criticizing these systematic abuses, Tryon did not go so far as to call for the abolition of slavery. (Few of his contemporaries ever did so publicly.) Instead, he believed that cleaning up the worst of the abuses would allow the system to proceed on a more humane basis. In particular, expanding slaves' allotted time for sleep and rest was "a thing worthy to be considered by our Masters," Tryon wrote, "for it would add much to their *Profit and our Health*, which is also their *Wealth*."

Tryon here sounds like one of those sleep management experts who have begun to crop up in today's world, advising companies about how to get the most work out of their workforce by striking the right balance between rest and labor. Many slaveholders would come to take such advice, often drawing on lessons learned from nineteenth-century industrialists to their north, who attempted to regiment their workers' lives in order to extract the most labor from them without wearing them out. One difference, of course, was that most of the southern slaves worked in the fields rather than in factories, and so their tasks tended to come in seasonal spurts as they neared harvest time, rather than in the orderly shifts marked by factory bells. But according to historian Mark Smith, this did not stop slaveholders from self-consciously borrowing from techniques of time management developed by their economic rivals in the North. One plantation owner calculated that "the difference between [slaves] rising at six and at eight, in the course of forty years, amounts to twenty thousand dollars." Some planters were guided primarily by natural rhythms (the sun rising and setting; seasonal adjustments); others insisted that slaves punch a clock, metaphorically speaking. One southern slaveholder wrote, "Their breakfast hour is eight o'clock. . . . I require them to retire at nine o'clock precisely. The foreman calls the roll at that hour, and two or three times during the night, to see that all are at their places." Another noted that the night horn "must be blown in winter at 8, in summer at 9 o'clock, after which no negro must be seen out of his house."

These schedules were enforced by the whip. Former Louisiana slave Solomon Northup wrote in his memoir *Twelve Years a Slave* of the severe whippings that resulted from oversleeping: "With a prayer that he may be on his feet and wide awake at the first sound of the horn, he sinks to his slumbers nightly." Indeed, sleep deprivation is a major theme in Northup's portrait of plantation life: at one point, he is hired to discipline other slaves who are engaged in grinding and boiling sugarcane, an unceasing task that affords him "no regular periods of rest," and he can catch only "a few moments of sleep at a time." Abolitionist writing is full of references to such treatment. The memoir of William Wells Brown, a former slave who went on to write one of the first novels by an African American author, described in heart-wrenching detail watching his mother being beaten mercilessly for oversleeping. And Frederick Law Olmsted, who was a journalist before he was a landscape architect, wrote of a girl's agonizing pleas while being whipped for missing the morning's work (presumably because of oversleeping): "Oh, don't, sir! Oh, please stop, master! Please, sir! Please, sir! Oh, that's enough, master! Oh, Lord! Oh, master, master! Oh, God master, do stop! Oh, God master! Oh, God master!" The spectacle of such beatings, accompanied by the sounds of the lash and the cries themselves, served not only as a warning to other slaves not to oversleep, but also as a demonstration of slaveholders' absolute control over slaves' bodies.

The issue was not simply extracting the maximum amount of work, which, as Thomas Tryon had argued, would have been a good impetus for ensuring that the workers were well-rested. For many reasons, a rested workforce was not always in the best interests of the slaveholders. In his 1784 book *Notes on the State of Virginia*, Thomas

Jefferson turned Tryon's plea for adequate downtime for slaves inside out, arguing that proper plantation management demanded *less* rather than *more* sleep for slaves.

In a passage of shockingly naked racism—shocking even for those who know of Jefferson's tangled position on race—the man who wrote that all men are created equal argued that blacks and whites were simply timed differently. For blacks, he wrote, "seem to require less sleep. A black, after hard labour through the day, will be induced by the slightest amusements to sit up till midnight, or later, though knowing he must be out with the first dawn of the morning. In general, their existence appears to participate more of sensation than reflection. To this must be ascribed their disposition to sleep when abstracted from their diversions, and unemployed in labour. An animal whose body is at rest, and who does not reflect, must be disposed to sleep of course."

Tryon saw the overwork and sleep deprivation of slaves as threats to the slaveholders' economic interests; but Jefferson saw them as biological and economic imperatives. For him, because of what he saw as natural differences between the races, slaves simply didn't need much rest and therefore should be worked to exhaustion. In a move that would be taken up with surprising frequency in the nineteenth century, Jefferson appealed to the sleeping state of the slave to justify unequal treatment. Because "negroes" tended to fall asleep at the drop of a hat while not laboring or being diverted by amusements, Jefferson concluded, they were deficient in "reflection"—a higher sentiment that impelled whites to feats of learning and creativity in their leisure hours. Without the ability to reflect, blacks had nothing to do with themselves when the day was done other than dance and sing or drop off immediately to sleep, whereas whites could stay up late reflecting, thinking, or creating art. Here Jefferson was drawing out the racial implications of a common eighteenth-century view that certain mental afflictions—a nervous sensitivity that might result in sleep loss—indicated a superior cast of mind; they were, in a sense, unfortunate byproducts of belonging to a superior race. Rather than seeing an obvious sign of exhaustion among laborers whose bodies were worn to the point of being "deprived of our natural Senses"—as Tryon put it—Jefferson concluded that black slaves were naturally prone to sleep less than whites. Their quick descent into sleep was a sign not of sleep deprivation but of inadequate powers of self-control and lack of intellectual inclination.

Former slave and abolitionist leader Frederick Douglass would have none of this. Writing in the 1840s and 1850s, he went further than Tryon in his complaints about the cruelty of the exhausting schedules. In a section of his 1855 autobiography, he devoted several pages to "Deprivation of Sleep," which he felt was intentionally induced:

> The sleeping apartments—if they may be called such—have little regard to comfort or decency. Old and young, male and female, married and single, drop down upon the common clay floor, each covering up with his or her blanket,—the only protection they have from cold or exposure. The night, however, is shortened at both ends. The slaves work often as long as they can see, and . . . at the first gray streak of morning, they are summoned to the field by the driver's horn.
>
> More slaves are whipped for oversleeping than for any other fault.

At issue for Douglass was both chronic sleep deprivation and tight regimentation of waking hours. In his memoir, he showed that this combination produced a kind of vegetative state during slaves' scant leisure time:

> Sunday was my only leisure time. I spent this in a sort of beast-like stupor, between sleep and wake, under some large tree. At times I would rise up, a flash of energetic freedom would dart through my soul, accompanied with a faint beam of hope, that flickered for a moment, and then vanished. I sank down again, mourning over my wretched condition.

One can imagine the usefulness of this "beast-like stupor" to the slaveholders—not in making money directly, but in breaking the will of potentially rebellious or noncompliant slaves. The slaves were worked to the point of exhaustion, and had just enough time to recover on Sundays, but they were so wiped out that they could not act on those flashes of "energetic freedom" that might lead them to "rise up." The historian Walter Johnson described such tactics of enforced sleep deprivation as torture. (In response to American use of sleep deprivation on prisoners in Afghanistan and Abu Ghraib, several international human rights agencies have ruled the technique a violation of the Geneva Convention on Human Rights.)

———

It was also important to slaveholders that the people they held in bondage stayed in bed at night. This was as much a matter of security as economics, for nighttime was good cover for runaways, thieves, and rebels. Slaveholders may have borrowed some time-management techniques for regularizing schedules from northern industrialists, but some degree of patterned irregularity was also necessary. As historian Smith noted, too much precision and regularity in their night watches could allow calculating slaves to evade surveillance that much more easily by feigning sleep at the expected time. In an implicit acknowledgment of his slaves' clever manipulations of the nighttime watch, one South Carolina slaveholder introduced a strategic unpredictability in his nocturnal surveillance of slaves. A plantation overseer, he wrote, "should not fall into a regular day or hour for his night visit, but should go so often and at such times that he may be expected anytime."

Such random spot-checks of slaves' sleeping quarters—a mode of surveillance also enamored of store and factory managers in the twentieth century as a means of keeping employees on their toes—were seen as matters of life and death, both for the enslaved and the enslavers. The most famous evasion of nighttime surveillance was the uprising of the rebel slave Nat Turner and his associates in Southampton, Virginia, in 1831. In addition to knowing how to read and write, Turner had a keen sense of clock time—an ability that, as literary scholar Daylanne English has shown, many whites assumed people of African descent lacked. Many slaveholders invested in large clocks, which they placed in central locations; this was apparently the case where Turner lived. Wherever the clocks were, Turner turned them to his advantage, telling his band of conspirators to meet at the big house at "about two hours in the night." They planned to murder the inhabitants while they slept. By planning the revolt for the middle of the night, Turner was depending on the slaves' capacity to frustrate their masters' attempts to control their sleep-wake cycles. The scores of dead whites were testimony to the slaves' self-mastery over their passage through time, precisely the quality that Thomas Jefferson was convinced they lacked.

So a great deal was at stake in controlling the sleep-wake cycle of an enslaved people: economics, control of an unwilling labor force, psychological domination, and physical security. To throw off the bonds of slavery was to retake control over one's body at the most elemental level, that of its daily and nightly rhythms. Tellingly, just as slaveholders were developing elaborate punishments for slaves who overslept—and methods to detect those who weren't sleeping at the right times—many white writers, and even medical men, were promoting the idea that blacks were constitutionally predisposed to sleep more than whites, or at least to drop off more easily. Jefferson had argued that blacks required less sleep, but in dozens of nineteenth-century novels, travelogues, and writings on health we find the reverse: the image of the black man who slept so heavily that he could barely be roused by the commotion around him. "You ought, if you are long acquainted with the South," says a southerner to a visitor from the North in one piece of magazine fiction, "to know that you may shake a Bear out of his winter nap than rouse a sleeping Negro." And pro-slavery novelist Caroline Lee Hentz wrote that "the negro's sleep" was so "deep and sound" that "he can sleep anywhere—reclining, sitting, standing, even walking. He can sleep, we verily believe, on the ridge-pole of a house, or the apex of a church dome." Rather than seeing signs of chronic exhaustion from overwork and poor sleeping conditions, such writers saw a supposedly natural distinction between the races that helped justify the dominion of one over the other.

A popular novel by the South Carolina writer William Gilmore Simms, published in 1835—just four years after Nat Turner's night-time raids—elaborates this idea most fully. In *The Yemassee*, a black slave named July is appointed to watch over a white woman at night during a frontier war with the Indians, who are plotting to massacre the whites in their sleep, and kidnap and perhaps rape the women. "We need scarcely add," the narrator interjects, "knowing the susceptibility of the black in this particular, that sleep was not slow in its approaches to the strongest tower in the citadel of his senses. The subtle deity soon mastered all his sentinels, and a snore . . . sent forth from the flattened but capacious nostrils, soon announced his entire conquest over the premises he had invaded." July, then, is a perfect illustration of Thomas Jefferson's assertion that blacks tend to fall asleep as soon as they stop working. For Jefferson, this tendency was an aspect of the "negro's" inability to reflect, to properly understand his place and function in the world, and therefore of his need to be governed by others. Of course, as the Indians sneak into the cabin and prepare to seize the fitfully slumbering white woman, July lies snoring. The woman is only saved by the fact that one of the Indians trips over July's sleeping body. When he awakes, he, "like most negroes suddenly awaking, was stupid and confused," and he has his skull split open by a hatchet.

The sleeping white woman is more fortunate, for her aged father had been sleepless in the next room, and is roused into immediate action by her screams. Insomnia was increasingly viewed in the nineteenth century in racial terms: it was an ailment of civilized whites, whose ceaseless mental activity could force their brains to stay awake mulling over the problems of the day even when the body began to wear down. This idea goes back at least as far as George Cheyne's influential tract *The English Malady*, which in 1733 explored the characteristic "nervous distemper" brought on by the English climate, diet, and occupations: its symptoms prominently included "*Inquietude* of Spirit, and want of natural *Sleep*." In America, medical theorists tended to stress the racial dimensions of this tendency. As nineteenth-century neurologist William Alexander Hammond put it, an increase in "morbid wakefulness or insomnia" was a byproduct of advanced civilization. Hammond explained that because mental activity leads to increased "wear and tear" of the brain, members of "advanced" civilizations were particularly susceptible to sleep loss.

Hammond's medical investigations into the causes, functions, and disturbances of sleep built upon new understandings of the brain's role in controlling sleep, specifically Johann Blumenbach's earlier theories that sleep was a function of the diminished flow of oxygenated blood to the brain. Hammond believed that during waking hours, blood flowed freely to the brain, impelled by a combination of muscular and mental activity, but as brain stimulation decreased and oxidation subsided, less blood was drawn into the brain, and sleep ensued. But problems sometimes arose, particularly because mental activity could force the capillaries open, giving the brain no opportunity to rest. And so insomnia was particularly prevalent among what would today be called knowledge workers and members of the creative class: stockbrokers, writers, and intellectuals. Such were the types that Thomas Jefferson had in mind when he wrote that only whites could stay up all night reading or composing philosophical treatises. The slave July, snoring lustily through the violent attack in Simms's novel, apparently lacked the burst of oxygen to the brain that would allow him, like the heroine's father, to start up from sleep in a moment of danger.

The southern physician Samuel Adolphus Cartwright turned a similar theory of sleep and oxygenation into a full-blown medical justification for race-based slavery. Cartwright, who was appointed by the Medical Association of Louisiana to study the diseases of slaves, saw his task as inquiring into the propriety of race-based slavery, as well as the best management practices for maintaining the slave system, from a medical point of view. In a frequently reprinted and widely cited set of articles published in a leading journal of southern thought in 1851, he wrote that the subject of the diseases and physical peculiarities of "the Negro race [had] a direct and practical bearing upon over three millions of people, and $2,000,000,000 of property!"

In his medical investigations of that human property, Cartwright returned again and again to the slave's sleeping body, trying to divine what the body at rest could tell him about its capacities while awake. After detailing distinctions between black and white in terms of skin tone, spine and pelvis curvature, facial angle, and the capacities for hearing and sight, he found that the main difference in the constitution of the races was a cardiopulmonary one: specifically, the amount of oxygen flowing to the brain during sleep. "Negroes," he wrote, were afflicted with "a deficiency of red blood in the pulmonary and arterial systems, from a defective atmospherization or arterialization of the blood in the lungs. . . . That is the true cause of that debasement of mind, which has rendered the people of Africa unable to take care of themselves."

This deficiency, Cartwright argued, resulted from the natural sleeping habits of blacks. Following Blumenbach's model of the respiratory function of sleep, and paralleling Hammond's elaboration of the connections among sleep, oxygenation of the brain, and "civilization," he outlined a theory that connected white supremacy to differences in sleep patterns. In childhood, the two races were basically equal in both sleep behaviors and intellectual capacity. Unlike adults, he argued, children of all races did not need full circulation of fresh air during sleep; instead, they instinctively would smother their faces in their mothers' bosoms or cover their heads with a blanket, thus inducing "re-breathing" of their own breath, which in turn led to a "hebetude [lethargy] of intellect from the defective vitalization of the blood distributed to the brain." However, white children eventually moved beyond this stage and breathed freely during sleep, he said, whereas blacks continued "covering their heads and faces, during sleep, with a blanket, or any kind of covering that they can get hold of." This propensity for warming the head indicated "an instinctive design to obstruct the entrance of the free external air into the lungs during sleep," causing black people to breathe in "heated air, loaded with carbonic acid and aqueous vapor."

The resulting restriction of oxygen in the brain, said Cartwright, led to a permanent intellectual state similar to that of a small white child. Trapped in this childlike state, blacks instinctively "love[d] those in authority over them, who minister[ed] to their wants and immediate necessities," and, like children, they required "government in every thing; food, clothing, exercise, sleep . . . or they will run into excess." Perhaps forgetting—or more accurately, repressing—the story of Nat Turner rising up in the night, he wrote that black people, with their brains weakened by nocturnal oxygen deficiency, were easily ruled over by white masters. Hence "the facility with which an hundred, even two or three hundred, able-bodied and vigorous negroes are kept in subjection by one white man, who sleeps in perfect security among them."

While Cartwright clearly intended to suggest that these differences in brain development justified an unyielding racial hierarchy, an attentive reader will notice that in his account, the supposed inferiority of blacks to whites is not completely innate: it depends on black and white children sleeping differently. Racial theory in the mid-nineteenth century was a curious amalgam of scientific, sociological, and even religious thinking, which generally did not conclude that biological difference was entirely determinative—as late nineteenth- and early twentieth-century theories often did. An egalitarian response to Cartwright's account would have been to find ways for blacks to stop breathing in "heated air," and thus bring their brain oxygen levels up to those of whites. But Cartwright had a ready defense against this proposition: it was widely believed that "negroes" were simply not constitutionally capable of surviving prolonged exposure to cold air, and so it was natural to assume that they would always gravitate toward fires, smoke, and other sources of warmth in their sleep. The need for heated air thus ensured that their brains would not develop properly. Because these nocturnal behaviors that stunted their development were a matter of survival, blacks would always depend on whites to provide "the kind of government which we call slavery, but which is actually an improvement on the government of their fathers."

Without this proper "government," slaves were liable to run amok. Cartwright is most famous today for developing several disease categories that pertained only to slaves—and troublesome slaves, in particular. Among these was "Drapetomania," or the tendency to run away; another was "Dysaesthesia Aethiopica, or hebetude of mind and obtuse sensibility of body," in which the slave became "like a person half asleep, that is with difficulty aroused and kept awake." Stumbling in this half-awake state, the slave lost all concern for his or her personal well-being and for the property of the master (which was more or less the same thing). Afflicted slaves tended to "break, waste and destroy everything they handle[d] . . . paying no attention to property." They would "wander about at night, and keep in a half nodding sleep during the day," mindlessly disrupting their communities like a "faulty automaton or senseless machine." Cartwright's remedy for these sleep disorders "peculiar to the Negro" resembled Jefferson's: more work. With masters putting the patient "to hard work in the open air and sunshine to expand his lungs," the result would be a happy slave and a well-run plantation.

Cartwright's theories about sleep and race gave medical legitimacy to the fast-developing stereotype of the "lazy Negro" that spread through the nineteenth and twentieth centuries through minstrel shows, early films, Jim Crow racist discourse, and even Reagan-era complaints about "strapping young bucks" who used food stamps to buy T-bone steaks and "welfare queens" who found it easier to chisel the system than to work. Under this medical rubric, the depressing, exhausting, and soul-killing aspects of enslavement, disenfranchisement, and poverty could simply be interpreted as aversion to work, inability to control the body's urges, and a need for imposed discipline.

And so controlling and interpreting sleep had important ramifications in a slaveholding society. Taking charge of the sleep-wake cycle was a way to break slaves, to make maximum profit, and to protect the white slaveholding class from retribution. Slaveholders had to strike a careful balance: they had to allow enough sleep for their captive workforce's labor to be profitable, yet not so much that they might be clear-eyed and energetic enough to escape. Slaveholders and their apologists, though, did not want to admit to others, or perhaps to themselves, that they were intentionally manipulating their human property in this way, and so they concocted various explanations for what Frederick Douglass called the "beast-like stupor" in which many slaves passed their bleary days: they belonged to a naturally lazy or sleep-inclined race; they couldn't control their bodies with their minds the way whites could; they never were capable of the full consciousness that led to the superior attainments of whites, and so must be kept in a subservient position.

Slavery's critics did not simply reject this picture—sometimes they turned it around. The sociologist Orlando Patterson in 1982 famously characterized the slaveholder as a "parasite" who fed off the labor of the slave but then camouflaged that dependence by describing the slave as the one who fed off of the master. Nineteenth-century writers who opposed slavery used sleeping patterns as an index of this cruel reversal. In 1835, Alexis de Tocqueville argued that slavery had led the slaveholders to lead the kinds of slothful lives of dissipation that they attributed to blacks in their natural state. Tocqueville claimed that the free labor system of the North created energetic bodies, whereas the slave system led to indolence—not of slaves, but of masters. In the North, he wrote, "the white extends his activity and his intelligence to all undertakings," but members of the southern master class were spoiled by having others labor for them. In the South, "you would say that society is asleep; man seems idle."

This picture of white southern somnolence was taken up with a vengeance by Harriet Beecher Stowe in *Uncle Tom's Cabin*, where slavery is shown to corrupt the morals and the work ethic of whites. The chief representatives of slavery's ability to sap the will of whites are the sickly, lethargic Augustine St. Claire and his hypochondriac, bedridden wife, Marie, who together run—or fail to run—a Louisiana plantation. Of Marie, Stowe wrote, "There was no end of her various complaints; but her principal forte appeared to lie in sick-headache which sometimes would confine her to her room three days out of six." Such writers combatted popular images of deep-sleeping, insensate slaves like those purveyed by novelists Simms and Hentz, as well as the more scientific-sounding conclusions offered by Jefferson and Cartwright about black people's inability to control their sleep-wake cycles, by depicting "the sleepy South" as a zone where black people did all the bone-wearying work and slaveholding whites lolled in indolent repose.

Think about the trains that Thoreau witnessed whipping through the Concord woods of the 1840s, deranging his countrymen's sense of time and disrupting the sleep cycles of those who had to adjust their lives according to the new schedules—and fast-forward a few decades. Later in the century, railroad companies made even further incursions across the boundary between sleeping and waking when the Pullman Company began to run the first trains with sleeping berths for passengers. The trains were something of a luxury for travelers, but who worked on them? From the time he started his company in 1867, founder George Pullman believed that former slaves emancipated during the Civil War were particularly suited to this kind of personal service, which included making beds, shining shoes, and polishing spittoons. By the 1920s, the Pullman Company was the largest employer of African Americans in the nation. Like steelworkers, these African American sleeping-car porters had extremely long hours on duty; making matters worse, they were expected to sleep in public places. A porter in 1903 estimated that members of his crew averaged less than four hours of sleep per night; echoing the punishments of oversleeping slaves, the company disciplined those who fell asleep on duty or in the wrong places, with suspensions that could last up to thirty days.

In 1925, the porters organized to create the first major national union by and for people of color: the Brotherhood of Sleeping Car Porters, with A. Philip Randolph as chief organizer and leader. (Randolph would go on to play a major role in the civil rights movement.) One of the union organizers' more clever tactics was to align their rhetoric with management's reliance on industrial efficiency: "It is a well-recognized principle in psychological physiology that fatigue destroys efficiency and lessens productivity." Initially, they demanded a 240-hour month, down from the 400 hours expected by the company; not until 1965 did the Brotherhood achieve a 40-hour week for its members. In addition to pushing for more humane schedules that would allow these guardians of white travelers' sleep to find some rest themselves, they focused on the spatial arrangements in which they were expected to catch their few hours of release from work. Porters were typically expected to sleep on couches in the restroom or smoking room, which were not only unsanitary and uncomfortable but also left them vulnerable to being thrown violently to the floor with a derailment or collision. These conditions, as well as the health implications of their punishing schedules, became a public matter when Pullman workers testified before the US Commission on Industrial Relations and several labor boards during their decades-long effort to improve working conditions. As historian Alan Derickson put it, these workers, with no training in biomedical sciences, contributed important knowledge about the effects of sleep deprivation on respiratory, cardiac, and mental health. Frederick Douglass, Solomon Northup, and others had protested the ways in which white slaveholders had pushed those they held in bondage outside the bounds of normal sleep and full awakening in order to control their bodies and dominate their minds. It is fitting that descendants of these chronically exhausted black men and women fought back to reclaim adequate sleep as a basic human right.

In American society today, sleep is still not distributed equally, and racial disparities are particularly stubborn. Public health researcher Lauren Hale of the State University of New York at Stony Brook, who investigates the socioeconomic forces behind sleep-related behaviors, discovered in a 2009 study of almost 33,000 people that African Americans were far more likely than other ethnic groups to find themselves sleeping outside the confines of the "normal" spectrum: that is, either fewer than six hours per night or more than nine. Hale hypothesized that such clustering of sleep at the poles resulted from stressful sleep environments, including noisy or dangerous sleep arrangements, irregular work shifts, and "an abundance of life stressors among racial minorities." Compounding the problem—an earlier study cited by Hale showed—was a finding that compared to whites, African Americans experienced significantly less slow-wave sleep—the heaviest part of slumber, which is essential to physical healing, growth, and optimal cognitive functioning. Unlike Cartwright, who nearly two centuries before had also connected differences in sleep to differences in cognition, Hale and her colleagues saw such differences as anything but innate. Rather than seeing sleeping differences—as so many white nineteenth-century observers did—as a sign of the superiority of one race over the other, Hale sees such differences as an effect of social domination. Leveling the playing field for sleepers, in her view, is as much a matter of social justice as is anything that occurs in the waking world.

No one would wish to revisit the dark nights of rough sleep experienced by blacks living under a system of racial slavery, but Joseph McGill, a museum professional from South Carolina, doesn't want to forget them, either. The founder of the Slave Dwelling Project, McGill leads groups of interested visitors on overnight stays in the existing slave quarters of old plantations—both South and North. His goal is "to wake up and deliver the message that the people who lived in these structures were not a footnote in American history." The groups he assembles—mostly, like himself, descendants of enslaved people, but also occasionally descendants of slaveholders—are generally not interested in re-creating misery; indeed, McGill writes in his blog of the camp-like feeling of gathering around the fire, swapping stories, and meeting new friends. But the experience of sleeping on the hard floor of these cabins honors, in a more visceral way than one can get from reading a book or watching a film, the experience of naked vulnerability that was impossible to avoid facing squarely at night. Describing one of these sleepovers, McGill wrote that after the simple meal had been eaten, the stories told, and the fire extinguished, the participants

eventually all retired to our chosen cabins for the night, but it wasn't until the morning that I began to process what the life of a slave must have felt like in real life. This feeling that I would never get from any slave narrative, no matter how telling. I awoke sore from sleeping on a hard, holey, wooden floor. I was more tired waking up than when I laid down to sleep. Because it was the end of winter, the creepy crawlers had yet to emerge, but the floorboards had gaps big enough for snakes to emerge. The bed had no mattress, but I imagine the mattresses were probably made of hay or moss. The cabins themselves were essentially duplexes, one room per place. The stoves shared a chimney.

Imagine what it was like to have up to 13 children and two parents living in a room and just on the other side of a thin wall, the same thing. There was only space enough for one bed. Now imagine being forced into these conditions at the end of a day that started with you being forced to wade in the stagnant waters of a rice plantation, sun up to sun down.

Waking history was not enough to tell him the story of the past that he was seeking. Only after struggling for sleep on these cold, rough floors could he say, "This was the life of a slave."

PART III

Rocking the Cradle

*I've more than once
screamed the title of this
book in my own head.*

—Anonymous reviewer on
Amazon's page for Adam
Mansbach's *Go the F**k to Sleep*

*This being married and
bringing up children is as
easy as can be—when you
learn how!*

—Charlotte Perkins Gilman

CHAPTER FIVE

Wild Things

From the perspective of many of the world's poor and outcast, being able to sleep in a room of one's own through the night must seem an almost unattainable ideal. And it's an ideal that those with sufficient means pursue almost obsessively, training their children to sleep in this way from an extremely early age, as if the children's lives—or the parents' sanity—depended on it. Solitary and uninterrupted childhood sleep is a crucial feature of middle-class Western family life, one that requires an enormous amount of micromanagement and psychic energy. Yet for millions of families, the frustrations and perils of childrearing often coalesce around a bedtime struggle that begins in early infancy and continues well into adolescence; one study shows that more parents seek pediatric advice about children's sleep than about any other topic. Nothing better expresses the anxiety associated with this essential incubator of middle-class normality than the 2011 runaway best-selling mock-bedtime book *Go the F**k to Sleep*, written in the voice of an exasperated parent who is about ready to give up on the enterprise and simply strangle his child. The book undeniably struck a nerve for readers, as comments on its Amazon product page attest: "I've more than once screamed the title of this book in my own head," one reader admits. "It's nice to know there are millions of other parents out there sharing our pain," writes another. "It totally made me feel better." Five stars from both.

Part of the problem, to be sure, is a matter of brain development. Children need more sleep than adults, largely because sleep helps promote the development of neural networks crucial for the brain's maturation. Children of different ages also have different needs. All of this means that at different ages, our bodies are timed differently. So some degree of tension around family sleep is probably inevitable.

But there's nothing in nature that says children should sleep through the night, or alone—and precious little in history, either. Trying to make this happen in a consistent way often generates a power struggle that brings out the worst in all parties involved: emotional terrorism, feelings of powerlessness and rage, and a host of anxieties about privacy, child development, sexuality, educational attainment, time management, and the parents' own productivity in the workplace. The hundreds of guidebooks written by pediatric sleep experts and self-help gurus (two overlapping categories), with their charts, graphs, and elaborate sleep-training systems—as well as the brisk market for baby sleep gizmos and even professional sleeping coaches—testify to the mess we have created around the child's bed. And debates about parental roles often expose or exacerbate gender conflicts within the household.

Beyond intergenerational psychological warfare and the battle of the sexes, the problem of children's sleep also has hidden environmental and economic dimensions. To be a middle-class family, particularly in the United States, one is practically required to have sufficient square footage to allow for separate bedrooms where children can learn to sleep alone in order to become self-reliant little Thoreaus of the night. This arrangement—parents amusing themselves in the main part of the house and then sleeping in a private bedroom, each child sleeping in another, straight through the night—is a historical anomaly of the West in the past century and a half. In fact, it's such a departure from the rest of human history that it might seem like child abuse in other times and places. And it's an arrangement that remains frankly unaffordable for most of the world's population, for whom American-style suburban sprawl seems an unachievable dream, a wasteful abomination, or both. Since solitary children's sleep is so costly and difficult to maintain and produces such anxiety and frustration—as well as being unusual in the broad scope of history—there must be powerful forces at work that make this arrangement such a central focus of parenting in our world. So how did this training ground for normal sleep take shape?

———

Before the industrial revolution, getting children to sleep could certainly be rough. Even in rural communities that timed themselves by the rise and fall of the sun and the passage of the seasons, rather than by factory bells or the rhythms of global corporate capitalism, children's sleep was still a burden to haggard parents. Poor women, especially, had their hands full, especially at night. A 1739 poem by the English "washer-woman" poet Mary Collier makes clear that women's labors, unlike men's, did not end when the sun went down. Writing back to a male working-class poet who had chided women for their frivolity and their tendency to chatter during work, she insisted that it was working women who bore the heaviest load:

> *We must make haste, for when we Home are come,*
> *Alas! We find our Work but just begun;*
> *So many Things for our Attendance call,*
> *Had we ten Hands, we could employ them all*
> *Our children put to Bed, with greatest Care*
> *We all Things for your coming Home prepare:*
> *You sup, and go to Bed without delay,*
> *And rest yourselves till the ensuing Day;*
> *While we, alas! But little Sleep can have,*
> *Because our forward Children cry and rave;*
> *Yet, without fail, soon as Day-light doth spring,*
> *We in the Field again our Work begin.*

Although "Children cry and rave" across the centuries, often driving their parents to a state of exhausted distraction in any age, much has changed from Collier's time to ours. The great labor historian E. P. Thompson cited Collier's poem as evidence of a different time-system for labor before the industrial revolution. Rather than worry about getting to the factory or office "on time," as measured by a clock and a scowling manager, Collier measures her day by tasks: washing or working in the field, obviously, but also making supper, mending clothing, making beds, feeding swine, pumping water, stoking fires—and, of course, tending to infants. Certainly it was a grueling routine: as Thompson noted, "the most arduous and prolonged work was that of the labourer's wife in the rural economy." Yet, although Collier's ordeal sounds exhausting, it lacks the psychological tension and anxiety, the maddening urgency that pervades the contemporary management of children's sleep.

Why is this tension missing? Many features of contemporary middle-class sleep management are absent from Collier's picture. There is no mention of a bedtime for the children, or different bedtimes for different children at different ages. There are no pharmaceutical aids—mother's potentially addictive little helpers—for the exhausted woman, who, she tells us, rises "often at midnight" to complete her chores, while her husband lies in oblivion. No sleep expert hovers in the background telling her how to get everyone on a schedule; no alarm clock rouses anyone in the morning. Nor is there any mention of helping the kids with homework, or nagging them about it, or, indeed, of sending anyone to school. There aren't any distractions to keep the kids up, either: no TV, no video games, no electricity to power them, maybe not even any books or magazines. And the kids themselves just cry—they don't whine and stall and argue. The parents are not itching to have "quality time" after the kids go to bed—either for entertainment or recreational sex. There are no separate bedrooms, as is now practically mandatory in all but the poorest households in North America and Europe; apparently the household does not even have separate *beds*, though there are multiple children. The extent of co-sleeping (do the parents retire to the same bed as the children?) is not detailed, but certainly the night is a time of bodily contact quite different from what we experience as the contemporary middle-class norm of sleep as an activity in which only consenting adults allow body parts to touch. This sense of intergenerational bodily contact continues into the working day on the fields:

> *To get a Living we so willing are,*
> *Our tender Babes into the Field we bear,*
> *And wrap them in our Cloaths to keep them warm,*
> *While round about we gather up the Corn.*

This is not to argue that Collier's predicament is less severe than yours or mine, or that her family was closer, or that they slept better, or even more naturally. It's simply to say that while tending to children's sleep was a hardship, it wasn't a *problem* as it is now in many parts of the world. In other words, putting children to bed was a chore, even an ordeal, but it didn't have so many vexing angles to consider: psychology, leisure, discipline, scheduling, cognitive development, and so on. Collier may have been as sleep-deprived as any harried office-working parent trying desperately to synchronize her child's sleep with the rhythms of her allotted place in global commerce and the child's place in the educational system, but she can't exactly be said to have experienced anxiety about them. Sleep could be rough, but it didn't have to be micromanaged and fussed over, dosed up, sprayed with expert wisdom, measured by clocks, protected from distractions, and shut off in a dark room to work its magic upon the child.

Consider now the narrator of the exhausted, frustrated parent of Adam Mansbach's *Go the F**k to Sleep*, a man who has apparently tried everything to get his child to sleep on time, only to be confronted by demands for a glass of water, a trip to the bathroom, another bedtime book, parental help with the stuffed animal arrangement, attempts at escape. Giving voice to the feelings of any parent who faces such truculent behavior, he explodes in frustration at the end of every stanza, offering endless nursery-rhyme variations on the book's obscene title. How did we get from there to here—from a weary mother who sees her children's crying and raving as a necessary burden to a man so desperate to have time to watch a movie with his wife that he can only splutter expletives at his child? E. P. Thompson's epochal shift from task-orientation to factory time is a large part of the story: once parents had to wake up at a standardized time to get to work, children had to be synchronized to the needs of parents and the educational system adults had devised, and a new zone of struggle around sleep and waking hours came into being. But as this chapter will show, there are other dimensions to the problem, involving lighting, electricity, leisure time, privacy, sexuality, living standards, medicine, commercialism, education, and changing sleeping arrangements—as well as philosophical conceptions of what childhood meant and what it was for. The child's bed, in other words, became a pot in which the stew of the world's problems was cooked.

———

Half a century before Mary Collier wrote "The Woman's Labour," the English philosopher John Locke penned a series of letters to a gentleman friend who wished to have some sustained advice about the proper rearing of children. Eventually Locke published these letters in book form, as *Some Thoughts Concerning Education* (1693). Here he offered a concrete, practical follow-up to his more abstract account of intellectual development in *An Essay Concerning Human Understanding* (1690), which had expounded his theory of the infant mind as a *tabula rasa*, or blank page, to be inscribed by experience and association. How to write on that page—to form the script for a proper gentlemanly upbringing—was his concern in *Some Thoughts*. With sections on scholastic curriculum (less Latin, more vernacular language training; more drawing, less poetry and music), discipline (less whipping, more shame and rewards), food, and clothing, the book became a classic of educational theory and remained so through the nineteenth century. It also set a precedent for generations of experts—whether self-appointed or professionally accredited—in terms of the range of topics appropriate to a treatise on parenting and child development. One of these topics, unsurprisingly, was children's sleep (sandwiched between sections on fruit and constipation).

Locke was the great theorist of nurture over nature: he believed that character arose from the influence of experience and environment, and could therefore be shaped by careful training. The surprise, however, is that this most famous theorist of *nurture* left most of sleep to *nature*. "Nothing is more to be indulg'd children, than *sleep*. In this alone they are to be permitted to have their full satisfaction; nothing contributing more to the growth and health of children, than *sleep*. All that is to be regulated in it, is, in what part of the twenty-four hours they should take it, which will easily be resolved, by only saying that it is of great use to accustom 'em to rise early in the morning." Of all the areas of a child's life, he wrote, sleep is the only one that should *not* be regulated: left to his or her own devices, the child will sleep as long as he or she needs to. The parent's only duty is to get the child to rise early, and then natural inclinations will lead the child to begin going to sleep at the appropriate time. There is some discussion about bedding (a hard mattress is preferable to a "down bed," because it will make it easier for children to travel if they are not used to luxury), but there is nothing about bottles, books, snuggling, or toys. Sleep, he wrote, is "the great cordial of nature," a resource that is allotted to each child in perfectly fitting measures by nature itself. The parents' or nurse's main duty is to get out of the way.

Locke's attitude concerning childhood sleep bears a surprising degree of resemblance to that of the writer who is usually considered his antagonist in theories of childhood, Jean-Jacques Rousseau. In his influential *Émile, or On Education* (1762), Rousseau developed the important romantic concept of childhood as a zone of innocence and extended play, which should be interfered with as little as possible. The idea extended to sleep. Going even farther than Locke, Rousseau held that *any* imposition of sleep discipline on the child—even waking a child up early—was dangerous: "The only habit the child should be allowed to contract is that of having no habits. . . . [L]et him not want to eat, sleep, or do anything at fixed hours, nor be unable to be left alone by day or night." The mild differences between Locke's and Rousseau's counsel on sleep schedules reflect competing aims in the cultivation of the child. Locke—who promoted training in correct behavior—believed that a child should be guided to form the habit of waking early, so that in later years he (and Locke does seem to worry mainly about boys) would be disinclined to stay up late and go carousing with unsavory characters in wine halls. Rousseau—who wanted to teach citizens how to rationally manage their political liberties—saw strict scheduling as habit-forming, something that could create emotional and physical dependencies that would limit freedom. For this democrat, sleeping late, rising early, and staying up all night were life choices that the child must learn to make independently.

Despite the broad philosophical differences between these thinkers—nurture vs. nature, training vs. self-cultivation—when it came to children's sleep, Locke and Rousseau agreed on far more than they disagreed on: Don't meddle too much. Appeal to the child's natural inclinations. Encourage flexibility over rigidity. As Rousseau put it, "when the child is put to bed and his nurse grows weary of his chatter, she says to him, 'Go to sleep.' That is much like saying 'get well,' when he is ill. The right way is to let him get tired of himself." This is not to say that their famously opposed systems of training and pedagogy bore some deep resemblance. Rather, it is to highlight the fact that children's sleep in the preindustrial early modern period was not yet experienced as a problem of much significance. This is to be expected of Rousseau, whose notions of the naturally innocent child mirrored his conception of the noble savage—leave them in a state of nature. But it is a surprise to encounter in Locke, whose name became synonymous with the call to train and refine the mind. It would take centuries before behavioral psychologists—the twentieth century's true heirs of Lockean systems of training—would identify sleep as part of their system of training and habit formation.

———

Through the eighteenth century and much of the nineteenth, the advice—or really anti-advice—of Locke and Rousseau was usually enough: beyond gently waking the child in the morning, let nature run its course, or simply help the child find the right amount of sleep and the right time for sleep on his or her own. Eighteenth-century medical advice added nuance, but nothing like the elaborate systems developed centuries later. Several eighteenth-century physicians, for instance, counseled against putting children down to sleep right after a meal. One, writing in 1763, offered some practical tips about when and how to breastfeed a child at night so that the mother's sleep would be least disrupted: "Supposing the Mother go to Bed at ten or eleven, if the Child should happen to be awake, let it be turn'd dry . . . and suckled again; and it will sleep soundly for six or seven Hours: perhaps now and then it will whimper a little, but if it is not touch'd it will fall asleep again immediately." Some offered thoughts about when to burp the child, and one wrote that if the child did not burp roundly after being patted on the back, "I would recommend a gentle Puke." Sleeping posture was also a general health concern. The author of *The Art of Nursing* (1733) warned that children should not sleep on their sides (unlike adults), as their bones may become damaged; it was much better for them to be laid on their backs in the cradle. And sixteenth-century physician Thomas Cogan wrote that lying on the side would draw phlegm and other toxic humors into the base of the brain, which would cause nightmares.

A few disputes did arise about children's sleep in the eighteenth century. One of these involved opium as a sleep aid for children. Cogan mentioned in the late sixteenth century that "the women of Salerne give their children white Poppie seeds with milk to cause them to sleep." (He also mentioned mixing opium with "Almonds and Hemp-seed"—a pretty potent combination that must have led to interesting dreams, whether the child was asleep or not.) But by 1731, Thomas Apperley was warning parents about nurses who, when they heard children crying in the night, rushed to give them "Doses of Meconium, or Syrup of White Poppies, in order to get them to sleep, and to keep them quiet." This, he wrote, "is a very pernicious and roguish Custom, and Parents can never be too cautious about it. . . . It is high time to keep an Eye on such a Nurse." He undercut his case, though, by simply recommending a concoction with a lower concentration of poppy syrup in it.

Another disagreement arose about the use of cradles vs. beds, in some ways foreshadowing contemporary debates about co-sleeping.

On the pro-cradle side, physician James Nelson warned of what today are called "catastrophic layovers" that may occur when an infant is left in bed with the parents: "There is always Danger more or less of the Child being overlaid. . . . Many Children have by this means been killed in one Night's time." On the other side was William Moss, who wrote in 1781 that sleeping in an adult's bed was far more comfortable and natural for a young child than being in a crib. As for the concerns about "the danger of a nurse's overlaying the child," he assured readers that "of this there is little to fear, if she has been accustomed to sleep with children; and is an accident that scarcely happens once in an age with those who have not been accustomed to it." He also mentions the objection that the child might "learn a custom it may hereafter be difficult to break him of: but this seems founded more upon surmise than reality; as it may be generally effected, with a little pains taking, at a proper season."

In general, though, discussions of children's sleeping patterns and spatial arrangements were offered in genial, non-alarmist tones, and where the authorities disagreed (except in the case of layovers), they did so in terms that were meant to instill comfort rather than fear of doing the wrong thing. But that began to change in the nineteenth century. Take the case of wake-up times. Benjamin Franklin's famous "early to bed, early to rise" dictum was already a commonplace when he uttered it; and one finds the early-to-rise nostrum regularly rehashed in popular health journals of the eighteenth and nineteenth centuries as "one of the strongest indications of health." Wealth and wisdom, Franklin mentioned, were additional benefits: adherent to the "early rising" movement included the famous minister John Wesley; and a "Young Men's Early Rising Association" was founded in New York in 1859, with members attributing "marked success in life" to their participation.

The primary goal of the early rising movement was to cultivate health and economic productivity. But a moral note also crept in, and here we can locate an emerging source of anxiety about children's sleep and bedtime activities. "Get up the moment you wake in the morning, for . . . drowsing in the morning, often induces the emissions," wrote the author of *Vital Force: How Wasted and How Pre-served* (1872). Fear of spontaneous ejaculations, and more broadly, autoerotic activity (whether consciously indulged in or not) gained traction in the eighteenth century and spread virally through the nineteenth, turning the child's bed into a zone that absorbed adult anxieties about sex.

The age of Enlightenment was also the age of anxiety about masturbation and other forms of "self-pollution." Beginning with the anonymous 1712 publication of *Onania, or the Heinous Sin of Self-Pollution, and Its Frightful Consequences in Both Sexes, Considered*, a steady stream of physicians, preachers, pedagogues, and other moralists fanned readers' fears about this common practice, show-ing that it was connected to infertility, birth defects, insanity, crime, prostitution, a host of physical ailments and infirmities, and virtually every other nasty thing one could imagine. Nineteenth-century asy-lum directors believed that many cases of insanity were caused by masturbation, and so they took extraordinary measures to prevent it within their institutions. The superintendent of McLean Asylum for the Insane in Massachusetts, Luther Bell, proposed beds with straps, active labor, and opium to induce sleep, and even a special masturbators' ward, where "a relay of guards should be so employed that a constant watch should be kept upon the sufferers at night, while by day, at their labors and amusements, the same precautions should be continued." Outside of the asylum, a cottage industry of anti-masturbation appliances—erection alarms, penis cases, sleeping mitts, and devices to keep girls from spreading their legs—grew up around the fear of self-abuse.

Why was this so? Historian of sexuality Thomas Laqueur aptly calls masturbation the "crack cocaine" of eighteenth- and nineteenth-century sexuality; it served as an all-purpose vice because it was the evil twin of the most valued Enlightenment ideals: pri-vacy, autonomy, and imagination. Where philosophers and states-men saw the proper cultivation of these qualities as the key to a well-regulated democratic society, masturbation made a mockery of them. "Masturbation," wrote Laqueur, "hijacked some of the central virtues of civil society and transformed them into evils; it was the dark underbelly of a new social and cultural order that seemed to threaten its very core." It was fanned, too, by the new commercialism of the industrial age that made soft pillows, private bedrooms, and racy reading material widely available. Supposedly counteracting this tendency, anti-masturbation tracts themselves soon became marketable commodities, but they were sometimes hard to distinguish from the stuff that provoked the solitary vice.

Autoerotic urges could be consummated in many locations, but none was more worrisome than the bedroom—the bedroom of the child, in particular. Warned Luther Bell, the combination of books and recumbency created an almost irresistible inducement to self-pollution. "To lay on the bed in the day time, not for the purpose of sleeping, but to gratify this feeling of weakness, to read in bed at night, and to continue in bed in the morning, after being awaked," inevitably led a child's imagination to "run riot," with fearsome consequences. Accordingly, guidebooks and health manuals urged parents to practice vigilance on children who had been trundled off to bed. The Enlightenment physician Samuel Auguste David Tissot first warned in 1759 about the developmental hazards of childhood masturbation; and in 1875, Pierre Larousse's *Grand Dictionnaire* announced, "We find in the annals of medicine plenty of cases of five-, six-, and eight-year-old children dead as a result of masturbation."

But a contradiction arose: if children were sleeping in their own beds, apart from their parents, wouldn't the solitary vice flourish in their private chambers? William Whitty Hall, the American physician who warned so fervently about the risks to health and well-being posed by co-sleeping, tried to have it both ways. In his book *Sleep*, which was published in at least five editions across the third quarter of the nineteenth century, he explained that rather than being a solitary vice, children learned masturbation by co-sleeping with each other, which is one of the reasons that he urged parents to place children in their own bedrooms by age seven. The risks became particularly acute in the teen years, when younger children might learn from older ones to indulge in those practices that "waste away the vigor and flesh and strength of the body, eventually impairing the mind itself." He counseled against sleepovers, too, because "your neighbor may be as pure and blameless as yourself, but never having had the attention directed to the point in question, may have been remiss in the matter of her children's associations." Yet he was also conscious that by counseling parents to make older children sleep alone, he might be creating conditions under which the child was afforded "the amplest opportunity of unbridled indulgence." Therefore, for parents who suspected their child of succumbing, he recommended spending a few nights awake in the child's room, carefully observing the child's behavior. If they detected anything untoward, they were to lecture the child the following morning. He offers a script for how parents might address the problem: "My child, I noticed something last night not uncommon with youth, and as you may not know the nature of it, perhaps it might be best for me to tell you all about it, because sometimes persons become deranged by it, or kill themselves."

By the age of Sigmund Freud, such wild fears had largely been tamed; masturbation was beginning to be accepted, or at least tolerated, as a universal and healthy expression of children's sexuality (albeit one that needed to be outgrown for healthy development of the personality). However, the nearly two-centuries-long panic over what happened in the bed of the child did not entirely vanish. Psychoanalysis simply redirected that fear of sexuality into the bedroom down the hall, where the child's parents might be engaging in nighttime behavior that would be traumatic for the child to witness. Freud's lurid 1918 case study of the floridly neurotic patient known as the "Wolf-Man" makes clear the troubles that could result from watching one's parents do unspeakable things to each other in the night. Moralists and physicians had already counseled keeping children apart from other children at night; now keeping the child out of the parents' bedroom seemed warranted as well.

———

Benjamin Spock, the massively influential mid-twentieth-century pediatrician, was one of the first children's health experts to assimilate Freudian theory into his medical worldview. His 1946 book *Baby and Child Care*—expanded and revised periodically through the 1990s—sold nearly a million copies in its first year, and a generation of children came be known as "Spock babies." Spock was in a sense a latter-day Rousseau, often regarded by conservatives as promoting permissiveness and giving in to "instant gratification" of children's desires. In the matter of *infants'* sleep routines, Spock is quite mellow: "As long as a baby is satisfied with his feedings, comfortable, gets plenty of fresh air, and sleeps in a cool place, you can leave it to him to take the amount of sleep he needs." But it is another story altogether after the age of six months, when it becomes imperative to get the child out of the parents' bedroom. Partly, this is for the sake of the parents' privacy, but the greatest danger is to the child's psychosexual development: "The young child may be upset by the parents' intercourse, which he misunderstands and which frightens him. Parents are apt to think there is no danger if they first make sure the child is asleep. But children's psychiatrists have found cases in which the child awakened and was much disturbed without the parents' ever being aware of it." Such shocks could reverberate for decades afterward, stunting the child's sexual development and ability to form healthy relationships with others. From Locke to Freud to Spock, childhood sleep had gone from the great "cordial of nature" to a psychological danger zone: the Oedipal complex might never be surmounted if the child were not physically separated from the parents at night.

The solution, of course, was to put the child firmly in its own bed and to make sure it stayed there through the night. To this end, in 1956 Spock recommended trapping the child in bed with an adapted badminton net. (It should be "cut in half and the two pieces sewed together side by side. Then it can be bound with firm cord to the top rail of the side of the crib next to the wall, and also part way along the top of the head and foot of the crib.") Draconian as this webbed cage sounds, it was still a relatively soft kind of restraint when compared to the behavioral psychologist B. F. Skinner's "baby-in-a-box" system, which he tried out on his own daughter. Skinner left the child in a climate-controlled "closed compartment about as spacious as a standard crib," with one wall made of safety glass. There the child had no need for clothing or bedding and could fall into a "natural" rhythm of sleeping and waking, feeding and defecating. (He did allow for a diaper.) The parents benefited, too, because the chamber muffled sound; so if the baby cries, said Skinner, "there is no reason why the family, and the whole neighborhood, must suffer."

Surprising as it may sound, Skinner, arguably the most famous psychologist of the mid-twentieth century, was a devotee of Thoreau. His baby-in-a-box method seems like a complete inversion of the freedom and naturalness that Thoreau sought at *Walden*. But in a weird way one can see how Skinner might have gotten the idea from reading Thoreau. (Skinner included it in his utopian novel *Walden Two*, which will be discussed in the next chapter.) In order to escape unnatural social pressures that wreaked havoc upon his rhythms of sleeping and waking, Thoreau had experimented on his own body in a little cabin in the woods. In a sense, Skinner brought that laboratory inside the home, where he kept it in a glass-enclosed box on a table. The baby, untethered from parents, learns independence and self-sufficiency. But in another sense it was the *baby* who was the source of the problems for the parents, not shrieking trains or materialism or the hectic pace of modern life. "The trouble," Skinner wrote, "is that a routine acceptable to the baby often conflicts with the schedule of the household." Putting baby in a box was not just good for the parents, though. Skinner used the box as a tool to create sturdy, self-sufficient individuals, who would learn not to look to their parents to gratify their every whim: the parents, after all, couldn't hear their cries. Like Thoreau, Skinner was also guided by an anti-consumerist impulse: in the climate-controlled box, babies would experience "freedom from clothes and bedding" and would learn to amuse themselves without a constant stream of diverting new toys. Thoreau's cabin had become a baby box designed by a behavioral engineer.

Skinner's baby box, Spock's net: these were two extreme manifestations of the widely felt need to form an impassable line between child and parent at night. While Skinner was no Freudian and had little interest in human sexuality, his vision served an age in which crossing that line represented a dangerous passage into the adult world where Oedipal terrors lurked. But staying in the bed, crib, or box had its own dangers. In Spock's safety-netted bed, the child was restrained from annoying the parents, but the old demon of self-pleasuring might well take hold within the webbed cage. Spock—in true Freudian fashion—counseled that while children should be directed away from masturbation, they should never be threatened or frightened: "The sensitive child takes [threats] to heart. He may develop such a morbid fear of anything sexual that he will grow up maladjusted, afraid, or unable to marry or have children." Anti-masturbation sermons and medical tracts of the nineteenth century had warned of insanity, debility, and sterility, but here it is the anxiety about masturbation, not masturbation itself, that stunts development.

So, in short, from the nineteenth century through the mid-twentieth, the child's bed remained sexualized and subject to surveillance and restraints, but the morality had shifted. Rather than fearing the autoerotic impulses of the child, parents were counseled to guard children from the twin threats of witnessing adult sexuality and experiencing repression of their own urges, and to safeguard their own privacy to pursue adult nocturnal behaviors. As a result, children's bedtime routines and practices became pressurized from new angles. Children's sleep had been a relatively simple moral equation through the turn of the twentieth century—early rising meant health and productivity; lingering meant dissipation and possible self-abuse; now one had to worry about where the child slept, how to keep him or her there, and what he or she could see if awakened. As well, parents had to walk a tightrope between directing children away from autoerotic explorations, on the one hand, and stunting their sexual development by making them feel ashamed or afraid of such urges, on the other. And so it wasn't just the Spockian child who was caught in a net: despite the good doctor's famed gentleness and reassuring manner (his most famous line to parents is "Trust yourself. You know more than you think you do"), his best-selling book helped entwine parents in a skein of anxiety.

Skinner's baby box was just one way out. The more common approach was, and still is, simply to train the child to stay in bed, in a separate room, all though the night. This arrangement is so pervasive in our contemporary middle-class households that parents who practice co-sleeping with their children are often considered weird, verging on incestuous. And the successful solitary sleeping child has become an idea enshrined by psychology and pediatrics. As the anthropologist Matthew Wolf-Meyer put it, a baby who sleeps well is often called a "good baby," and the "responsible, lone sleeper" is the model against which early states of development are measured.

———

There are exceptions, of course. In a class on sleep that I taught at Emory, my co-teacher David Rye and I asked students to indicate whether they had slept in their own beds by age six. All but three of them raised their hands. Of those three, two were African American and the other had grown up in India. The solitary sleepers were either white or Asian American. In many places around the world, autonomous childhood sleeping is not practiced or even contemplated. In India, China, Indonesia, and Egypt, for example, private sleeping rooms are the exception rather than the rule. All available historical and cross-cultural evidence suggests that solitary sleeping for children is an anomaly of the modern, industrialized West. No ethnographic research has found a widespread tradition of infants sleeping outside of the mother's room anywhere else.

At least as much as changing theories of children's psychosocial development, and changing ideas about the sexual morality of family life, new domestic arrangements explain how children's sleep became such a problem. As with most shifts in human social behavior, there is no precise date when parents in Europe and North America began to put their children into separate beds within specially appointed rooms during the night. Historian of childhood Philippe Ariès cited an example of seventeenth-century French bishops who "prohibited—with a vehemence that gives one pause—the practice of having children sleep in the beds of their parents." A health manual published in 1781 recommended that children be put in beds apart from parents early in infancy, which would allow the sleeping child's body to regulate its own temperature and reduce the risk of the child being smothered by a sleeping parent rolling over in the night. Clearly, though, there were limits to how far away one could put the child. Most early modern European homes had only two or three rooms, and prior to the mid-seventeenth century the hallway was usually the chief sleeping space.

Most scholars of childhood cite the nineteenth and twentieth centuries as the crucial period for the rise of solitary childhood sleep. According to historians Peter Stearns, Perrin Rowland, and Lori Giarnella, in the mid-nineteenth-century United States, middle- and upper-middle-class children usually slept near a nurse in infancy and then shared a bed with same-sex siblings (Henry David Thoreau, for instance, in the trundle bed with his brother John). By the 1890s, as cribs began to replace cradles, even very young children were separated from their parents at night, and by the early twentieth century many middle-class homes had separate bedrooms for each child. The behavioral psychologist John Watson—who argued that too much coddling could stunt a child's development—wrote in 1928 that "when the 25 million American homes come to realize that the child has a right to a separate room and adequate psychological care there will not be nearly so may children born"; and an article in a 1920s family magazine asked children: "Do you sleep in a bed all by yourself? It is much better to sleep by yourself. You can rest better and breathe fresher air if you have a bed all your own."

Whether Freudian psychology was a result of this spatial arrangement or a cause of it is impossible to say. Suffice it to say that if little Oedipus had slept in the same room as mother and father, it's hard to imagine his famous complex taking hold. How could the idea of parental sex be a scandal, and how could little Wolf-Man be so scarred by witnessing it, in a society in which children stayed in the same room as the parents well past infancy, maybe even into adolescence? But Stearns and his colleagues suggest a number of other plausible causes for the new sleeping arrangements beyond sexual anxiety. Children needed their own sleeping space as homes became noisier with the invention of vacuum cleaners, sewing machines, and radios. Similarly, more powerful artificial lighting made certain regions of the home poor environments for children to fall asleep in. Adding to the sonic and optical challenges to sleep in the bourgeois household, increasing wealth in the industrial age afforded parents more opportunities to socialize in the home after hours; having children around would be an inconvenience. This wealth also made it possible to own a home with separate bedrooms for each child, especially in an era when birth control limited the size of families. The growing emphasis on the child as an "individual" also contributed to the new spatial arrangements. And so, as Stearns and colleagues put it, "Sleep was a new issue because families and children were getting accustomed to very novel, and in terms of historical traditions counterintuitive, arrangements." The washerwoman poet Mary Collier and her children could hardly have imagined these developments.

How did children respond to the new demands to sleep through the night by themselves? Not well, apparently. Children don't write history, but a number of adult writers captured the fright, anxiety, and simmering resentment that children directed toward the parents who shuffled them off to bed alone. Robert Louis Stevenson's 1884 collection of children's poetry, *A Child's Garden of Verses*, included several poems expressing children's bedtime worries, but it also included some where parents are subtly trying to manage them. "Escape at Bedtime," for instance, is written from the point of view of a child who pops out of bed to look at the night sky and fantasize about the stars, which the parents cannot see, as "the lights from the parlour and kitchen shone out / Through the blinds and the windows and bars." But the parents catch on that he is playing out a nocturnal game, for "They saw me at last, and they chased me with cries, / And they soon had me packed into bed." In another poem, "North-West Passage," the child learns the strict discipline necessary to go off into nighttime exile from the parents' world: "Must we to bed indeed? Well then, / Let us arise and go like men, / And face with an undaunted tread / The long black passage up to bed." Stevenson's adult ventriloquism of a child's voice is imperfect: arising and going off to bed like men—soldiers, really—is easier to imagine as the goal of an adult who wants separation from children than as a goal of the children themselves. The poem is actually a command masquerading as an expression of sympathy. One can imagine a parent reading it to a child and then gently pushing the child (the fuck) upstairs.

More poignant, but also more psychologically treacherous, are the opening bedtime scenes in the first volume of Marcel Proust's *Remembrance of Things Past* (1913). The narrator of Proust's epic feat of literary memory describes minutely the childhood feeling of his cheeks rubbing against a pillow, drifting off while reading, the patterns of moonlight streaming in through his window, and the reverse vertigo of the room coming into focus as he wakes up. But these sensations begin to coalesce into a scenario of anxiety: "Long before the time when I should have to go to bed and lie there unsleeping, far from my mother and grandmother, my bedroom became the fixed point on which my melancholy and anxious thoughts were centered." This is because during long summer nights, his parents send him up to his room alone while they remain in the parlor below talking or entertaining guests. His mother comes up each night to offer him a good-night kiss, an interchange so charged for young Marcel that he contrives to keep her away as long as possible, "so as to prolong the time of respite during which Mamma would not yet have appeared." On nights when guests are present, the pain is doubled, for he needs to receive his kiss down below, and when he begs her to accompany him to his room, his father lays down the law: "Leave your mother alone. You've said good night to one another, that's enough. These exhibitions are absurd. Go on upstairs." Which he does, but because Proust will be Proust, the scent of varnish on the staircase haunts him into adulthood.

One night, feeling particularly agitated about his mother's exiling him to bed, Marcel rushes out of his room when he sees his mother's candle in the hallway and throws himself on her. She is furious, refusing to speak to him, but he implores her to give him another kiss. To Marcel's great surprise, his father takes his side, urging his wife to stay in the boy's room for a while. "'But, my dear,' my mother answered timidly. . . . 'We mustn't let the child get into the habit.'" The father insists, and the mother stays in his room through the night. But rather than feeling triumph, or even relief, what he experiences is crushing guilt:

> I ought to have been happy; I was not. It struck me that my mother had just made a first concession which must have been painful to her, that it was a first abdication on her part from the ideal she had formed for me, and that for the first time she who was so brave had to confess herself beaten. It struck me that if I had just won a victory it was over her, that I had succeeded, as sickness or sorrow or age might have succeeded, in relaxing her will, in undermining her judgment; and that this evening opened a new era, would remain a black date in the calendar.

Proust claimed not to have read Freud, but the son's rivalry with the father for a chance at bedding with the mother, and the ensuing guilt, make this scene a perfect Oedipal scenario. And in truth, in Proust's own life, his relationship with his mother mirrors the intimacy and power struggles depicted in the fiction: his biographer tells us that Proust's mother demanded, well into his early thirties, that he write home with details about his daily activities, including what time he went to bed and woke up. The fictional child's mother seems concerned primarily with her own desire to stay up late without being interrupted by her son's demands for kisses and cuddling, but she also reflects an old concern going back to Rousseau that "we mustn't let the child get into the habit." The habit in question is not simply rigid adherence to a schedule, as Rousseau had warned against, but a psychosexual Freudian stew of dependence, domination, and physical desire. Spock and Skinner would have known what to do with such a child. ("Into the box, you!")

———

By the late twentieth century, two kinds of books were being produced to help parents negotiate the fraught passage into children's solitary sleep. One kind they read and talked about among themselves; the other they read to children. First was the pediatric sleep hygiene book, usually, but not always, written by prominent medical professionals who had given special attention to children's sleep. Such titles included Marc Weissbluth's *Healthy Sleep Habits, Healthy Child* (1987, 1999, 2003); Jodi A. Mindell's *Sleeping Through the Night: How Infants, Toddlers and Parents Can Get a Good Night's Sleep* (1997, 2005); Tracy Hogg's *Secrets of the Baby Whisperer* (2001); and Harvey Karp's *The Happiest Baby on the Block: The New Way to Calm Crying and Help Your Baby Sleep Longer* (2002). These books mixed psychological, medical, managerial, and moral instruction in friendly, soothing tones, selling expert reassurance to frazzled parents who wanted to know that they could soldier their children off to bed without turning the house into a chaos zone and without turning themselves into exhausted, impatient, hectoring somnambulists who resented their children. These experts had charts for feeding, nursing, sleeping, napping, and crying, and they provided diagnostic criteria whereby parents could judge whether their children's sleep problems were "normal" or needed medical treatment.

The differences among the books, though, were so great as to add to the parents' confusion rather than abate it. Cribs, cradles, or family beds? Side, stomach, or back? Bottle or breast? Pacifiers? How much comforting should the parent offer at bedtime or through the night? At what age is bedwetting a problem? Could the wrong kind of sleep arrangement stunt your child's development? Or even kill the poor thing? The conflicting answers to these questions are offered with equal certainty and a welter of empirical data and compelling anecdotes. The approaches befit medical entrepreneurs trying to distinguish their products from others on the market, but taken in the mass, they could only add layers of worry—even panic—to the desperate parents who were the primary audience for such books.

No issue divides these experts, whose books are still popular, like the "cry-it-out" versus the "no-cry" methods, which are connected to solitary sleep arrangements and co-sleeping ones, respectively. In fairness, "cry-it-out" is not a label that any renowned pediatric sleep expert has advocated in print. Skinner said of his mechanical baby-tender that "it was never our policy to use the compartment in order to let the baby 'cry it out,'" although this was a logical assumption to make about putting a child in a Plexiglas-enclosed box. (It wasn't soundproof, but it definitely reduced baby-related noise.) The charge was later leveled with particular ferocity at Richard Ferber, the author of *Solve Your Child's Sleep Problems* (1985; rev. 2006). Ferber is sometimes referred to as "the sleep Nazi"—a cruel hyperbole, but one that points to the emotional stakes of the argument. Like the authors of most such books, Ferber begins with a description of the bewildering contradictory advice one can get from "family, friends, and health professionals": let the child cry, lock the child in his or her own room, sleep with the child, change the child's diet, increase nighttime feedings, offer warm milk or a pacifier, rock the child to sleep, turn on a radio or white noise generator, drive the child in a car at bedtime, eliminate naps, switch to a water bed, administer sleep medicine. But amid this noise, Ferber promises that most children's sleep problems can be eliminated "by simple, straightforward measures"; all healthy babies, he says, can sleep through the night by the age of six months.

Lest his reassuring manner and promise of simplicity make one think that Ferber is posing as a latter-day Rousseau, the book quickly pivots to describing a System. Ferber's method entails developing elaborate routines that are to be followed as consistently as possible: children, he tells us, should have rigidly enforced schedules for changing into pajamas, brushing teeth, getting into bed, and reading. The routine culminates, not surprisingly, in the child being put to bed—alone: "Bedtime means separation." And what if the child can't sleep? For this, Ferber developed the famous method that came to be known popularly as "Ferberizing." Let your child cry in the crib for five minutes before returning to the room, then reassure him or her that you're there. But don't, by any means, pick the child up, which may lead to the child's falling asleep in your arms, a pleasure that will soon turn to habit. When the child (inevitably) resumes crying, wait ten minutes, and repeat; then fifteen; then twenty, the maximum. The next night, start at ten-minute intervals. Eventually your child will get the message that being picked up and cuddled is not going to happen anytime soon and will learn to sleep alone.

For my family, Ferberizing was a disaster. Our son, Isaac, was an especially finicky sleeper, and we tried the method on him somewhere around his first birthday. I practically had to restrain Devora from running to the room to respond to his cries, but after a few days he was sleeping for long stretches. Devora and I had our first sound sleep in a year. Then, a week or two later, he suddenly reverted to form, crying out and thrashing practically every hour. It turned out he had an ear infection, the first of about ten over the next year. Each time, we'd give him antibiotics, and when his ears cleared we'd Ferberize him again. By about the fifth try, we felt battered, and we worried that we were doing more harm than good by insisting on taming his sleep in this way. (Once we put tubes in his ears and he no longer suffered from ear infections, the system magically took hold without struggle.)

Yet for many families, Ferberizing does work—enough to ensure superstar status for Ferber and sales figures for his book in the hundreds of thousands. The rationale for this grueling treatment is that it ultimately improves sleep quality and that it is important for the psychological development of the child. Ferber cites evidence that solitary sleepers have fewer interruptions during the night than co-sleepers do, but above all, he sounds the note of psychological independence. Sleeping alone, he writes, helps the child "to see himself as an independent individual," whereas sleeping in the parents' bed can make the child "confused and anxious." This is because he may get the sense that he is "separating the two of you," which will make him feel—like young Marcel in *Remembrance of Things Past*—"too powerful"; after all, the child wants to know that the parents are in control.

Ferber is no Freudian, but sex is part of the equation for him, too. Benjamin Spock had stressed the psychosexual trauma that might develop if the child were to witness the parents having sex, but Ferber's concern is that sleeping in the parents' bed could *prevent* sex. One might assume that this is more of a problem for the parents than for the child, but Ferber assures his readers that the child will suffer, too. For instance, if one parent sleeps with the child and the other takes the child's bed, the child "may begin to worry that he will cause the two of you to separate, and if you ever do he may feel responsible. . . . And if as a single parent you begin a new relationship, your child will certainly resent being displaced in your bed by this 'intruder.'" Some parents like sleeping with their kids, but he hints that this may be an expression of adult hang-ups: "If you find that you actually prefer to have your child in your bed, you should examine your own feelings very carefully." Parents sometimes take a child into bed because of loneliness, or to create a buffer from a spouse with whom one is having conflicts. "As such a pattern continues, your child, and your whole family, will suffer." The basic pitch, then, is: do it the Ferber way, or everyone will be massively screwed up.

In fairness to Ferber, he left the above passages denigrating co-sleeping out of his 2006 revision to *Solve Your Child's Sleep Problems*, telling an interviewer for *Newsweek*, "That's one sentence [it was actually many sentences] I wish I never wrote. . . . [I]t was describing the general thinking of the time, but it was not describing my own experience or philosophy." Falling back on a Spockian bromide, he continued, "Whatever you want to do, whatever you feel comfortable doing, is the right thing to do, as long as it works." And yet in all crucial respects he sticks to his guns, continuing to counsel that parents should have a plan—the Ferber method—to get the child to sleep on its own by six months.

This valuation of solitary and consolidated sleep for children— you're not healthy unless you do it alone, and stay knocked out through the night—is at odds with most of global history. As anthropologists Carol Worthman and James McKenna have shown, there is no evidence that people living in societies in which co-sleeping is the norm experience greater difficulty in sleeping; nor does co-sleeping stunt the psychosexual development of the child. In fact, Worthman and another colleague, Ryan Brown, have shown that among some non-Western societies in which co-sleeping is the norm, family structures tend to be tighter and more intimate than in much of the West. Writer Anne Fadiman, in her extraordinary study of cross-cultural conflicts involving a Hmong family's encounters with the medical system in California, reports that "in Laos, a baby was never apart from its mother, sleeping in her arms all night and riding on her back all day." The babies, medical studies showed, tended "to be less irritable and more securely attached to their mothers than Caucasian infants"; mothers, in turn, were "'exquisitely attuned' to their children's signals." Children's sleep, in such scenarios, is not a solitary "downtime" enforced by parental rules and demands, but—as Worthman and Brown argue—an important aspect of the "mutual recognition" of family members, who learn to knit together their responsibilities and to synchronize their schedules. Yet as we have seen, health experts and colonial authorities from the nineteenth century onward tried actively to stamp out such practices, labeling them backward, morally degrading, and unsanitary. Such efforts continue: in 2005, health officials in Nunavut, the northernmost territory in Canada, launched a campaign to end Inuit traditional parental practices of sharing a bed with infants under the age of one. Such arrangements, they argued, increased the risk of Sudden Infant Death Syndrome (SIDS), especially since the Inuit people now were sleeping on softer surfaces than in times past, which might suffocate the child if he or she rolled over. A member of the Pauktuutit Inuit Women of Canada pushed back: "You know it's an Inuit tradition. . . . I'm sure you know if they take proper precautions, then there shouldn't be [any] danger."

Despite such efforts to stamp out co-sleeping globally, the practice has made something of a comeback in the United States: a 2003 study by the National Institutes of Health concluded that 45 percent of all parents routinely shared a bed with an infant. A spate of books argued that Ferber's aggressive program for separating parents and young children at night created its own risks: such "detachment parenting" would create psychological problems, wrote pediatrician William Sears. Sears's protégé and parent educator Elizabeth Pantley wrote that the Ferber technique was "a simplistic and harsh way to treat another human being." Sears was advocating co-sleeping arrangements by the mid-1990s, and Pantley soon followed suit. The position was gaining market ascendancy as the new century approached. Some feminists, however, challenged co-sleeping and other aspects of "attachment parenting," arguing that it tethered women more tightly to traditional maternal and housewifely roles, making it almost impossible to attain the separation from children's needs necessary to succeed in the workplace.

Ferber's revision of his book in 2006 made allowances for both the historical record and the current climate, offering what appears to be a balanced tally sheet of the advantages and disadvantages of co-sleeping. However, his sympathies are never really in doubt. Despite assuring readers that "you are free to choose the way that best suits you," he reminds them that co-sleeping societies tend to "remain economically and socially 'primitive'"—playing to old associations of collective sleeping with supposedly inferior or backward cultures. And as a final kicker, he cites evidence that unexpected sudden death—either from SIDS or from a drunken or heavy parent rolling over on the child (catastrophic layovers)—increase when adults share a bed with children. This was in total contrast to James McKenna and Thomas McDade's finding that SIDS and other nocturnal catastrophes are far more likely to occur when the child is in a separate room. You may be free to choose, these experts tell us, but the wrong choice may kill your child.

———

Despite co-sleeping's persistence in the West—especially among immigrant and racial minority families—spatial separation of parents and children remains the norm. And yet in many families it is a norm that is hotly contested on any given night: the parents want the child to go to bed, the child doesn't want to. Once the child is in bed, she feels alone, perhaps frightened, abandoned. She asks for water, a snuggle, rearranged bedding, a nightlight, a menagerie of toys; maybe she even sneaks out to jump into the parents' bed if she is old enough. The whole routine is enough of an ordeal that elaborate bedtime rituals are invented to smooth the transition. The most prevalent of these is the reading of the bedtime story, an activity that has spawned entire walls full of board books in the few brick-and-mortar bookstores that remain. And what are these books about? One thing above all: going to bed, alone, and staying there.

168 I WILD NIGHTS

The evergreen of this genre is *Goodnight Moon* (1947), written by Margaret Wise Brown and illustrated by Clement Hurd. This story of a young bunny spending his final minutes in a "great green room" before going off to bed is a wonderfully peaceful, tranquil staging of the child's detachment from the adult waking world. "Goodnight moon . . . goodnight air. Goodnight noises everywhere." Millions of children have been lulled to sleep by the murmuring sounds of Wise's words and the twilight tones of Hurd's illustrations. But as children's literature scholar Mary Galbraith argues, for all the book's subtlety and gentleness, it remains a tool of manipulation: it is, she writes, the paramount example of a book that offers a model for the child of "how to behave and what to feel, even as the separation is imminent." Over the course of the book's pages—or boards— the little bunny repeats a mantra of farewells directed at all of the objects in the room (clock, stuffed bears, furniture, paintings, etc.), and finally at the "old lady" who stays in her rocking chair while the child goes off to sleep. Implicitly, the child being read to is being coaxed through a series of detachments concluding with the detachment from the parent.

If *Goodnight Moon* creates an aura of enchantment around the transition to bed, other bedtime books are more overt about the tenuousness of the parental agenda and potential blowback from the child. Maurice Sendak's *Where the Wild Things Are* and *In the Night Kitchen* seem to amplify children's nighttime fears about being left in the dark, conjuring up either a chaotic and alluring world below stairs or a realm of grotesque (if ultimately friendly) monsters outside the window. When *Where the Wild Things Are* was first published in 1963, psychologist Bruno Bettelheim castigated Sendak for fanning the "basic anxiety" of children: desertion by their parents. Reading such books to children, in other words, might upset the fragile intergenerational peace about solitary sleep for children. Other books pictured this rebellion explicitly. In Russell Hoban's *Bedtime for Frances* (1960), the child makes numerous requests to remain in the parents' world—asking for milk, TV, and piggyback rides. Only when she crawls into her parents' bed in the middle of the night do her parents finally lay down the law, threatening her with a spanking. And Peggy Rathmann's *Goodnight Gorilla* (1994) features zoo animals that crawl into bed with the zookeeper and his wife only to be led time after time back to the cage.

Which brings us to *Go the F**k to Sleep*, which was only the most popular of a string of mock-parenting books, which included *The Three-Martini Playdate* (2004), *Raising the Perfect Child Through Guilt and Manipulation* (2009), *Let's Panic About Babies* (2011), and *Toddlers Are Assholes* (2015)—as well as twisted picture books like *Monsters Eat Whiny Children* (2010), *Baby Mix Me a Drink* (2005), and *Pat the Zombie* (2011). This highly self-referential genre turns expert advice, best practices, and cloying paeans to childhood comfort on their heads, offering burnt-out parents the cathartic experience of releasing their submerged anger at the little people who—in the subtitle of one book—"ruin your body and destroy your life." All the picture books in the world, all the Ferber techniques, Spockian nets, and Skinner boxes (to say nothing of the bottles, blankets, pacifiers, stuffed animals, songs, threats, music boxes, and white noise machines), can't give Daddy and especially Mommy the peace they need. Sendak's wild things, in the child's imagination, were downstairs or outside. Mansbach's monsters are the creations of the parents, and they're all too real, coming at you from upstairs or down the hall.

———

The twentieth-century struggle over children's solitary sleep clearly has its psychic consequences for both sides. Parents ultimately know that their children will grow out of it—that is, if they're not found dead in their cribs or permanently scarred by sneaking out of bed and witnessing parental sex. But for children, the parents' command to stay in solitary confinement may feel as authoritarian as any dictator's decree. It's not too much to speculate that this nightly power struggle—brought about by nineteenth- and twentieth-century shifts in sleeping arrangements, economic conditions, theories of childhood and sexuality, and increasing demands on chronological regularity—may have been one of the hidden sources of the rebellious youth movements that marked the late twentieth century. As historians Stearns, Rowland, and Giarnella put it, "sleep became one of those areas where children might be heedlessly bossed about," a situation that only increased children's desire to flout authority by staying up late. Back in 1693, John Locke was worried that if children became too well-acquainted with the midnight hour, they might ultimately gravitate toward wine halls populated by unsavory characters. Little did he know that staying up all night—whether for sex, drugs, or rock and roll—would become the chief way for young people to get back at their parents.

Parents, too, were once children, and the ingrained expectation for solitary, consolidated sleep has no doubt led to long-term consequences for all of us. Could it be that the explosion of sleep disorders and sleep obsessiveness is partly the result of growing up with so much pressure put on one's sleeping habits? In particular, the command that we fall asleep on our own, in a darkened, sealed room, would seem to make it more difficult to tolerate the behavior of bedmates for those of us who acquire them. If you were brought up sleeping with others, would your partner's snoring, rolling over, or midnight trip to the bathroom trigger your own midnight insomnia, or would you just accept it as the part of the natural environment of sleep?

The demand for solitary sleep is affecting the environment in other subtle ways. A 2007 report by the National Association of Homebuilders showed that couples were starting to prefer homes with separate master bedrooms, which would allow them to control their own sleep environments rather than having to put up with a partner's annoying sounds and movements. Suburban spreads, it seems, are going to have to spread a little wider to accommodate the desire for absolute separation of family members at night. In his little cabin in the woods, with its narrow cot and three chairs, Thoreau railed against big houses and their wastefulness. But the individualism he preached has found a home in them. He advocated solitude, but maybe the best way to honor his environmental vision of making do with less is to learn, again, how to sleep together.

CHAPTER SIX

Utopian Sleepers

Since the rules governing modern sleep have functioned so badly for so many people, why doesn't someone do something about it? There are certainly plenty of tinkerers: school boards that adjust start times to account for the circadian rhythms of particular age groups, enlightened business owners and managers who allow or even encourage nap times for workers, parents who share a family bed with children or try some other unorthodox sleeping arrangement.

But if sleep patterns are so deeply connected to social structures, and so few of us are happy with the role that sleep plays in our world, where's the revolution? A few people in fact have imagined one, and some have even tried to overthrow the old order or create utopian sleep communities in its midst. This chapter will look at some of the more far-reaching, even outlandish—yet sometimes inspiring—attempts to find a different place and rhythm for sleep in modern life. Religious visionaries, feminists, socialists, communards, behaviorists, novelists, scientists, and futurists of various stripes have all proposed, and sometimes attempted to build, utopian societies—and with surprising regularity, many of these systems have tried to rewrite the rules for human sleep. That few of these attempts have lasted does not diminish their capacity to inspire us to think differently about our own possible futures.

———

But let's start with the present. The idea of a sleep revolution has some popular currency, thanks largely to digital media maven and sleep proselytizer Arianna Huffington, whose best-selling 2016 book *The Sleep Revolution* proclaims that we are in the midst of a "sleep crisis" that will trigger a radical reclamation of sleep as a central component of the good life. After detailing the health and public safety risks of catastrophic sleep loss (including her own blackout, in which her head slammed on her desk and she awoke in a pool of blood), she points to developments in technology and the corporate world that augur a "renaissance of sleep." Mostly, the ones who are ushering in this renaissance turn out to be the enlightened executives who have begun to testify in public about the benefit of allowing naps into their hectic schedules, many of whom have consulted with Huffington herself. Some of these titans are even restructuring office life to allow midday power napping for their workers. (I'm reminded of Thomas Tryon's 1684 advice to slaveholders to give their slaves more time to rest, "for it would add much to their *Profit.*") Huffington approvingly cites early twentieth-century labor activists' efforts to secure adequate rest for workers, a movement safely in the past—yet her vision of the contemporary sleep movement is strikingly top-down. The end of her book contains a "sleep wish list": all politicians should develop policies on improving sleep health, a congressional committee should set an agenda for the Centers for Disease Control and Prevention to promote healthy sleep, and so on. Salutary as these developments may be, though, they hardly feel revolutionary, and not just because her revolution appears to be led by billionaires and government officials. Much of the book is given over to touting the benefits of meditation, exercise, warm baths, herbal sleep aids, peaceful routines, and planning for sleep, all of which sounds like many other sleep hygiene books. She slides over into commercialism when she provides appendices listing the best hotel chains and mattresses for obtaining a comfortable night's sleep. Huffington herself has a line of sleep products, including organic cotton sheets, virgin wool duvets, lavender- or eucalyptus-scented pillows, and the like. And perhaps product tie-ins with Marriott: in a recent hotel stay, I found in the drawer of a bedtable not a Gideon's Bible, but a card with "Arianna Huffington's 8 tips for better sleep," featuring an image of her book cover.

On a broader scale—and in a more scientific vein—a team of chronobiologists in Germany is experimenting with optimizing the sleep patterns of one community. In Bad Kissingen, a town in the south-central region of the country, these sleep scientists, led by Thomas Kantermann, are conducting a civic experiment with the goal of promoting "optimal sleep and recuperation in everyday life." Residents of the town will be equipped with a wearable device out-fitted with a sophisticated app that tracks sleep in relation to a myriad of waking variables: work, exercise, diet, mood, screen use, social activities, and so on. The goal is to obtain "significant insights into the interactions between chronobiology and the manifold structures of the society" and "to design innovative and directly applicable solutions" to problems involving collective sleep disturbance. Such information will guide specific recommendations, including: start and end times for schools based on peak alertness periods for students at any given age; timing of treatment for patients in the hospital synchronized with patients' optimal times for healing and caregivers' own maximum alertness; gradual changes in the intensity of public lighting to mimic the transition from dusk to dawn; and the distribution of "intelligent alarm clocks" that will be timed to go off within a thirty- to sixty-minute period corresponding with the lightest phase of an individual's sleep. In addition, the app on the wearable device will provide feedback to individual residents who seek to adjust their own sleep routines based on crowdsourced information provided by others who experience similar issues. The project is billed as the world's first "Chrono City."

The ambition of team Chrono City is grand—it amounts to redressing some of the basic ills of modernity through technology, city planning, and scientific expertise. As the project's promotional materials put it, because the "modern 24/7 lifestyle introduces light at non-optimal times and thus interferes with circadian synchronisation and the timing of sleep . . . circadian misalignment results."

The benefits would not just accrue to individual sleepers, but to the entire town and its environment. New lighting technologies would save energy, reduce the town's carbon footprint, and even benefit wildlife. Development of a "starlight park" on the town's edge— where light emitted from populated areas does not penetrate—will attract dark sky tourism. Businesses will become more efficient and profitable, and the research team's presence may even help to draw new business ventures "related to chronobiology technologies."

As scientific/social experiments go, this one has far-reaching ambitions. As Kantermann put it to me in an email, quoting his colleague Michael Wieden, their broadest aim is "to wrap work around humans, and not to wrap humans around work." The project is just getting off the ground, so it is too soon to know its outcome: whether businesses will be more efficient, kids smarter, patients healthier, birds chirpier, residents happier.

Yet for all of this ambition, Chrono City seems to me to be an attempt to reform sleep and its environments rather than to overthrow the old order. In a way, Chrono City is reminiscent of approaches to climate change that feature technological solutions to problems created by technology, such as capturing carbon underground rather than steering society toward a break from carbon dependence, or, even more challengingly, toward a break from its fixation with technology. Similarly, the chronobiologists involved in the project are attempting to repair broken sleep with some of the tools that broke it: alarm clocks, all-seeing screens, hovering experts, mountains of data and advice, concerns about productivity, and new rules and new reasons to obsess.

———

For centuries, though, the utopian imagination has devised better ways to sleep, both in patently fictional scenarios and in real-life planned communities. In these scenarios, casting aside the rules for sleep means rearranging the society that created them. Sir Thomas More's *Utopia*, the 1516 prose work that inaugurated the utopian fiction tradition, offered a very early version of the twentieth-century labor cry of "eight hours for work, eight hours for rest, eight hours for what you will." Key to this vision was the democratization of sleep and labor. In More's ideal world, every adult in the community—including every woman—is required to work, but for no more than six hours a day. Because *everyone* works—as opposed to societies in which the wealthy, "the great lazy gang of priests," and beggars who feign lameness are exempt—there is a surplus of time for rest and leisure. "They work three hours before noon, when they go to dinner. After dinner they rest for a couple of hours, then go to work for another three hours. Then they have supper, and at eight o'clock . . . they go to bed and sleep eight hours. The other hours of the day, when they are not working, eating, or sleeping, are left to each man's individual discretion." More's sixteenth-century vision of shared, gender-neutral work and sleep was astonishingly forward-looking: in the imperfect world, he wrote, "hardly any of the women, who are a full half of the population, work; or, if they do, then as a rule their husbands lie snoring in the bed." Yet he ignores that women really did work in imperfect, decidedly nonutopian early modern England: cooking, cleaning, mending clothes, and—above all—raising children. How these tasks would be performed was left unimagined in his narrative, although he does mention that slaves would be on hand.

In late eighteenth-century New England, a group of Protestant reformers attempted to form a kingdom of heaven on Earth that would go even further in overturning gender roles. The Shakers were led by an English textile worker from the factory town of Manchester named Ann Lee. Lee had grown up poor in a family that slept six to a room; after she married a blacksmith, she suffered through many painful pregnancies and brought four children to term, all of whom died. Not surprisingly, Lee developed an aversion to sex. In the religious visions that made her famous, she learned that the original sin committed by Adam and Eve was not biting a piece of fruit from the tree of knowledge, but the sexual act that preceded that bite. Accordingly, in the utopian community she led in the New World, sex was outlawed. (However, one of many reasons the group was viewed with suspicion was that they were said to favor nude prayer meetings featuring the violent, spasmic dancing for which they were given their name. Even more vicious rumors spread that members of the group practiced infanticide to cover over the results of breaking their code of abstinence.) The movement was devoted to forming a communal way of life that rejected the notion of a biological family.

It may seem a minor point in relation to such a radical sect, but the Shakers also slept quite oddly. In their first communal home outside of Albany, New York, women slept together in a downstairs great room, and the men upstairs. As new members joined and brought their families with them, children were raised collectively in order to break filial ties, and dormitory rooms were shared by groups of same-sex members. The group was also devoted to an artisanal way of life that rejected America's growing industrialism, and they became famous for their well-crafted furniture. The irony is that their group sleeping took place in crowded quarters that in some ways resembled Ann Lee's impoverished childhood circumstances in industrial Manchester, the world she was trying to overthrow.

The nineteenth-century United States spawned numerous utopian societies, all of which rejected the commercialism, mechanization, and materialism of an emerging industrial capitalist society. And like the Shakers before them, almost all presented alternatives to the biological family as the main unit of socialization and private property as the sacrosanct value; perhaps not surprisingly, their communalism generally extended to sleep. The "phalansteries" inspired by French socialist Charles Fourier featured dormitory-style sleeping similar to that of the Shaker community. In the most famous such community, at Brook Farm in West Roxbury, Massachusetts—run by Ralph Waldo Emerson's friend George Ripley—members each did a fraction of the necessary labor of farming, cooking, and cleaning in order to avoid the competitiveness of the outside world; each adult member, in turn, was allowed time for artistic activity, continuing education, and the joys of fellowship. In such an atmosphere, it seemed to some that the rules of sleep could be completely rewritten: one visitor said "he had not slept for a year," according to a new study of utopian societies; he attempted to convince the society's members that sleep was completely unnecessary. Only slightly less radical in vision, the Brook Farmers planned to construct a Fourier-style communal sleeping hall, but they were unable to achieve this before the community collapsed in the wake of financial shortfalls and a disastrous fire. Thoreau himself was apparently invited to join Brook Farm in 1841, and despite the fact that many of New England's leading intellectuals joined up (including Nathaniel Hawthorne, who later satirized Brook Farm in his novel *The Blithedale Romance*), Thoreau demurred. Writing in his journal, he declared that he would rather sleep in a bachelor's hall in hell than board (presumably with others) in heaven. One could say that he did eventually join such a utopian community at Walden Pond, but it consisted of only one member.

The utopian movement peaked in the years before the American Civil War, whose carnage stood in stark contrast to the boundless optimism (and naïveté) of these social revolutionaries. But writers, reformers, and other dreamers never entirely gave up Thomas More's dream of a perfect society. One such dreamer was the feminist icon Charlotte Perkins Gilman, arguably the best-known female intellectual of the nineteenth century, who initially achieved fame by writing a story about a woman cruelly confined to bed. "The Yellow Wall-paper" (1892) endures as a masterpiece both of gothic writing and of feminist thought, but it is also relevant to the history of sleep in that it shows how the bed became a battleground for the control of troublesome bodies, in this case women's. In later writings on the politics of domestic arrangements, Gilman went from being an inert, prone victim in the struggle to control her own body to a social engineer who would reinvent structures of marriage, parenting, and work in order to allow women to reach their full potential. The revolution that she imagined began in the bedroom and the nursery; the changes she proposed had surprising currency in real-life twentieth-century settings, far from the pages of her fiction.

Charlotte's troubles with sleep began early in life. According to her biographer Helen Lefkowitz Horowitz, as a young girl raised by a single mother, whom she later blamed for withholding affection from her, Charlotte would often "pretend to fall asleep in order to get the kiss her mother denied her when she was awake." Her attempts to control her own sleep-wake cycle became more concerted in her teens and early adulthood. An athletic young woman, she took to regulating her own body rhythms somewhat obsessively, noting in her journal each day the times that she rose and went to bed, and avoiding "corsets, tea, coffee, late hours and other known evils" that might weaken her self-control. Charlotte became attracted to the ideas of British philosopher Herbert Spencer, who believed that conservation of energy was the route toward health and the improvement of the human species, and that ignoring bodily sensations such as hunger or fatigue could endanger both bodily and mental health.

Nonetheless, sleep began to elude her control. The warning signs for Charlotte came during her tumultuous courtship with the man who would become her first husband, the chronically down-at-heels and somewhat emotionally domineering artist Walter Stetson. Describing the downside of her roller-coaster relationship with him, she wrote, "Isn't catalepsy something like this? A trance state? My heart is asleep—numb—gone." Marriage and motherhood only made the condition worse. During pregnancy, Walter tried to prevent her from attending lectures and other stimulating activities, reflecting the fear common in medical circles of the late nineteenth century that sudden jolts to the expectant mother's brain might disturb the prenatal development of the child. Nonetheless, he wrote in his journal, "She is more sensitive and easily fatigued both physically & mentally & at times despondent." The reason for her despondency was her fear that motherhood might unfit her for the writing life she had dreamed of; Walter's concern, increasingly, was that mental strain would unsuit her for housekeeping and motherhood.

With the help of his father, a dealer in patent medicines, Walter put her on a course of bromides—a leading sedative of the day (along with opium), often used as a remedy for insomnia and jangled nerves. After the birth of her daughter Katharine, Charlotte alternated between doses of cocaine mixed with alcohol to stimulate her waking hours and morphine to send her to sleep. (These concoctions were sold over the counter under such innocuous names as

"Dr. Buckland's Essence of Oats.") Her brain doped but her nerves still raw, she wrote of her anxiety about putting her child to bed: "Get hysterical in the evening while putting K to sleep. When I am nervous she never does sleep easily." On the advice of a close friend, she wrote to the great nerve specialist Silas Weir Mitchell, describing how her long efforts to discipline her brain and body had led her to overestimate her capacity to withstand strain. Practicing "constant self supervision and restraint," she wrote, "I never rested." Now, she was constantly afflicted with "agony of mind," prone to extended bouts of weeping, and suffered from nervous exhaustion. "People tire me frightfully," her letter concluded. "I am running down like a clock."

Silas Weir Mitchell was, as Charlotte recognized, the foremost authority on nervous disorders in the nineteenth century—so famous that some of his supporters urged him to run for president. However, she probably did not know about his views on gender. In his medical memoir, *Doctor and Patient* (1888), he wrote that "the woman's desire to be on a level of competition with men and to assume his duties is, I am sure, making mischief, for it is my belief that no length of generations of change in her education and modes of activity will ever really alter her characteristics." Women whose minds were strained by excess mental activity were subjected to his famous "rest cure," administered in his Philadelphia clinic, to which he accepted Charlotte as a patient in 1887. The cure involved six to eight weeks of absolute rest and isolation from family and friends, a carefully controlled diet featuring copious amounts of milk to increase body weight, and massage and electrotherapeutics to keep the muscles stimulated. He had developed this protocol in response to the Civil War, when he had treated exhausted and emotionally traumatized soldiers in this way. These men, he found, were "tired by much marching, gave out suddenly at the end of some unusual exertion, and remained for weeks, perhaps months, in a pitiable state of what we should call today, Neurasthenia." Neurasthenia, a term coined by the New York electrotherapist George Beard—covered an enormous range of symptoms, many of which had previously been covered by the diagnostic category of hysteria: fainting, tics, depression, insomnia, eating disorders, and temporary paralysis. All of these were understood as symptoms of a nervous system that was weakened by strain. By the end of the nineteenth century, it was the most modish of all diagnoses, with even Sigmund Freud considering many patients—himself included—to be neurasthenics. Among the panoply of symptoms it covered (one physician referred to it as "a diagnostic wastebasket"), it almost always featured fatigue and sleep disturbance.

Mitchell's contribution to the theory of neurasthenia is his 1871 book *Wear and Tear*. "Wear," he wrote, was "a natural and legitimate result of lawful use" of an organ—in this case, the brain—whereas "tear" was an unnatural or overlong taxation of the organ, from "long strain, or the sudden demand of strength from weakness. . . . Wear comes of use, tear of abuse." Like many inquirers into mental maladies of his day, he blamed modern life for tearing the brains of so many patients; he pointed specifically to economic competition, the taxing habits of business life, the unnatural pace of social and economic activity induced by the railway and the telegraph, and "the overeducation and overstraining of our young people" as causes of nervous ailments. Manual laborers were generally spared the disease, because their work sent blood rushing to the brain, causing a feeling of fatigue, which then warned or even forced the worker to rest. Those who lived by "brain-work," in contrast, did not feel "any sensation referable to the organ itself which warns him that he has taxed it enough." Women, he felt, were more susceptible to such straining of the brain and nervous system, because their "organic development . . . renders them remarkably sensitive," and "over-use, or even a very steady use, of the brain is dangerous to health and to every probability of future womanly usefulness." By this he meant primarily motherhood, because "if the mothers of a people are sickly and weak, the sad inheritance falls upon their offspring." Mitchell's concern thus dovetailed more closely with Walter Stetson's than with his wife Charlotte's: the woman must be protected from her own intellectual ambitions for the sake of her children. Mitchell's diagnosis of Charlotte was "nervous prostration," a somewhat lesser form of neurasthenia that had also been used as a diagnosis for Emily Dickinson.

Despite the fact that he developed his theory of neurasthenia by observing and treating chronically fatigued Civil War soldiers, Mitchell's postwar clinic catered overwhelmingly to women. By putting them on bed rest and isolation for extended periods and restricting, if not eliminating, their mental stimulation, he opened himself up to charges of misogyny by feminist critics (first and most famous among them being Charlotte Perkins Gilman herself in time). Before we rush to agreement with this conclusion, however, it is important to view the rest cure in the context of other treatments of women's nervous ailments during the era. Because "pelvic lesions" were often thought to be the source of much nervous strain in women, for example, gynecological surgery was often the remedy. And so, although the rest cure may deserve its reputation as a sexist method—one that attempted to control troublesome women by putting them to bed—it at least had the virtue of not involving the knife. And it held its own attraction for many women—Charlotte included—who saw in it a way to escape the trials and strains of household management, a 24/7 task that in the popular adage "is never done." Historian Carroll Smith-Rosenberg even goes so far as to suggest that women could experience extended periods of bed rest as a sort of vacation from their stressful roles as mothers and homemakers: it offered one of the few opportunities for married women to be catered to and relieved of the constant burden of caring for others.

When Charlotte wrote to Mitchell, then, she had high hopes of being treated in as humane and respectful a way as possible. It is not clear precisely what happened while she was in his care, but within a few years, she chose to portray the rest cure in a way that ensured it would pass into infamy. First came "The Yellow Wall-paper," an 1892 story of motherhood, madness, and revenge that has justly become one of the most read and interpreted works in American literature. The story is narrated by an aspiring woman writer who is married to a physician named John (perhaps a conflation of Charlotte's husband Walter and Dr. Mitchell). John confines her to bed for a summer in their rented "colonial mansion"—which the narrator mentions may be "haunted"—to treat her "temporary nervous depression" that has been brought about by the birth of her daughter. He forbids her to work until she is "well again," although the narrator believes that "work, with excitement and change, would do me good." In bed, all she can do is to fixate on her room's "smouldering unclean yellow" wallpaper, which is marked by "sprawling flamboyant patterns committing every artistic sin."

Thus confined, the narrator begins to imagine that the paper contains "absurd, unblinking eyes" that watch her every move, and occasionally she catches a glimpse of "a strange, provoking, formless sort of figure" to which the eyes belong: it is "like a woman stooping down and creeping about behind that pattern." Occasionally the narrator gets out of bed to see if she can follow the woman in her creeping. John always puts her back into bed, however, with the admonition that she needs to sleep as much as possible. In an effort to flout John's control, the narrator only feigns sleep as she continues to puzzle out the wallpaper's meanings: "I don't sleep much at night, for it is so interesting to watch developments," she says, "but I sleep a good deal in the daytime," especially when the company of John and his sister Jennie becomes "tiresome and perplexing." Meanwhile, the woman camouflaged in the pattern is busy creeping "all over the house" and even across the yard, all the while emitting a terrible smell that makes the narrator want to burn down the house. Eventually, she becomes convinced that there are many women trapped under the paper trying to get out, and that her duty is to get behind the pattern—whether to liberate the women or to join them is not clear. On the last night of the couple's gothic nightmare vacation, she locks John out of her room. When he is finally able to enter, he finds her crawling about the floor, having pulled off most of the wallpaper. "Now why should that man have fainted?" she asks at the story's end. "But he did, and right across my path by the wall, so that I had to creep over him every time!"

Gilman eventually produced a magazine called *The Forerunner*, which she published monthly from 1909 until 1916, writing every article and story it contained. In a brief essay in this magazine that appeared over twenty years after she wrote the story, Gilman explicitly links it to her treatment in Mitchell's clinic, suggesting that in having the narrator creep over her fallen husband, the writer was really thinking of trampling her own medical tormentor. In "Why I Wrote the Yellow Wallpaper?" (1913), she describes him as "the physician who so nearly drove me mad." He had told her when sending her home to "live as domestic a life as far as possible" and "never to touch pen, brush, or pencil again as long as I lived." Contemporary scholars question whether Mitchell ever advocated anything so draconian, but in her essay Gilman paints him as a foil to her own intellectual ambition: "I cast the noted specialist's advice to the winds and went to work again—work, the normal life of every human being; work, in which is joy and growth and service, without which one is a pauper and a parasite." She notes that despite the concerns of the medical and literary establishments about the story's implications (one correspondent said, "[It] ought not to be written . . . ; it was enough to drive anyone mad to read it"), "The Yellow Wallpaper" ultimately "saved one woman from a similar fate." It even convinced Silas Weir Mitchell to "alter . . . his treatment of neurasthenia."

The battleground in the story is ostensibly the bed: a woman is told to sleep in order to stop thinking, but she stays awake to frustrate her male captor, pretending to sleep while being lectured on her proper place. The real battleground, though, is her mind, which is simultaneously drug-addled (she is given "phosphates or phosphites"—probably a form of codeine), stressed and exhausted from childbirth, and repressed from her inclination toward thinking and writing. The men around her—like those around Charlotte in her own life—clearly want to control her mind and refocus it on childrearing, a task that over the course of her career she saw as inimical to pursuing the life of the mind. Literary scholar Clare Eby has called Gilman the "foremost feminist theorist in her time," mainly for her penetrating analyses of marriage as an economic institution. A woman, Gilman showed, was unpaid for doing the most grueling labor around the home in order to secure her husband's right to make money outside of it.

Central to the wife's economic function within marriage was her willingness to work the night shift, and in much of her writing, Gilman devised strategies for protecting women from the assault on their sleep-wake cycles made by little creatures. Some of this advice was simply to double down on her society's increasing demand to end co-sleeping arrangements. In her 1900 book *Concerning Children*, she included an anecdote about a thirteen-year-old girl who slept in bed with her mother, whom she wakened several times during the night to adjust the covers. "There was no reason why her tired mother should lose sleep for this purpose," she wrote. As a corrective, she suggested that the mother turn the tables and "waken the child with the same demand," as a way of demonstrating its unreasonableness. But in the same year that she published "Why I Wrote The Yellow Wallpaper?" Gilman published another, lesser-known story that combined issues of sleep, time, creativity, labor, and motherhood in a very different way. In "Making a Change," she imagined a world in which husband and wife could *both* work, without either parent being burdened by the necessity of child care and its disruptions to sleep. Rather than pitting the woman as mad rebel against male authority, she portrays a relationship in which women convince men to remake the family in the name of efficiency. The change, not surprisingly, involves altered sleeping arrangements.

The story begins with another young mother being driven mad after childbirth, this time by a baby who keeps her "awake nearly all night, and for many nights." Julia Gordins is a music teacher with the "hypersensitive" ears of a musician who has given up her career in order to serve her husband. She is initially flooded with happiness upon becoming a mother, but she lacks talent for household management, and her impulsive artistic temperament does not afford her the patience needed to withstand the baby's incessant cries. As a result, she is "nearly crazy" with sleep deprivation, "a form of torture" that leads her to "wild visions of separation, of secret flight—even of self-destruction." For "Sleep—Sleep—Sleep—that was the one thing she wanted." Her husband, Frank—a well-meaning electrical engineer—is also increasingly unhinged by the household turmoil; he thinks to himself, "This being married—and bringing up children—is not what it's cracked up to be." In his distracted and exhausted state, he has trouble supporting his young family.

Fortunately, the Gordins household also includes Frank's mother, an eminently practical and efficient person who suggests that the child's care should be left to her. After heroically saving the sleeping Julia from certain death (Julia had carelessly left the radiator spewing gas with the pilot unlit), she realizes that it is time—as the title suggests—to make a change. Without informing her son, she not only takes charge of the infant (whom she quickly trains to sleep at length and in regular intervals), but also opens a child day-care center in the house's upper flat, where she promptly puts most of the neighborhood children on a proper schedule of naps and playtime. By taking in forty dollars a month, she is able to hire an attentive household servant, refurnish the home, and start a rooftop garden. Her help, in turn, frees Julia to offer music lessons, which not only yield additional income but also restore her zest for life. Frank is initially astonished to learn of these developments, but he is won over by Julia's declaration that "I love my home, I love my work, I love my mother, I love you. And as to children—I wish I had six!" Years later, he is overheard to remark, "This being married and bringing up children is as easy as can be—when you learn how!"

In this story, Gilman offers hints of a systematic solution to the hopeless nervous exhaustion of the young mother in "The Yellow Wall-paper." She would take the suggestion even further in her future political and fictional writings, in which she imagined a social transformation that would essentially blow up the nuclear family in order to free women to pursue their talents and passions. What enabled her to think on such a broad scale was her exposure to a strand of socialist thought that called for fundamental changes to society. Specifically, her involvement in the Nationalist movement inspired by the novelist and social reformer Edward Bellamy prompted her to think about the underlying structures behind particular social problems—such as women's nervous exhaustion at home. The movement got its start with the publication of Bellamy's 1888 utopian novel, *Looking Backward: 2000–1887*. Bellamy imagines a futuristic society in which the government controls all industry and enormous economies of scale eradicate inefficiencies in production and distribution. There are huge "armies" of workers, with each person doing the work best suited to him or her, and the monetary system has been eliminated (it is replaced by a system of "credit cards" that are calibrated to meet each person's needs). Individual competition and labor strife are flushed from the system, as are crime, poverty, mental illness, and other infirmities. Although Bellamy does not dwell at length on domestic arrangements or women's place within them, he does include in his ideal world a special industrial army that is "under exclusively feminine regime." This army is exempted from the most physically grueling work, but it still operates under the theory that each woman should be given "the kind of occupation . . . she is best adapted to." This development, the protagonist concludes, overcomes the "root of [women's] disability," that is, "her personal dependence upon man for her livelihood."

Within a few years of the publication of *Looking Backward*, Bellamy found himself at the head of a movement—Nationalism—inspired by his novel: by 1890, there were 162 Bellamy Clubs in twenty-seven states developing proposals and calls to action based on his ideas. Charlotte Perkins Gilman was a member of the branch in Pasadena, California. By this point, she was much in demand as a speaker, and her lectures sounded Nationalist themes, such as advocating government control of banking and railways. But she offered her own feminist slant, too, by proposing specific social and economic reforms geared toward eliminating economic inequality between men and women. Gilman expanded on these ideas in her political tract *Women and Economics* (1898), and she wrote a utopian novel of her own, *Herland* (1915). Bellamy imagined that the women's army would be paternalistically established by men ("We have given them a world of their own"), but Gilman pictured a world apart, in which a tribe of women manages to survive a volcanic eruption that has killed off all the men, and has magically acquired the ability to reproduce via parthenogenesis. In this woman-only world, children are raised in collective nurseries and comport themselves with perfect sweetness, as if raised by a tribe of Mrs. Gordinses. As the male narrator who stumbles upon this world amazedly puts it: "The youngest ones, rosy fatlings in their mothers' arms, or sleeping lightly in the flower-sweet air, seemed natural enough, save that they never cried. . . . If I feared at first the effects of a too intensive culture, that fear was dissipated by seeing the long sunny days of pure physical merriment and natural sleep in which these heavenly babies passed their first years."

Perhaps it would be too much to claim that the utopian vision animating Gilman's work revolved around sleep. But getting children to sleep on their own so that their mothers would be free to work and enjoy life was a powerful motif in this political phase of her career. The social reform of sleeping arrangements that she pictured in her work connected her own childhood concern with disciplining her body, her early (and famous) writing on women's psychosexual vulnerability to the demands of mothering, and her later vision of social engineering. In order to untether women from the tyrannical demands of a colicky or sleepless baby, she had to imagine another world.

———

Such imagining may seem far-fetched, but I spent six months living in another socialist community, founded at about the same time as Gilman wrote *Herland*, that tried something quite similar. In 1987, like many young Jews around the world, I decided, somewhat impulsively, to spend some time in Israel living on a kibbutz—mainly because I wasn't sure what I wanted to do with myself, and living on a collective farm in a foreign country that I had been brought up to identify with seemed like a romantic adventure. Plus, the whole thing was free: room, board, language lessons, tours of the country, the whole deal; it seemed like more than a fair trade for picking avocados, or whatever, for a few hours a week.

The Israeli kibbutz movement, a socialist-Zionist enterprise in collective living, was founded not only on ideas of eradicating private property and class distinctions among Jews, but also on the principle of women's equality with men. And this meant destroying the institution of the nuclear family. As the famous Austrian-born child psychologist Bruno Bettelheim put it in his 1968 study of kibbutz childrearing practices, *The Children of the Dream*, kibbutzniks wished to create a world in which the peer group, rather than the nuclear family, was the primary social unit. When the original founders of the movement began to have children, a crisis ensued: How could women continue to work, socialize, and run their society shoulder-to-shoulder with men if they were expected—like Charlotte Perkins Gilman's poor Mrs. Gordins—to tend all day and night to their children? As a founding member of the first kibbutz, Degania—founded in 1910—put it to Bettelheim, "The women wouldn't hear of giving up their share of the communal work and life. . . . Somebody proposed that the kibbutz should hire a nurse. . . . [W]e didn't hire a nurse, but we chose one girl to look after the lot of them and we put aside a house where they could spend the day while the mothers were at work." Before long, the children were sleeping in this house, which eventually became standard practice at virtually all the kibbutzim.

The more doctrinaire among the kibbutzim insisted on absolute separation of children from their parents at bedtime; and through most of the next half-century, children were raised and put to bed in nurseries, where *metaplot* (caregivers) watched over them in the night in isolation from their parents, but in the company of their peers. Parents were typically given a brief time to spend with their children before they sent them off to the nursery for the night. During this time, they were encouraged to read to the children—but not the traditional bourgeois bedtime stories in which children (or bunnies) snuggled with parents before being sent off to bed alone. Instead, special children's books were produced that told inspiring stories about socialist values and the importance of the children's social group. Parents and their living spaces were generally absent from these narratives. According to Israeli child studies scholar Yael Darr, although some authors deviated from this script, in general "the going-to-bed scene, which in western children's literature revolves around a loving parent attending to a child, here reflects just the opposite: it serves to emphasize the independence of the children's society."

The kibbutz movement was, according to one of its most prominent scholars, the largest utopian experiment in history, with 125,000 members living on over 200 kibbutzim by 1990. When I stayed on one in the 1980s, though, I found a community rapidly transforming, and losing much of its original, utopian drive. At the edge of the farmland where chickens and cows were raised, avocados plucked, and grains harvested, there was a factory that made air-conditioning parts. About half of the assembly line in this factory consisted of paid workers from the outside. Property was all held communally, and town-hall-style decisions still ruled, but I sensed that the younger members of the kibbutz were more interested on a day-to-day level in the swimming pool and the discotheque than in socialist politics. (Although, to be honest, so was I, so I may have missed out on some of the more idealistic strains.) A certain materialism was creeping in, countering the asceticism of the founding generation. When a family that I got to know learned that my parents were coming for a visit, the father was intent on having them bring a very specific kind of television set that was difficult to obtain in Israel. One key feature of the collective enterprise was still intact, though: the children were raised communally, by *metaplot*. The term uses a feminine noun, and I noted that despite the kibbutz movement's rhetoric of gender equality, all of the caregivers were women.

The changes that I witnessed accelerated across the 1980s and 1990s, gradually chipping away at the core values of the collective enterprise. Many kibbutzim, driven by members' hunger for a higher standard of living, began to allow members to retain outside income, to hold private funds and property and pass them along through inheritance, and even to charge for meals in the collective dining halls. Some of the kibbutz factories and agribusinesses hired outside managers who weren't bound by the community's rules. The final straw for many traditionalists was the decision to abandon collective childrearing in favor of "family sleeping"—a decision that old-timers and purists saw as the "end of the kibbutz." By the 1990s, virtually every kibbutz had given up on the idea of collective childhood sleeping. With this linchpin of communal living gone, by the end of the century one could argue that kibbutzim resembled suburban planned communities at least as much as they resembled the founders' dream societies.

The kibbutz where I lived in 1987 still clung to the idea of collective child-care and the sleeping arrangements that made it possible. How did this tenet affect the life of the community? As I look back, I would characterize the adults as better rested than the harried professionals I had grown up with; certainly they were better rested than the few young parents I knew at the time. Not having to commute to work or the grocery store must have had something to do with this, too. But it seems likely that for young parents, especially, outsourcing nighttime child-care contributed to maintaining high energy levels through the day. I didn't get to know any of the children who were being put to bed each night by *meta-plot*, but I did spend much of my free time with young adults who had been brought up in this way. They certainly had life stressors that I couldn't imagine—compulsory army service and the stirrings of the first Palestinian *intifada* chief among them. But parents and their neuroses played a surprisingly minor role in their lives, as did conflicts among peers. The group bond between the members of the cohort was simply assumed; there were disagreements and petty quarrels, to be sure, but being raised as a peer group probably contributed to the less noticeable cliques and social fault lines than I had experienced growing up.

As for sleep, I was struck by the fact that the young men and women who returned exhausted during breaks from army service seemed to be able to drop off anywhere. During a kibbutz cultural event that I attended, one of these young men grew tired. He put his rucksack on the floor, amid a group of a hundred people, and simply napped. Army life must have toughened him up to rough sleeping environments, but his childhood sleep environment also made this conspicuously public snooze more acceptable. Weren't non-kibbutzniks more likely to feel embarrassed about sleeping out in the open like this? No one teased him or even commented when he arose and rejoined the event. The experience of being raised among dozens of other sleepers, night after night, may well have spared him the inhibitions that people who associate sleep with privacy experience. And it may have inured him to the sounds of the waking world that would have made sleeping difficult for those who are brought up sleeping in solitary, noise-free chambers.

Different rules for sleep affected ideas of privacy in waking life as well. One small detail of life on the kibbutz struck me as particularly odd, indeed uncomfortable. A close friend I had made during the year, an eighteen-year-old aspiring artist who was about to begin his military service, never knocked on my door in the volunteers' quarters when he wanted to find me—he just barged in. After this happened a few times, I politely explained to him that sometimes I wanted privacy. He looked at me quizzically, and he tried to honor my request to knock first, but it seemed to me that a small cultural line had sprung up between us: the utopian collective sleeper versus the neurotic American used to his private fortress.

———

While the kibbutz movement presented a highly unusual sleeping environment, especially for children and young parents, I could have found similar collective sleeping arrangements back in the States if I had tried. The idea of communal living, and particularly of communal childrearing and the utopian sleeping conditions that parents might experience, took root in several utopian schemes from the 1960s onward. Oddly enough, the most durable of these schemes owes its inspiration to Henry David Thoreau as much as it does to the kibbutz movement.

Thoreau's cabin in the woods was in a sense a utopia of one, but how could his attempt to recalibrate his daily rhythms to those of the natural world be a model for an entire society? This was the impetus behind a very strange piece of fiction—one that inspired numerous real-world imitators—by B. F. Skinner, the behavioral psychologist whose "mechanical baby tender" was introduced in the previous chapter. The baby box makes an appearance in *Walden Two*, Skinner's 1948 utopian novel in which he pictures a planned community run by experts who manage rational systems of labor, education, entertainment, and child care. As far removed as this scenario seems from Thoreau's unwitting prequel ("How deep the ruts of conformity!" Thoreau wrote; and "I suspect any enterprise in which two were engaged together"), Skinner fancied himself a latter-day Thoreau. Following the lead of his nineteenth-century predecessor, Skinner designed an imaginary community that would consume the minimum amount of resources using the minimum amount of labor necessary to promote a good life. The main vision behind the novel was to rationalize labor through a system of work-credits instead of money—more credits for less desirable work, meaning more time for leisure and culture. But in order to create a thoroughly rational community, each member must be fully alert, and so "the cardinal piece of engineering," he wrote, was ensuring that everyone gets a good night's sleep. Too many people on the outside, says the society's founder, "never know what it's like to be rested. They never have a chance to discover . . . how well they could work otherwise, or what brilliant flashes they might have."

The novel tells the story of Burris, a psychology professor, who heads a small group that visits a utopian community established by a former classmate of his, Frazier. This community is called Walden Two, and Frazier fancies himself "a sort of second Thoreau." But this world inspired by the transcendentalist critic of group-think, institutional authority, and worship of technology is a bit peculiar: Frazier's bedrock belief is that "any group of people could secure economic self-sufficiency with the help of modern technology, and the psychological problems of group living could be solved with available principles of 'behavioral engineering.'" This egghead techno-utopia has nearly a thousand members living in low-cost, multifamily, mixed-use buildings. Everything, including clothing styles, food, leisure activities, education, and exercise, is planned by a committee of social-scientist experts in order to maximize efficiency, minimize waste, prevent social conflict, and allow everyone time for intellectually and morally elevating pursuits.

As in Israeli *kibbutzim* (and Mrs. Gordins's upstairs nursery), children at Walden Two are raised largely apart from their parents by professional caregivers. Parents can afford to work on their own schedules because "they have no reason to wait for the day's work to

be over, or the children put to bed." The earliest sleeping arrangements, though, are not exactly communal: the key is separating the
children from the parents. Recalling Skinner's "baby in a box," the
story has the babies kept in isolated, temperature-controlled cubicles, where they can be free of bedding and clothes, save a diaper.
Children from one to three years old sleep in small sleeping rooms
that are essentially larger versions of the boxes; a few are in training pants, but the rest are naked. At around age four, they graduate
to small cots in a dormitory and begin wearing clothing, and they
gradually are accorded more individual space up until age thirteen,
at which time they take temporary rooms in the adult building. Not
long thereafter, they are paired off in marriage, in order to avoid
"pathological aberrations" that follow from sexual frustration. The
nighttime separation of parents from each other also improves
matters. "Living in a separate room not only made the individual
happier and better adjusted, it tended to strengthen the affection of
husband and wife," Skinner wrote.

The novel shares its predecessor's commitment to simplicity, to
preserving time, to renouncing consumerism, and to marrying labor
with life of the mind. But it is almost shocking that Skinner saw
no contradiction in this top-down scheme, in which every major
decision in the community is made by a board of managers, with
Thoreau's radical anti-hierarchical thinking, or between the behaviorist's overt appeal to social conformism and engineering and the
transcendentalist's militant rejection of convention. Despite Skinner's somewhat forward-thinking conservationist ethic, there is
practically no space for nature, and certainly none of the "wildness"
Thoreau promoted. There is also no room for eccentricity, free
play, or spiritual reflection. And worst of all, no irony. *Walden Two*
is a crushingly, deadeningly self-serious production. Skinner never
plays with language, or with ideas, or with evanescent thoughts and
impressions such as those that enliven Thoreau's work. Skinner was
also well-known for inventing a "teaching machine," another box-
like structure, which automated children's instruction. *Walden Two*
reads as if it were written by one of those boxes. And yet there is

something impressive about the moral certainty expressed in the book, an almost inhuman, persistent rigidity and self-assurance that somehow resists being boring.

As terrible as the novel is, as a cultural document it fascinates. *Walden Two* sold over 2.5 million copies before 1990, most of those in the 1960s and 1970s. One might suppose that some of these sales were made to readers who would better know their enemy; in general, the countercultural movements of the time considered Skinner the antithesis of the freedom and radical self-actualization that guided protest politics. Critics on the left called him an apologist for totalitarianism or fascism, a proponent of mind control worthy of Stalin and Hitler. His faith in technology as a solution to social problems didn't help: his famous teaching machine became a symbol of an oppressive and impersonal "automated mass society"; some readers compared it to something out of Aldous Huxley's *Brave New World* or George Orwell's *1984*. The folk singer Pete Seeger's song "Little Boxes," about the mind-numbing conformism of suburban life, might just as well have referred to the mechanical baby tender, the teaching machine, and the general squareness that Skinner came to represent.

But one hippie's bad trip is another's visionary experience. A countercurrent within the counterculture embraced Skinner just as fervently as others rejected him. To these radical stepchildren of the great behaviorist, *Walden Two* served as a model for creating a society free of consumerism and conflict and promoting equality and communal values. In 1965, a group in Washington, DC, attempted to begin a Skinner-inspired intentional community called Walden House; the organization quickly fell apart, but some of its members joined forces with an Atlanta community called Walden Pool, and together they began to plan a viable utopian enterprise. In June 1967, the Twin Oaks Community was founded on a farm in rural Virginia. Its eight founding members used Skinner's variable labor credit system to reward undesirable work, but disagreements soon arose about how much credit to give each task. One member explained that they abandoned it after about a year because "there were always people who figured out how to manipulate it for their own benefit." Yet Twin Oaks still made work assignments largely based on individual interests, and the members of the community found that intrinsic work satisfaction seemed sufficient to enable them to accomplish most of the goals of variable labor credits without using the credits themselves. As in Skinner's novel, a board of "Planners" made general community decisions, and managers were appointed for farming, child care, kitchen work, construction, and receiving visitors. Decisions by managers could be overruled by Planners, and Planners could be overruled by the community as a whole.

In Skinner's novel, Frazier articulates the rationale for communal parenting—and for separating out the generations at bedtime. Rejecting the special nature of maternal love, he explains: "We go in for father love, too—for everybody's love—community love if you wish. Our children are treated with affection by everyone." At Twin Oaks, child care was part of the initial labor credit system, and a "child manager" made all substantive decisions about their upbringing. Young children up to age five slept in a building called Degania after the first kibbutz, where one baby was raised in a mechanical baby tender (or air crib) as an experiment. At around age five, children graduated either to their own rooms or shared a room with another child; by age nine each child had his or her own room in the same building as at least one parent. Yet the program ultimately sputtered: within a few years, several parents left the community when they could not bear to hand over childrearing to the child manager, and the collective arrangements were discontinued not long afterward. Today, Twin Oaks is still in operation, with about ninety adults and fifteen children. It is still run as a collective, with all income from its hammock-making, book-indexing, and heirloom vegetable seed-growing enterprises shared among members. But the communal sleeping arrangements for children are gone.

What can we take away from these failed—or at least abandoned—efforts to revolutionize sleep? We can start with their partiality: they address only those who are willing to join a collective enterprise; they don't seem to address the problems of race and poverty that have contributed to an unequal distribution of sleep; and, while they boldly address the sleeping patterns of parents and young children, they hardly change those of sleepers at different points of the human life span. For all these limitations, the effort that goes into wrapping society around sleep rather than the other way around is still pretty impressive. Many of us can tinker with our own sleep rhythms, and a few can make radical changes at an individual level. (Retirees, trustafarians, and professors on sabbatical come to mind.) But to really overhaul the system, even within a family, seems to require massive social change on a level that so far hasn't seemed entirely sustainable, even among the dreamers. Perhaps the failures of these schemes can remind us of sleep's stubborn power, its resistance to our determined efforts to bend it to our own wills, or even to the collective will. Thoreau saw this unconquerable wildness as a basic fact of nature: we could pollute sleep, batter it with rules and chemical substances, try to tame it with social standards—but it would still run its wild course. Not even a revolution seems entirely able to tame sleep.

On a more positive note, the utopian schemers might send the message that for all its dissatisfactions, the way we sleep is, in the end, an arrangement of our own making. They each valued sleep enough to try to reengineer it to their own satisfaction in an entirely new society. We may not choose to lie in the beds these dreamers made, but why should we continue to toss and turn in ours?

PART IV

Global Weirding

The future is already here; it's just not very evenly distributed.

—William Gibson

CHAPTER SEVEN

Beyond Normal

With or without the help of utopian dreamers, cracks are beginning to appear in the rules of normal sleep, that rickety contraption
devised early in the industrial age. For a few hundred years, most of
us have lived under the reign of a fairly rigid set of rules and expectations governing sleep, and enforcing them seems ever more tenu-
ous. Those who can't afford the private spaces and regular routines
required for normal sleep face health risks and social stigmas. And
those of us who struggle to maintain the rules batter our sleep-wake
cycle with an ever-expanding arsenal of drugs and devices, consult
guidebooks and sleep coaches to get ourselves and our children on
the right schedule, and monitor ourselves and each other in sleep
clinics or at home with wearable electronic devices—all in the name
of attaining a mode of sleep that is increasingly ill-suited to the
lives many of us lead. Yet this version of normality seems unlikely to
withstand the various futures that are barreling down on it. We have
technological tools of unprecedented power and nuance to peer into
sleep and detect its tremors and disturbances, but we have other,
even more powerful tools that are keeping us up at night. In a wider
context, changes in the global economy have led to a restructuring
of the way we experience time, including the internal time that regulates our bodies' systems involved in sleeping and waking.

On one level, established Western sleep patterns seem to be gaining ground rather than losing it, as they are increasingly becoming global norms. Almost as soon as Thomas Edison's incandescent light bulbs became widely available, physicians warned of their sleep-deranging effects. As we have seen, historians and anthropologists have documented the erosion of traditional sleeping patterns worldwide wherever electric lighting was introduced; but television has also taken its share of blame for global sleep disruptions. For instance, not long after television was introduced into Yemen in the 1970s, an anthropologist found that most people would stay up watching until the signal went off at 11 p.m.; many viewers then had trouble getting up the following morning.

The idea—or even the reality—that electronic technology is disturbing sleep is hardly original to our age. Edison himself bragged about his limited need for sleep, and later in his career he referred to his research team as an "insomnia squad" because in their quest to perfect a phonographic machine in the 1910s, they slept as little as possible. What's new in our world today are the global circuits that link capitalists, workers, and consumers in patterns of sleep and waking that have virtually nothing to do with either the diurnal rhythms of day and night or the rules of any particular society. When I have a software glitch, I might call a support center and speak to someone named "Mike" who lives halfway around the world; in the process, I am depending on someone else being awake on a regular basis at 3 a.m. in order to cater to my technical ineptitude. In turn, Mike helps keep me satisfied with a product that inarguably disturbs my own sleep patterns, and especially those of my teenaged kids. Deepening our bond of weird sleep, we are communicating via a commercial infrastructure that never shuts down, offering us both opportunities to buy and sell whatever we want or need at any moment—although, in this case, my convenience is underwritten by Mike's anti-circadian work schedule. "Eight hours for work, eight hours for rest, eight hours for what you will" seems like a quaint slogan from a bygone era under these circumstances.

Outside of offices like Mike's call center, on the streets of cities like Delhi, the situation is even more dire for those who have not found a secure niche in the global workplace. In the vast homeless encampments of Delhi, the need for sleep is so severe that entrepreneurs have figured out how to profit from it. A "sleep mafia" has sprung up, renting mats, quilts, rickshaw cushions, and other minimal protections against the elements to those who can afford them; the prices go up in wintertime. In a sense, this is a shadow market of the sleep-products and sleep-services industry that has experienced such an astonishing rise among more privileged sectors of the economy. The medical and technological wings of the sleep-hygiene industry generate billions of dollars for pharmaceutical companies, sleep researchers, and clinicians. While the privileged few are seeking gourmet sleep in such markets, those on the streets are paying what they can for table scraps.

In a way, "sleep change" is running parallel to "climate change." Some environmentalists prefer the term "global weirding" to "global warming," because the changes taking place in the earth's climate go far beyond a uniform, steady warming of temperatures: they also involve floods, droughts, and pockets of intense cold. Similarly, changes to sleep are moving in several directions at once—but the common denominator—as with climate—is change. The arrangement whereby my consumerist impulses are linked to an anonymous stranger's sleep deprivation thousands of miles away is just one bit of strange weather in the world of sleep. For instance, enlightened American executives may be bringing power napping into the workplace, as Arianna Huffington's *The Sleep Revolution* pointed out, but at the same time many traditional napping cultures are being pressured to abandon the practice. It is well known that China, Spain, Greece, and many other countries have customary napping periods at different points in the day—but now government officials and business groups who want to "modernize" their economies are trying to eradicate napping. The pressure became particularly urgent after Spain's economic crisis began in 2008. "We need a more efficient culture," said Ignacio Buqueras y Bach, president of the National Commission for the Rationalization of Spanish Times. "Spain has to break the bad habits it has accumulated over the past forty or fifty years." In 2006, government offices in Spain adopted a

9-to-5 workday, eliminating the late-afternoon siesta break, and the consolidated model seems to be taking hold in many other napping cultures, too. In a global economy, consolidated sleeping seems to be equated with economic might, even as the economically mighty are finding that strategic napping might actually serve productivity rather than impede it.

———

The global weirding of sleep is also affecting family life in the United States and elsewhere. As any parent can tell you, the digital age has affected children's sleep profoundly, and this is one area in which the reign of "normal" seems to be particularly unsustainable. One of the fastest-growing areas of sleep research involves the effects of exposure to screens on the sleep-wake cycle. Upward of two hours of exposure to screens at night, researchers have found, can significantly affect sleep onset and duration, and the danger is most extreme for children. Yet the average American child now spends upward of seven hours staring at glowing electronic screens. The problem is not only that kids delay going to bed because they have trouble turning off their devices; the blue light that our screens emit reduces our melatonin levels, so that long after we've turned off the machines, our brains continue to behave as if it were daytime.

Putting children whose eyes and brains are bathed in blue light on a proper sleep schedule can be extremely challenging. Since at least the late nineteenth century, as detailed in Chapter Five, parents have been enjoined to put their young on a rigid schedule in order to raise them to be hearty, independent, well-adjusted sleepers capable of staying knocked out on their own through the night. (It was this set of sleep rules, as Chapters Five and Six showed, that pediatricians were most intent on enforcing and utopian thinkers were most intent on overthrowing.) Part of the impetus for the sleep-training systems that sprang up around this central feature of normal sleep was that children had to learn to wake up in order to clock in at school, where attendance was a newly universal requirement in the late nineteenth century. In this way, children's rhythms would also suit the needs of their parents, who were increasingly working outside of the home at jobs that required them to be on a similar schedule.

Yet now, thanks to the clamor for preparing students to enter the global workforce fully adept at manipulating the latest technological gadgetry, many school systems are unintentionally undermining parents' efforts to produce the kind of well-regulated childhood sleep necessary for optimum, or even basic, functioning in school. Before the twenty-first century, doing homework generally meant burying one's head in a book, working out problems on a sheet of paper, or trying to make baking soda erupt out of a clay volcano; now it usually means sitting in front of a computer screen or a tablet. Assignments often involve looking up information on the Internet (this is now referred to as "research"); students are encouraged to communicate with each other and with their teachers through online chat forums; and finished work is often submitted online. Not only does all of this online activity require students to submit their optical nerves to melatonin-suppressing blue light, but only the most motivated and self-disciplined kids can resist the urge to surf the Web for videos, play games, and "like" each other's social media updates while the homework is supposed to be happening. As many parents can attest, this nightly routine opens up a new zone of intergenerational struggle—often a losing one for parents, who can no longer enforce a division between recreational screen use and homework. Sane bedtimes often hang in the balance, as protestations of "But I'm doing homework!" extend late into the night, with inevitable drowsiness and irritability following the next day. (Predictably, a whole new line of technological gadgets has recently appeared on the market, promising parents the means to control this dynamic by filtering out certain types of screen activity at given hours.)

Children's sleep is far from the only temporal pattern being disrupted by our obsession with gadgetry. Thoreau warned about humans becoming tools of our tools; he might have been speaking to our sleeping selves as well as our waking ones. Take, for example, the case of Apple's iPhone 5c, the dinky little machine I use, or that uses me, to obsessively check emails or place phone calls while I walk my dog, or to navigate the streets and highways of a city I've lived in for ten years, but whose roadways I've never really had to learn for myself. In fact, I'm using it even as I write these words to stream music based on a complex algorithm of my tastes. That magical, maddening little wafer has generated a worldwide web of altered sleeping arrangements.

Everyone complains about how tempting it is to reach for a smartphone in the middle of the night and how easy it is to get sucked into an orgy of social-media bingeing; it's especially tempting to do so if you use your phone as an alarm clock and keep it by your bed. But few contemplate how the thing is made. A 2013 investigation by China Labor Watch revealed that, among other abuses, the factories in which the 5c was assembled were responsible for offenses against sleep: they demanded that workers stay at the job for 11.5 consecutive hours, with only a thirty-minute meal break. Day-shift and night-shift workers in the plant were made to sleep eight to a dorm room, stacked on hard, narrow cots, where they suffered inevitable interruptions of sleep as their roommates came and went on different schedules. Said one worker on the night shift at the plant, "Since my sleep in the daytime was not very good, I really needed to get as much sleep as possible on the bus, otherwise I would not be able to stand up for the entire 12-hour shift this night."

If such conditions seem eerily similar to those in American steel plants and other heavy industrial sites of the early twentieth century, it's a similarity by design: in order to evade workers' protections of their right to rest, corporations have outsourced labor to places where circadian cycles can be manipulated or disregarded without consequence—other than to workers' health and well-being. Such disruptions in the nineteenth-century United States paradoxically helped spread the demand for rules to govern normal sleep as workers agitated for their right to an eight-hour workday. Their successes were not only the result of labor activism: eventually, factory managers came to understand that allowing workers sufficient rest was an important factor in creating an efficient workforce. One wonders whether Chinese factory workers will ever demand similar protections, and whether the version of normal sleep that emerges will mirror the twentieth-century Western one.

On the global level, severe disruptions to circadian cycles do not just take place on the floors of Indian technology call centers and in Chinese factories, but also in a host of other settings. Other kinds of technological outsourcing have similar effects on workers' sleep rhythms. The "business process outsourcing industry"— which involves contracting third-party sources to perform specific operations for a given business—affects the circadian rhythms of computer animators and software developers in the Philippines. Meanwhile, radiologists in India and Australia often read the medical CAT scans of US patients, with around-the-clock service to provide the information as quickly as possible for patients facing emergency situations. Even sleep labs themselves are increasingly outsourcing the scoring of patient records, sometimes to workers overseas. The disrupted sleep that follows, researchers have found, has serious health consequences, ranging from depression and chronic fatigue to predisposition toward infections. As the anthropologist Kevin Birth put it, such technology-mediated disturbances in circadian cycles arise from "conflicts between global and local schedules and between the timing of global relationships and the cycles of one's locally embedded biological rhythms." Or, to put it more plainly, much of the world's population is being taught to sleep globally, even as their internal clocks are still set locally.

Yet technology also promises to correct such imbalances. To return to the smartphone and its derangement of sleep cycles worldwide: if your screen use, your work schedule, your health, or your anxiety about any of the above has disrupted your sleep patterns, you can outfit your phone to produce highly detailed records of your every sleep-related activity, rivaling the "actigraphy" used by sleep professionals. With this information, you can perhaps self-diagnose a sleep disorder, the one that was caused by the very device you're using to measure your sleep, or by how much you're freaking out about what you read on it. (Such smartphone-based sleep-monitoring apps, though, are being supplanted by smaller, wearable devices that can measure your sleep and its interruptions.) Many sleep apnea masks and dental devices that set the jaw for better air-flow during sleep now also come outfitted with digital data collection devices. With all of these derangements and recalibrations of sleep patterns, we are experiencing a more and more complicated relationship with our technology; and our sleep, like the environment in which it occurs, is now subject to global weirding. Yet, as with climate change, some areas will be harder hit than others. The conflicts between the pressures of circadian, diurnal, and global rhythms, according to anthropologist Birth, tend to be resolved in favor of those living in time zones where the most economically advantaged people live.

These developments have a history that long predates the development of the smartphone or the personal computer. It's hardly a new idea that machines are distorting sleep patterns—in fact, this concern extends back at least as far as the nineteenth century, when trains and telegraphs were also said to produce a frantic pace in people's lives that led to unnatural sleep. Then as now, novel technology was thought to be both the cause of and cure for insomnia. Victorian scientists and lay commentators often used the telegraph as a metaphor for understanding how the nervous system worked, much as today we speak of the brain being "hardwired" in the manner of a computer. According to one late nineteenth-century Anglo-Irish physician, when modern man pushed himself too hard, to the point of fatigue or nervous exhaustion, he ran the risk of "the battery of the brain [being] destroyed altogether." Today we complain about our electronic products ruining our sleep, yet we turn to sleep apps, sleep masks that practice surveillance on their wearers, and smart beds to counteract those effects; in a sense, we are simply recycling Victorian attempts to counteract neuro-electrical meltdown with more electricity. As cultural historian Lee Scrivner writes, Victorians deployed all manner of electrified sleep gadgetry, including belts, rods, brushes, and even a vibrating helmet to induce the sleep that seemed so difficult to attain in their frantic, hyperconnected world. Today we have refined some of these Victorian gadgets: for $149.99 you can buy a Sleep Shepherd Biofeedback Sleep Hat, which measures electrical activity in your brain as you crawl into bed, then emits pulsing tones mimicking the frequency of your brain waves. As the Sleep Shepherd's pulses gradually slow down, so, too—the manufacturers promise—will your racing brain.

Not surprisingly, the market for sleeping aids and wakefulness-promoting agents is now a global one, too—and this has a deep history as well. Historian Daniel Lord Smail suggests that the effort to alter brain chemistry via addictive or alluring substances was a driver of human history from the millennia-old agricultural revolution onward. As soon as the first hoe tilled a row of potatoes, surplus calories were suddenly available, and all sorts of food products were popularized not so much because they were life-sustaining, but because they produced desirable effects on brain chemistry. The production and consumption of such mind-altering substances really heated up in the eighteenth century with the spread of caffeine and chocolate, at the same time that other kinds of neural stimulation—from newspapers to racy novels—were also finding wider markets.

The long history of sleeping aids (from the judicious placement of sheep's lungs on the sides of the head, to poppy juice dripping into leech-bored holes behind the ears, to a simple Ambien down the hatch) and wakefulness extenders (from caffeine to cocaine to modafinil) suggests that human attempts to manipulate states of alertness and repose has long constituted a significant slice of the market for brain-chemistry-manipulating substances. There was never a great market for sheep's lungs, but wars have been fought over the economic control of caffeine, cocaine, and opium. And yet the market for substances that manipulate the sleep-wake cycle chemically has entered a new phase since the late twentieth century, as economic incentives for producing new products has increased. Despite its disastrously addictive properties, opium had a millennia-long reign; nowadays, new products chase down old ones as soon as profitability wanes. After decades of multibillion-dollar traffic worldwide, sales of such drugs as Ambien and Lunesta began to level off when cheap generic substitutes became available in the mid-2010s. At this writing, the newest wonder drug, suvorexant (marketed as Belsomra), is poised to generate new cash flows in the sleep market—in part by promising fewer side effects than its rivals (such as some older drugs' reported pesky tendency to cause those under their influence to raid the refrigerator or drive a car while chemically unconscious). Belsomra also addresses insomnia in a novel way neurologically: instead of inducing sleep directly, it works to deactivate orexins, the chemical that keeps people awake. It's not lack of sleep that's the problem in this vision peddled by a global pharmaceutical corporation—it's being awake when you don't want to be.

Of course, many people want to be more awake rather than less, and so a fiercely competitive—even violent—market for stimulants has developed over the centuries, even millennia. Armed forces have long sought to gain a competitive edge through altered brain chemistry. Examples include the ancient Greek use of a physically enervating mixture of opium, wine, and honey to inspire courage in their warriors, as well as to relieve their pains after battle. Inca warriors used coca to stimulate extreme battlefield exertions, and twentieth-century European and American armies used amphetamines. The military is now a driver of new commercial products, not just a consumer of them. In 2002, the US Defense Advanced Research Projects Agency (DARPA) made research into optimizing sleep and wakefulness a priority via its Preventing Sleep Deprivation program. "The capability to operate effectively, without sleep, is no less than a 21st century revolution in military affairs," the agency's website proclaimed. In 2007 DARPA set a goal of extending effective wakefulness for up to one hundred hours (so far, to no avail). But several products emerged from this research. The US Defense Department, for instance, developed a highly caffeinated gum that is now being marketed to the general public as Military Energy Gum; its manufacturer promises that this "military spec caffeine gum" will allow chewers to "maintain vigilance performance across a single night without sleep." Other DARPA projects have looked into such rewarmed Victorian ideas as the use of electrical stimulation to counteract the adverse effects of sleeplessness on cognition; or investigated newer ideas, like whether a nasal spray containing orexin might be developed to increase wakefulness; or studied the potential for ideas even further out on the cutting edge of sleep research, such as how the migratory sleeplessness of sparrows might give us clues about human sleep-wake patterns, and how the brain might be manipulated to function similarly without loss of function.

The most successful product to be rolled out by the military is now in wide use for a variety of purposes: modafinil, marketed under the trade name Provigil and Nuvigil in the United States, Alertec in Canada, and Modiodol in France. Originally used to suppress the sudden micro-sleeps produced by narcolepsy, the drug was soon found to promote wakefulness in general. The research got a kickstart from funding by the French Ministry of Defense. Said a spokesman for the ministry: "If there is a war in Europe . . . it will be carried [out] during the night as well as daytime. Hence we need armies capable of maneuvering at any time, for three or four days, nonstop, without diminishing performance." Modafinil was used extensively during bombing raids in the Iraq War, but defense analysts now question its efficacy. Especially concerning is that modafinil use increases irritability; it also tends to promote overconfidence—so that a person who takes it is likelier than one who has not to offer wrong answers to questions and to act upon misperceptions with unearned certainty, sometimes with disastrous results. Some new military sleep-efficiency efforts are therefore turning away from pharmaceuticals and toward products that encourage a more flexible, catch-as-catch-can sleep pattern for warriors, especially those who never know quite what their long-range bombing schedule might be. The Somneo Sleep Trainer, for instance, is a mask that gently warms the areas around the eyes and blots out ambient noise and visual distractions to encourage sleep, and then gently awakens the wearer with subtle increments of blue light. With such devices, a new generation of fighters is being taught to sleep for an hour or two when time permits, rather than to ward off sleep altogether.

Yet modafinil has a robust post-military life among civilians. Provigil generated a whopping $1.4 billion in global sales in 2010; availability of cheaper generic versions had cut into that dollar figure substantially by 2012, but the number of units sold continued to rise. It was still officially prescribed for narcolepsy, but now new disorders were being identified that the drug could help to manage, such as shift-work sleep disorder and excessive daytime sleepiness.

The drug's developer, neurologist Michel Jouvet, predicted yet other uses, such as helping sleepy children stay awake in class, and he reported benefiting from its use himself. Through the 1990s and 2000s, it began to be used off-label to treat fibromyalgia, chronic fatigue syndrome, fatigue stemming from Parkinson's disease, and a host of other disturbances involving sleepiness and wavering alertness; the on-label uses were expanded to sleep apnea and shift-work sleep disorder. Gradually it became known as a wonder drug, prompting illicit traffic among students cramming for exams and others looking for a neurological edge—or what came to be known as "neuroenhancement." Even parents got in on the act: a 2009 poll conducted by the journal *Nature* found that one out of three readers would give their children "smart drugs" if they learned that other parents were doing so.

Modafinil's penetration into the culture sparked a debate among bioethicists about the benefits and hazards of neural enhancement—also sometimes called "cosmetic neurology"—in which drugs are used not to treat or cure harmful conditions, but to optimize performance well beyond normal functioning. Should such attempts to optimize cognitive functioning be legal? Encouraged? Subsidized through insurance? Restricted? Much of the debate focused on these questions in the abstract, but for those who are intent on gaining an edge in a competitive global marketplace, pressure to use such drugs often feels less like an exercise in ethics than a compulsion. As an executive of a firm that advises investors on neuro-technology said, "if you're a fifty-five-year-old in Boston, you have to compete with a twenty-six-year-old from Mumbai now, and those kinds of pressures are only going to grow.'" The implication is not only that you have to be smarter in such a world—with less room for the cognitive slips that might come with age—but that you need to rewire your brain to overcome its default circadian settings. The global weirding of sleep shows in a way that twenty-first-century capitalism has not just changed patterns of commerce and labor, but also basic physiological processes.

So where is sleep heading? This question has begun to preoccupy professional prognosticators in the media, where you can find articles and science shows with titles like "The Future of Sleep" and "7 Reasons Why the Future of Sleep Could Be Wilder than Your Wildest Dreams." According to these would-be oracles, we might soon be genetically modified in ways that reduce our need for sleep; we might come closer to inducing "cryogenic" sleep or human hibernation; dreams might be more effectively harnessed to promote learning; and we might even see the marketing of "smart pajamas" that offer total-body monitoring of our physiological particularities during sleep. Academics, too, have gotten into the act, but as in most things, they disagree. Sociologist Simon Williams, for instance, sees an increasing biomedical fine-tuning of sleep that will increasingly put sleep into the control of corporations and the military. In a more optimistic view, anthropologist Matthew Wolf-Meyer sees a future marked increasingly by openness to flexible sleep arrangements that "accept the disorderly as human variation rather than medical pathology."

In short, although there is no clear single direction for sleep, all roads point away from the norms we've inherited from the efforts of labor management, sleep hygienists, self-help gurus, pediatricians, psychologists, and other assorted experts over the past two centuries. Some of the same digital technologies that are said to be keeping us up are also providing us with the tools to diagnose sleep problems with a view toward quicker and more accessible cures: we have pills to put us to sleep for four, six, or eight hours, or perhaps much longer, but we now also have newer pills to keep us up for extended periods with minimal loss of function; we have patterns of work that derange sleep schedules worldwide, but we now also are exploring patterns with more flexibility that might accommodate those who could never adjust to the eight-hour lie-down-and-die norm.

Whatever new patterns, configurations, and technologies emerge for sleep, conflicts are sure to remain as long as there is money to be made: some will be able to afford high-quality sleep, and some won't. Even work environments that allow for naps and other flexible time arrangements, such as those favored by Arianna Huffington, generally favor white-collar workers: lower-level office workers and blue-collar workers generally are afforded much less control over their working arrangements. At the university where I teach, the employee code of conduct states that "sleeping on the job" can result in disciplinary suspension or firing. Although this is offered as a blanket policy, it would only seem to apply to office staff, lab technicians, and maintenance crews, rather than including professors and upper-level administrators. Indeed, several of my colleagues confess to arranging for midday naps in their offices, and for this purpose they stash pillows and sleeping pads in their filing cabinets. So flexible sleep times, amounting to what sociologist Simon Williams calls the "customization" of sleep, often only widen class divides, with flexible sleep granted to some, while others remain subject to chaotic and unforgiving schedules.

———

Although the utopian dreamers we met in Chapter Six saw the demise of normal sleep as a consummation devoutly to be wished, many contemporary cultural observers see it as a disaster. As the old norms collapse under the weight of changing historical circumstance and the development of new sleep-manipulating technologies, a certain panic about sleep has crept into our public conversations—from alarmist popular proclamations of a "war on sleep" to highbrow art and criticism that portrays sleep as a vanishing natural resource. As in so much of our culture, utopian impulses have given way to dystopian or apocalyptic imaginings. Cultural commentators have bemoaned the loss of a utopian impulse, which they attribute to the spread of a fatalistic acceptance of free markets and capitalist globalization, the same forces that are altering sleep patterns worldwide. As cultural theorist Fredric Jameson put it, "it is easier to imagine the end of the world than the end of capitalism." It's easier to imagine the end of sleep, too. "There is no alternative," was the rallying cry for Margaret Thatcher's Conservative Party and its headlong embrace of privatization and free markets. Perhaps not coincidentally, Thatcher boasted of her ability to get by on next to no sleep: a 1997 satirical novel by Jonathan Coe called *The House of Sleep* features a Thatcher-loving mad scientist who wants to abolish sleep altogether.

In several recent works, disturbances of sleep have come to stand in for the fear of a new world economic order that depends on systematically disrupting sleep cycles worldwide, in the process ruining sleep just as it has disturbed so many other natural processes. Cultural critic Jonathan Crary, in his harrowing book *24/7: Late Capitalism and the Ends of Sleep*, pictures a global system in which the entire planet has become "a non-stop work site or an always open shopping mall of infinite choices, tasks, selections, and digressions." Because sleep is such a terrible blank space in a society in which everything is supposed to be for sale at any time, global capitalism has even figured out ways to turn sleep into something one must buy. Just as drinking water has been despoiled by pollution, made scarce by privatization, and then purified, repackaged, and sold in bottles—so sleep has first been "injured" by a nonstop global consumer economy, and then marketed as a commodity in pill form. Crary regards the soaring use of hypnotics over the past few decades as a sign that global capital has conquered the final frontier, the one we all cross when we drift out of consciousness. Like all good dystopian fiction, Crary's book pictures a world only slightly more terrible than the one we actually inhabit. His work is a rather extreme polemic, but it captures a prevailing attitude toward sleep as a once freely available resource that can now be bought, sold, or stolen.

Novelist Karen Russell takes Crary's dystopian portrait one step further. In her 2014 novella *Sleep Donation*, she pictures a future in which sleep has literally become impossible, thanks to a deadly plague of insomnia that circles the globe. Like Crary's vision, *Sleep Donation* offers theories of sleep's demise that are connected to environmental catastrophe and media saturation: experts offer competing explanations for the plague, ranging from polluted waterways to overexposure to electronic screens. (In a sly irony no doubt not lost on the author, the book is available only in electronic format.) Conventional pharmaceutical measures are helpless in the face of this horrifying "Insomnia Crisis," and so scientists devise a way to extract surplus sleep from those who are still unaffected by the epidemic and distribute it to insomniacs via intravenous transfusion. Of course, black marketers soon rush in, preying on babies, who still possess the deepest reserves of unpolluted sleep. Crary saw sleeping pills as a way to market sleep to a populace that had been deprived of it; Russell's dastardly profiteers cut out the middlemen and sell sleep itself. In an age when body organs, blood, eggs, sperm, and even DNA fragments can be detached from individual bodies, stored in "biobanks," and turned into commodities, Russell's vision of a market for stolen aggregate sleep—like Crary's—is only slightly fantastical.

Like these other two works, filmmaker Christopher Nolan's 2010 smash hit *Inception* treats sleep as fertile ground for economic exploitation. In this science-fiction thriller, corporate spies infiltrate the dream-worlds of their competitors in order to extract information or implant ruinous ideas that would give them a competitive edge. Hacking dreams is treated as the ultimate trespass against private property, since dreams represent a storehouse of ideas and information that is even more safely guarded than a bank account or a corporate database. Crary's *24/7* and Russell's *Sleep Donation* held up mass insomnia as a metaphor for the fate of citizens in an era of global commerce; *Inception* plays on our fears that even if we *can* sleep, our downtime might be a resource in the game of capital.

One might argue that both utopian dreamers and these purveyors of dystopian nightmares portray modern sleep as worse than it really is. Kibbutzniks and other communards failed to consider that the dreamers might actually *want* to put their kids to bed in the context of a nuclear nighttime family. And by picturing the world as hurtling toward "the end of sleep," the dystopian view catastrophizes contemporary sleep without taking into account that in some pockets of the global system, sleep is actually improving. As mentioned in the first chapter, those of us with the means to avoid the roughest kinds of sleep that come with poverty, war, and natural disaster have certain undeniable historical advantages that are unaccounted for in these dark visions. General improvements in public health, nighttime policing, fireproof materials, hygienic sleeping accoutrements, climate control, and nourishment all arguably have made refreshing sleep easier to obtain in the past century or so than at any other time in history. Labor laws in economically dominant nations provide some protection against the economic forces that would rob citizens of the opportunity to get sufficient sleep, and we do at least have the physical capacity to turn off those glowing screens and to resist the pills, no matter how they insinuate themselves into our lives.

Yet the anxieties identified so alarmingly in these works (with a generous helping of absurdist humor, in the case of Russell, and astonishing visuals, in the case of *Inception*) are real enough. What's useful about them is that they present contemporary sleep troubles not as a personal problem to be managed by pills and experts, but as a social, economic, and environmental one. In all their dark imaginings, they give shape to the anxieties many of us feel when we are confronted by information overload, manipulative corporate messaging, and looming ecological catastrophe. They can help us to see that human sleep has become inseparable from commerce, technology, environmental despoliation, and the damaging illusion that humans can exist in a realm apart from the natural world. The way we buy and sell sleep, after all, links us to unseen economic forces and environmental disturbances. Where do the chemicals in those little pills come from, anyway? What happens when their residue is sent back into the water supply the next morning? And what about those glowing machines that keep us up at night, or the ones that we use to monitor our sleep—what's their footprint, carbon or otherwise, on the natural world? The environmentalist Bill McKibben referred to a world in which no essence (air, rain, oceans) is uncontaminated by human presence as the "end of nature." Crary's subtitle hints at the ways we've been ransacking the natural world in our war on sleep by playing on McKibben's phrase: instead of "the end of nature," he writes of "the ends of sleep."

Under these circumstances, can the idea of "natural sleep"—the elusive entity that so many sleep researchers have tried to capture and analyze in their caves, bunkers, labs, and clinics—survive? Is there a default mode of human sleep to which we can return, some primordial, unspoiled nighttime ooze of unconsciousness? Or in seeking to break out of our current sleep predicaments, will we only fall into a new set of constricting rules that are devised to extract maximum profit out of or in spite of our downtime? Sociologist

Nikolas Rose writes skeptically of the longing that many of us feel for recovering "natural" states of health, which he regards as a kind of fantasy. "Humans have never been 'natural,'" according to Rose: we've always tried to manipulate our physical and psychological states by whatever means we could obtain. Even Thoreau might have agreed with that. After all, he didn't try to live as some kind of nineteenth-century Paleo type, slaughtering animals and roasting his fresh kills over an open flame. Instead, he kept himself largely to a fairly fastidious vegetarian diet, which for him was a triumph over his own animal nature rather than an acceptance of it. It's this kind of self-control that allowed him to sleep and rise according to his own "genius," rather than simply listening to some natural, animalistic alarm bell within himself. He may have wanted his sleep to run wild—but paradoxically, this took a great deal of discipline, not entirely unlike the regimens counseled in sleep-hygiene books and other self-help manuals.

So even if there's no "nature" to go back to at night, no God- or Darwin-given standard from which we've deviated, something particularly strange and perhaps unprecedented does seem to be happening to sleep: biomedical attempts to control it are intensifying, competing economic interests are pulling it this way and that, and a sense that the rules governing sleep in much of the West are coming undone is growing. Most people until recently have accepted the rules dictating "normal" sleep unquestioningly, because they have taken them for granted. But the rules are being unwritten, and sleep talk suddenly seems to be everywhere in our culture. The Internet, that rough beast that is blamed for killing sleep, is also awash with stories about sleep research, sleep medication, sleep ailments, and sleep oddities. As are our newspapers and magazines: in today's news alone, from the *New York Times* and *Tech Insider*, there are stories about the connection between sleeping and getting a cold, and about which sleeping positions might lead to nightmares. More things to worry about, for sure. But some of the verbiage we throw at sleep points to new openings.

A good counterweight to the dystopian visions of sleep's end being peddled in some corners of our culture is a new fascination in literature with simply describing sleep and sleep disruptions—a more difficult task than meets the eye. Sleep would seem to be resistant to literary treatment, because nothing "happens" while we sleep, and in a sense we're not even "there" to have anything happen to us. Yet a new consciousness of sleep as a subject worth addressing in the stories we tell about ourselves and our world seems to be emerging, especially in literary memoirs. In our confessional age, memoirists have been writing for decades of once-taboo topics like incest, addiction, and madness; but only recently have they started to peel back the coverlet over sleep, the most intimate aspect of our private lives—so private that we can barely access it ourselves. A spate of books by major-league insomniacs, with titles like *Wide Awake*, *Sleep Demons*, and (my candidate for best bad-book-title ever) *Desperately Seeking Snoozin'*, has made sleep, or the search for it, central to the story of a life rather than an interruption of it. These works don't make enough of a collective noise to count as a new genre of literature, and insomnia memoirs aren't really creating a sense of collective identity among insomniacs, or inspiring social activism among those who deviate from "normal" in terms of sleeping. So they are not like the popular disability memoirs that have been springing up, for example, which show how the experience of going blind or using a wheelchair has led to an author's political awakening, based on a new awareness of the social conditions of people with disabilities. This is strange, in a way, because some severe sleep disorders are classified as disabilities, and the Americans with Disabilities Act protects those who experience them from discrimination and requires employers and schools to provide them reasonable accommodation.

The most comparable literary record of a political awakening of crappy sleepers is *Insomniac* (2008), by the poet and critic Gayle Greene, who writes out of a deep frustration at the ways in which primary insomnia (that is, insomnia that is not a byproduct or symptom of some other condition) is typically blamed on the psychology of the sufferer, whereas other, generally rarer and more exotic sleep disorders receive millions in research dollars. She becomes an intrepid reporter and dogged researcher herself, following the money trail to show why professionally ambitious sleep experts build clinics and develop elaborate machinery to treat other disorders, while insomniacs like herself are generally given a pill and some advice about setting routines from a primary physician. By the end of the book, she is a one-woman lobbying force, advocating for reallocation of funds in sleep research. And she calls for insomniacs to form activist networks that are free from corporate influence to advocate for neurophysiological research into the root causes of primary insomnia. Despite Greene's efforts, the book stops short of calling for a social revolution. Greene, like me, is an English professor, so there is enough built-in flexibility in her schedule that she has been able to move forward in her own successful career, albeit often in a groggy state, despite her titanic bouts of sleeplessness. A memoir that leads insomniacs to stagger into the streets protesting our society's oppressive rules for sleeping and waking has yet to appear.

The sleep(less) memoir most interesting to me is less political and more poetical: a strange, hallucinatory 2011 work by the experimental novelist Blake Butler called *Nothing: A Portrait of Insomnia*. Butler's story proceeds from a mind-blowing 129-hour bout of insomnia that opens a literary wormhole into another dimension of thought. First came warped sensations: "Panels of color began to appear over my bed and beyond my doorway, floating scrims of ghosting color that would dissipate as I moved toward them in my flesh," and "space became not a system of dimensions but a kind of substance one could mold." Lest this sound heroic or even transcendental, Butler also details the daily grind of insomnia: the aphasia, the frustration, the "overall slurring" that comes with sleeplessness. This condition generates occasional bursts of poetry or philosophy. His insomnia amounts to "hypersensitivity to the condition of being alive," and he ominously describes "the self appearing in a blacking sphere around the brain." But more often his mind is dragged downward rather than upward. He writes of the obsessive, looping thoughts that come unbidden in the middle of the night: "The backlog at work will build because I can't concentrate. . . . I won't be nice company," and so on. These voices contribute to a general deterioration of identity that almost approaches the nothingness of sleep itself, except for a kind of gluey mental and physical presence that simply won't go away: "Often the clog just wants more clog."

As an accomplished insomniac myself, I found myself nodding in recognition at much of Butler's writing. But I also wished for an equally precise and poetic rendering of sleep, rather than of its stubborn refusal to come when bidden. Obviously, it's impossible to describe the condition of *being* asleep. French philosopher Jean-Luc Nancy gamely gave it a try in his 2007 book *The Fall of Sleep*. "By falling asleep," he wrote, "I fall inside myself: from my exhaustion, from my boredom, from my exhausted pleasure or from my exhausting pain. . . . I myself become the abyss and the plunge. . . . I fall to where I am no longer separated from the world by a demarcation that still belongs to me all through my waking state and that I myself am. . . . I pass that line of distinction, I slip entire into the innermost and outermost part of myself." He falls, and then the screen goes blank.

Sleep itself can only be described as it happens to someone else—but even that has its built-in limitations. Andy Warhol's famous 1963 film *Sleep*, which consisted solely of his friend John Giorno sleeping for five hours and twenty minutes, has its avant-garde admirers, but even those who love it admit that they can barely stay awake to the end. The filmmaker and writer Lena Dunham, discussing her plans to do a remake of the film starring herself, confessed, "I fell asleep 25 minutes into it, but I was watching it in my dreams." (Her fascination with the subject may well have grown out of her own distinctly abnormal childhood sleep environment: in a magazine profile, she recounted co-sleeping with her parents until age twelve.)

The epic boringness of Warhol's film achieves a kind of sublimity, if you have stamina; the little twitches, heaves, and deflations of Giorno's body come to seem like heroic antidotes to Hollywood's promotion of high-budget action films. Students in my class on sleep could only take about five minutes of it before they began murmuring, checking their phones, and eventually demanding that I switch it off.

While Warhol's film is almost impossible to watch, it's almost equally impossible *not* to watch a contemporary work that draws heavily on its method: iconic rapper and performance artist Kanye West's notorious video "Famous." West once said, or shouted, in an interview, "I am Warhol! I am the number one most impactful artist of our generation." (He proceeded to explain that he was also "Shakespeare in the flesh," as well as Nike and Google.) Even discounting such self-inflations, it's likely that no one has done more to bring weird sleep into public view recently than West, although this isn't necessarily a good thing. His first brush with sleeping in public came when his wife, Kim Kardashian West, surreptitiously photographed him taking a snooze in a furniture store during an afternoon of shopping; the image generated a viral meme in which West's oblivious sleeping self could be found atop a dinosaur skeleton, on the set of a talk show, in the front row of a Taylor Swift concert, in a meeting with the pope, and in the jaws of a bear.

The accidental notoriety of West's knocked-out alter-ego was nothing compared to the spectacle of collective unconsciousness that he dropped on the public in June 2016. Taking his cue from visual artist Vincent Desiderio's painting *Sleep*—an eight-by-twenty-four-foot tableau depicting twelve naked sleeping bodies twisted among bedsheets, as seen from above—as well as from Warhol's *Sleep*, the rapper concocted a stunningly bizarre video to accompany his controversial song "Famous." In the song, West takes a crass shot at Swift, with whom he had been publicly feuding for years, boasting that one day she would sleep with him because his spat with her had made her famous. But there she is with him, lying naked along with ten other famous people, fast asleep, tangled in a stormy sea of white sheets, while "Famous" practically undresses her again with its insulting lyrics. Among the other naked people in the bed are Rihanna, Bill Cosby, George W. Bush, Caitlyn Jenner, Donald Trump, and Kardashian West, her famous derriere prominently mooning the viewer. (Trump's presence is particularly ironic: he has frequently claimed to get by on only three or four hours of sleep, a pattern that several political commentators have tied to his erratic public behavior and irrational thought processes.) Or so it seems. The hyperreal figures lying inert on the bed are actually made of wax.

What is sleep doing in this strange mash-up of voyeurism, misogynistic bravado, artistic homage, and noisy beats? *Nothing*, and conspicuously so. About midway through the video, the music stops, and the camera zooms in on individual bodies, or really body parts, while the soundtrack cuts to the noises made by the sleepers: obstructed breathing, snoring, occasional moaning. And there we stay, for an excruciatingly weird four minutes and ten seconds, in the company of inert boobs, butts, and nostrils that are the fleshly components of these famous personae. The nakedness and immobility of the bodies—underscored when the Jenner figure's hands twitch at one point—seems to be a reminder of the fragility and vulnerability of even the most powerful and wealthy members of society. Yet the video itself shamelessly trades on and even accentuates their fame; in contrast to the blurry and anonymous faces in Desiderio's painting, we can never miss Trump's orange tresses or Kardashian West's endlessly discussed posterior. Fame, it seems, survives sleep; in fact, this particular bit of public, collective sleeping practically sacralizes fame. West reported that when he premiered the video to a number of famous friends who didn't appear onscreen, the response was unanimous: "They want to be in the bed."

West's video is a study in contradictions: quiet and booming, shocking and boring, worshipful and demeaning, tender and brutal, artistic and trashy, hyperreal and fake. One of the most puzzling aspects to contemplate is whether sleep humanizes these notorious icons or mocks them. Desiderio commented on his own work that "as I was doing my painting, I wasn't feeling a tremendous amount of empathy for the people. I actually thought of them as slumbering idiots." As he fell deeper into the project, though, he underwent a transformation. "I felt a spark of empathy—not really for them, it was for the world." Similarly, one can feel disgust for the figures in West's video, and even for West himself (Lena Dunham, never one to miss out on the party, called "Famous" a disturbing violation of women's privacy and even went so far as to say it was made of "the stuff of snuff films"), and yet also be moved by the cocoon of nothingness they each crawl into at night. If we empathize with the slumbering idiots in the video, it's not as individuals, but as slabs of human meat, bound together most clearly when they lose all the attributes that make them who they, and others, think they are. Sleep marks the lowest common denominator not only of individuals, but—as Aristotle said—of animals and vegetables as well.

Collectively, the recent works discussed in this chapter may be turning sleep from a private affair into a public arena for confession, debate, wonder, revelation, exhibitionism, curiosity, advocacy, speculation, complaint, worry, advice, experimentation, exploitation, and even celebration. Such a proliferation of perspectives can only weaken the rules that are meant to tuck us all into the standard model of sleep. Yet these new visions are not necessarily restful ones. As sleep fully enters the digital age, in which everything we do is subject to public view, new avenues for exploitation emerge. We're already partway there, with our electronic sleep-monitoring devices, Internet sleep therapy sessions, and online shopping for sleep gear providing new ways to generate data from this most intimate portion of our lives to feed into the digital maw. Once there, our sleep is put to work, selling stuff to us.

In a strange sense, we've figured out a new way to lose sleep—it's now outside of us, in a sense staring at us. Just as the entire universe seems able to know what kind of shoes we were looking for last night, so our sleep—that most intimate experience of daily life—is in danger of becoming hacked. West's "Famous" video, like Nolan's film *Inception*, gives us a creepy vision of how the erosion of sleep's privacy might be experienced as an invasion of our innermost selves. One can only imagine how Taylor Swift felt about seeing her nude sleeping body represented on the screen; reportedly, she deliberately refrained from responding in order not to draw more publicity toward it. In abandoning the old rules in search of a better, less restrictive kind of sleep, we might seek to recapture the tranquility of Thoreau's cabin. But instead, we might find ourselves in bed with Kanye.

Three Chairs

At first I thought I might try to sleep there myself: the little cabin in the New England woods with its thin mattress supported by a bed with rattan cane slats. That actual cabin no longer exists, but a replica does, and Thoreau enthusiasts come from around the world to see it. The idea quickly became absurd when I realized that virtually no sleeping environment could mimic Thoreau's *less* than spending a night or two at Walden. Far from a secluded outpost between town and wilderness, Walden Pond is now a booming tourist destination. Its perimeter has been ringed with fine sand, making it a popular summer swimming and sunbathing spot. The cabin itself sits just off the main parking lot for Walden Pond State Reservation. Even if I could have talked my way into sleeping in the tiny architectural simulacrum, I would more likely have been awakened by the sound of cars entering and tourists taking selfies than by birdcall or the sound of my own genius, whatever that is.

Even discounting all that, the idea was ridiculous on its own merits. I couldn't come anywhere near replicating Thoreau's experiment, given our different circumstances. He had two years to practice sleeping and waking on his own terms, to the beat of his own particular drummer. I have a family and a house of my own, which means carpools, grocery runs, bills to pay, yardwork, and other responsibilities that usually can't be put off for more than a weekend. Others have followed in Thoreau's footsteps much more faithfully than I ever could, finding their own equivalents of Walden Pond in the remote regions of Alaska and California, in a secondhand RV, or in campsites or open spaces around the world. Thoreau tells us not to mimic him anyway, suggesting that each person should seek a different path outside of the conventions, rules, and expectations that create a conformist society. To follow his way too closely would be simply to create a new set of standards that would harden into another conventional way of life, a new normal. Or even worse, it would be a cheap and shopworn literary gimmick.

So I looked for opportunities within my own life, in my own house, to un-tame my sleep. In writing this book, I was fortunate enough to have a fellowship that released me from teaching and many of the other usual academic responsibilities for a year, which did allow me significant leeway in how I managed my time and attended to my own need to sleep. I generally had to be up at 6:30 a.m. to drive a school carpool, and consequently, I had to go to bed at a fairly standard hour, around 11 or 11:30 p.m. That's ordinarily a good recipe for insomnia for me, but knowing that naps were an option in the middle of the day made me worry less about those nights when I couldn't drop off immediately, or when I got up in the middle of the night and couldn't get back to sleep. Often I used those wakeful interludes to read or write, then napped in the afternoon. It was like finding a little tropical island in my own bedroom: I came to relish those moments when I could drop off after lunch, often with my amazingly soothing dog, Pepper, by my side, and then wake up feeling fresh warm breezes in my mind. There's nothing heroic about this, and probably nothing interesting or particularly unusual—except that so few people are afforded this very limited flexibility in how they manage their sleep. Hardly wild nights, but I suppose it's a start.

In the end, though, more significant to me than any private adjustment of my sleep patterns was how my work on this book changed my relationships with other people. Of course, any author becomes fixated on his or her own material and will usually want to talk about it with others. I've written other books, and held forth plenty, but never has the mention of my topic and a few words about my approach tapped such a response in people I meet. Something about becoming the Sleep Guy seems to have made me a magnet for interesting divulgences and unusual conversations. I once hiked up a mountain with my daughter's Girl Scout troop, walking most of the way next to a woman whom I'd not met before, the mother of one of my daughter's friends. She said she'd heard I was a writer and asked what I was working on. When I told her, she asked a few questions about it, and then began to talk about her own sleep troubles and the sleeping arrangements in her family, asking how they fit in with what I was finding in my research. We were soon joined by another Scout parent who eagerly added her perspectives, and before we knew it, we were at the top of the mountain, and it felt like I'd known them for years. In a Denver bar—at a sleep conference no less—I pulled up next to a friendly couple, also visiting, who asked what I was doing in town. Two hours later, the fellow was sharing tidbits from his dream journal with his wife and me, sending us into convulsive laughter over the image of him trying to hit someone in the face with a fist made of Jell-O.

I've had similar experiences with friends and other strangers, from Uber drivers to academic colleagues to people I meet at dinner parties—even one guy I hired, appropriately enough, to help me put together an Ikea bed. (My lack of handiness is one of the many ways in which I'm completely unlike Thoreau.) Sometimes these people turn to me as if I'm an expert who might solve their problems, and I quickly divest them of that notion; more often they just want to tell me their stories, sometimes requesting that I put them in my book. For most of us, sleep is the most private and mysterious thing we do, and yet it always occupies some part of our minds. Encountering an author who is trying to bring that private activity out into the light of day seems liberating for many people—it's as if they are suddenly free to acknowledge a part of their lives that they've hidden from public view. (And, of course, it's not as risky or degrading to talk about it openly as it would be to talk about other bodily functions.) The topic seems to create an instant bond, as we are all reduced—like the figures in Kanye West's bed—to a common denominator: no matter our differences in profession, status, religion, race, or political leanings, we all share the problem of how to incorporate this inconvenient need to shut down for hours at a time into our lives. It can be a source of shared mystery, frustration, humor, astonishment, pleasure, and embarrassment—but most of all, of shared humanity.

My most memorable experience of sleep's potential for sociability is an unlikely conversation I had with former president Jimmy Carter. In addition to his work for the Carter Center, where for decades he has been overseeing remarkable efforts to address problems in human rights, to monitor elections, and to eradicate deadly diseases worldwide, Carter is a faculty member at my university, Emory. Every month or so, he arranges to have lunch with a small group of faculty members at the Carter Center in order to learn about their work and to share with them the latest news of the center. In the final stages of writing this book, I was invited, along with three colleagues—all virtual strangers to me and to each other—to meet with this ninety-one-year-old eminence.

The meeting almost didn't happen: Carter was presumed to be dying only a few short months earlier, but had only recently announced that his stage IV melanoma—which had spread to his brain and liver—was in remission, thanks to his use of a new immunotherapy drug. I was amazed and slightly awed to be greeted warmly in the lobby by a hale-looking man with a steady gait and a familiar gentle face. As he escorted us toward the cafeteria, he walked assuredly down the Carter Center's winding staircase, then loaded up his own tray with food and carried it to his private dining room. After explaining the significance of the paintings on the wall—all done by himself ("I regret that I never had a chance to do one of Begin and Sadat")—he turned to me and began asking in great detail about my interest in sleep, how it connected to my work as a literature professor and to my other research projects, how I had found and used my evidence, what sorts of conclusions I was drawing, and what I thought were the biggest changes in human sleep over time. He even asked me about my interest in Thoreau, and something about this made me notice a special quality of attention: it turns out he'd thought deeply and even written a little bit about Thoreau in his own nature book, *An Outdoor Journal*. (He found *Walden* beautiful but was rather startled by Thoreau's aversion to steady work and his flouting of religion.) His questions were as sharp as any I've ever had about my work, and he followed my answers with as much curiosity and engagement as I could ever hope to find in a reader, colleague, student, or auditor.

After a few rounds of questioning, I decided to turn the tables. "How did you sleep as a child?" I asked him. "Did you have your own bedroom?"

He laughed and said that yes, he was fortunate to have had his own bedroom from an early age, but his sisters had shared one. "Our sleep was different then," he added. "We didn't have electricity until I was twelve, so we all went to bed when the sun went down. But then when I got my first radio, I would stay up late—till nine o'clock!—listening to the Glenn Miller Orchestra's radio hour." He paused for a moment. "I guess I did some co-sleeping later in life, though, with Hamilton Jordan"—referring to his campaign strategist and eventual White House chief of staff. "We had a shoestring budget for our campaign and didn't want to waste money on separate hotel rooms." The table burst out in boisterous laughter, and the ice was broken. We were no longer four somewhat nervous academics in the presence of a famous world leader, but five people who were sharing the pleasures of one elemental activity, eating, while talking about another, sleeping.

The moment was a great example of sleep's power of social leveling, which poets have been writing about for centuries. For Sir Philip Sidney, writing in the sixteenth century, sleep is "the poor man's wealth, the prisoner's release, / Th'indifferent judge between the high and low." This line of thinking has a decidedly more morbid connotation in what was likely its first recorded utterance, in the Book of Job. Job, lamenting his miserable lot in life, wishes he'd never been born: "For now I would be lying down in peace; I would be asleep and at rest / With kings and counselors." Closer to Thoreau's time, Herman Melville echoed this morbid equality of sleepers in his story "Bartleby, the Scrivener." After the passive-aggressive, maddeningly reticent clerk is sent to prison for refusing to leave his workplace when his employer moves, he dies alone, and the warden tells his former employer that "he sleeps with kings and counselors."

But around the same time, Walt Whitman revivified the democratic possibilities of sleeping with kings and counselors in a beautiful poem called "The Sleepers." Not just the poor and the wealthy, but convicts and freemen, lunatics and drunkards, married couples and masturbators, the blind and the deaf, the famous and the obscure, travelers and fugitives, scholars and the illiterate are all bound by the human need to sleep. Throughout the poem, Whitman's poetic persona hovers over a globe populated by such beautiful sleepers, declaring: "I swear they are averaged now—one is no better than the other, / The night and sleep have liken'd them and restored them." Whitman's ambition was to invent a mode of writing that would express the possibilities of democracy and the equality of all citizens. Here he found his perfect subject: that aspect of life in which none is more powerful than the other, none can judge and none can be judged. And you don't have to wait until you're dead to get there, as seems to be the implication for Job and Bartleby.

Much of *Wild Nights* has chronicled the opposite: how social inequities are reproduced and sometimes even magnified in sleep. The slaveholder and the captive both need sleep, to be sure, but it's hard to say that they are "averaged" or "liken'd" to each other when one sleeps in the big house and the other on a floor, maybe even chained to others. So, too, neither the lunatic in the asylum, nor the beggar on the city street, nor the displaced person on a convention center floor is in a position to follow the rules that the orderly, even finicky sleepers in their comfortable lodgings set for themselves and their families. And even in those comfortable family spaces, the war between parents and children over bedtime rages. There is no averaging, no leveling: sleep or refusal to sleep means something quite different to the wild thing and to the parent trying to tame it. So while sleep itself may be a common denominator in our lives, it also exposes the social fault lines that allow some to protect and comfort themselves while others are left defenseless against the terrors of the night. And as an inherently unruly activity, it is subject to systems of control in which some set the rules and others are made to obey.

So why is it that in my conversations with friends, neighbors, strangers, and even a president, sleep magically turned into a Whitman-esque level playing field, allowing for a bond of mutual recognition that momentarily made us forget all that divided us? The key is the inherent vulnerability of sleep, which we all share, and which accounts for the tenderness of Whitman's poem. The divisions come when some are better able to protect against sleep's defenselessness than others. Letting down our guard and acknowledging this shared vulnerability, even in the presence of strangers, is oddly liberating. We are vulnerable in sleep not just because we cannot move and cannot react to stimuli, but because we have all in some way covered over this aspect of our lives with a dense cloak of privacy—a cloak that often hides us even from ourselves. Who "we" are seems nearly to vanish when we sleep. And so we need to share these stories with others to grasp this hidden dimension of our lives, and when we do, we're surprised by the connections we can make, even in recounting our differences, our frustrations, our strangeness even unto ourselves.

Thoreau's little cabin had one narrow bed, but it also had three chairs. The author welcomed friends and strangers who were willing to make the trek to sit with him and talk, at least until the sun fell and they had to find their way home. Perhaps it's one of those chairs I want to sit in, rather than lying in the bed. Pulling sleep back into the social world might contribute, in a small way, to finding our common humanity.

ACKNOWLEDGMENTS

Sleeping and writing a book are two activities that no one else can do for you, but that doesn't mean no one else is involved. I've built this book on the solid foundation of research by other scholars who have explored sleep's sociohistorical dimensions. Several of them have been extremely generous in sharing their time and their ideas with me. Especially important to me have been Roger Ekirch, who offered wisdom and support at regular intervals along the way; and Hannah Ahlheim, who organized a fascinating conference on the history of sleep in Göttingen, Germany. (Thanks to Dan and Katerina Mayer for hosting me in Berlin.) Sasha Handley and Matthew Wolf-Meyer kindly shared their manuscripts with me before they reached print. I also benefited from speaking or corresponding with Michael Greaney, Gayle Greene, Lee Scrivner, Garrett Sullivan, and my Emory colleague Carol Worthman, a pioneer in the cross-cultural analysis of sleep whose work has not been surpassed in quality.

Outside of this small world of humanistic sleep studies, this book developed significantly out of conversations, correspondence, friendship, and/or moral support provided by Rachel Adams, Sari Altschuler, Lawrence Buell, Leonard Cassuto, Joe Crespino, Michael Davidson, Clare Eby, Michael Elliott, Ann Fabian, Yoshiaki Furui, Brett Gadsden, George Gordon-Smith, Lindsey Grubbs, David Henkin, Joe Johnson, Walter Kalaidjian, Paul Kelleher, Eunjung Kim, Stephen Krewson, Howard Kushner, Aruni Mahapatra, Maureen McCarthy, Bob McCauley, Sean Meighoo, Stephen Mihm, Michelle Neely, Adam Newman, Emily Ogden, Laura Otis, John

Plotz, Leah Price, Susan Rabiner, Rick Rambuss, Joel Reynolds, Carlo Rotella, Deboleena Roy, Ellen Samuels, Jen Sarrett, Ralph Savarese, David Serlin, Caleb Smith, Natasha Trethewey, Paul Wallace, Kevin Young, and David Zimmerman. I cannot begin to express my gratitude to Rosemarie Garland-Thomson, with whom I have worked closely for ten years, and whose work has influenced my own for twice that span.

A wonderful surprise to me was the openness of researchers in the sciences to hearing news from the humanities. My colleague Sander Gilman—long a model for me in how humanities can speak to health- and science-related issues, and vice versa—helped get me started by sizing up my project and setting me up with the neurologist David Rye, who co-taught a rewarding seminar with me. David has been a sounding board and collaborator ever since, and Sander has continued to offer guidance and support. Through David, I also got to know Carlos Schenck, who let me bend his ear on several aspects of this project and was wonderfully supportive. My Emory colleague Sherman James read a portion of the manuscript and offered invaluable feedback. Lauren Hale provided me an opportunity to try out some of my ideas in *Sleep Health* and connected me to the community that makes it go; her own research provided several fascinating pieces of the puzzle that I have assembled here. Kelly Drew and Thomas Kantermann also responded quickly, generously, and extremely helpfully to inquiries from a total stranger.

At Basic Books, I have been most fortunate to work with Ben Platt, a gifted, sympathetic, and insightful editor. Kathy Streckfus is not only a crackerjack copy editor, but she also pointed me to the Kanye West video that insisted on taking over the ending of my final chapter. Thanks also to Collin Tracy for overseeing the process, Allison MacKeen for bringing me on board, and Lara Heimert for her support throughout. My agent Wendy Strothman had faith in the project from the beginning, and she helped as much as anyone to give it a satisfying shape.

The writing of *Wild Nights* was supported by a fellowship year afforded by the John Simon Guggenheim Memorial Foundation. The project was earlier incubated during a National Endowment for the Humanities summer fellowship and a senior fellowship at Emory's Fox Center for Humanistic Inquiry. The Fox Center gathered a lively community of scholars, many of whom helped me sharpen my ideas—especially Elizabeth Bouldin, Roberto Franzosi, Walt Reed, and Randall Strahan. Randy was as gracious and exacting an interlocutor as one could hope for; his death cut short a burgeoning friendship that developed during our year together at the Fox Center.

Devora Reiss was with me every step of the way, in sleeping and in waking. She read drafts, talked me through snags and doubts, and made me laugh as no one else can. If she lost patience by my five hundredth text message about a subtitle, she never showed it. The bedrooms across the hall will be empty before long, but I'm lucky to have watched Sophie and Isaac vanish into them and stumble out of them—a little more grown up each time—for all these years.

A version of Chapter Two appeared in different form in the journal *American Literature*, and portions of Chapter Three appeared in *Common-place*. I thank the editors of those journals and the anonymous readers for their suggestions and support.

NOTES

Notes to Introduction

2 **expectations and social rules** Important studies of the cross-cultural dimensions of human sleeping patterns include Simon J. Williams, *Sleep and Society: Sociological Ventures into the (Un)known* (London: Routledge, 2005); Lodewijk Brunt and Brigitte Steger, eds., *Worlds of Sleep* (Leipzig, Germany: Frank and Timme, 2008); Katie Glaskin and Richard Chenhall, eds., *Sleep Around the World: Anthropological Perspectives* (London: Palgrave Macmillan, 2013). See also the work of Carol M. Worthman.

3 **Every species has a way** Jim Horne, *Sleepfaring: A Journey Through the Science of Sleep* (Oxford: Oxford University Press, 2006), 2–4. For a good overview of current sleep science, see also David K. Randall, *Dreamland: Adventures in the Strange Science of Sleep* (New York: W. W. Norton, 2012).

5 **"So many of the people . . . "** "Barbara Bush Calls Evacuees Better Off," *New York Times*, September 7, 2005.

5 **"sleep-industrial complex"** Jon Mooallem, "The Sleep-Industrial Complex," *New York Times Magazine*, November 18, 2007, www .nytimes.com/2007/11/18/magazine/18sleep-t.html.

6 **National Sleep Foundation poll** National Sleep Foundation, "2009 Sleep in America Poll: Highlights and Key Findings," 2009, https:// sleepfoundation.org/sites/default/files/2009%20POLL%20HIGH LIGHTS.pdf.

6 **More systematic research** Kristen L. Knutson, Eve Van Cauter, Paul J. Rathouz, Thomas DeLeire, and Diane S. Lauderdale, "Trends in the Prevalence of Short Sleepers in the USA: 1975–2006," *Sleep* 33, no. 1 (2010): 37–45; Yu Su Bin, Nathaniel S. Marshall, and Nick Glozier, "Secular Trends in Adult Sleep Duration: A Systematic Review," *Sleep Medicine Reviews* 16 (2012): 223–230.

8   **massive changes in technology and the organization of labor**
      Important work on the history of sleep analyzing these shifts
      includes A. Roger Ekirch, *At Day's Close: Night in Times Past* (New
      York: W. W. Norton, 2005); Matthew Wolf-Meyer, *The Slumbering
      Masses: Sleep, Medicine, and Modern American Life* (Minneapolis: University
      of Minnesota Press, 2012); Jonathan Crary, *24/7: Late Capitalism
      and the Ends of Sleep* (London: Verso, 2013); Alan Derickson,
      Dangerously Sleepy: Overworked Americans and the Cult of Manly Wakefulness
      (Philadelphia: University of Pennsylvania Press, 2014); Hannah
      Ahlheim, ed., *Die Geschichte des Schlafs in der Moderne* (Frankfurt:
      Campus Verlag, 2014); Lee Scrivner, *Becoming Insomniac: How Sleeplessness
      Alarmed Modernity* (London: Palgrave Macmillan, 2014). For
      an illuminating study of European sleep patterns on the cusp of
      these shifts, see Sasha Handley, *Sleep in Early Modern Europe* (New
      Haven, CT: Yale University Press, 2016).

9   **Sleep science emerged as a profound response to the industrial
      age** For an excellent account of the rise of sleep science, see Kenton
      Kroker, *The Sleep of Others and the Transformation of Sleep Research*
      (Toronto: University of Toronto Press, 2007). See also Wolf-Meyer,
      Slumbering Masses, 27–78.

9   **most societies that have not experienced the introduction of
      electricity** See Carol M. Worthman, "After Dark: The Evolutionary
      Ecology of Human Sleep," in *Evolutionary Medicine and Health*, eds.
      Wenda R. Trevathan, E. O. Smith, and James J. McKenna (Oxford:
      Oxford University Press, 2008), 291–313; Carol M. Worthman and
      Ryan A. Brown, "Companionable Sleep: Social Regulation of Sleep
      and Cosleeping in Egyptian Families," *Journal of Family Psychology*
      21, no. 1 (2007): 124–135.

9   **Historian Roger Ekirch's influential argument** Ekirch, *At Day's
      Close: Night in Times Past*, 300–323; A. Roger Ekirch, "The Modernization
      of Western Sleep; or, Does Insomnia Have a History?," *Past
      & Present* 226, no. 1 (February 1, 2015): 149–192. This thesis has its
      skeptics, as I will explain in Chapter One.

10   **Information overload** Scrivner, *Becoming Insomniac*, esp. 14–33.

10   **parents, given access** Peter N. Stearns, Perrin Rowland, and Lori
      Giarnella, "Children's Sleep: Sketching Historical Change," *Journal
      of Social History* 30, no. 2 (1996): 345–366.

11   **The sociologist Norbert Elias** Norbert Elias, *The History of Manners*,
      trans. Edmund Jephcott, vol. 1, *The Civilizing Process* (New
      York: Pantheon, 1978), 160–168.

13   **"You could sit up as late . . . "** Henry David Thoreau, *Walden and
      Other Writings* (New York: Random House, 1992), 27.

13   **"Only that day dawns . . . "** Ibid., 312.

14   **"mass of men . . . "** Ibid., 8.

14   **"restless, nervous, bustling . . . "** Ibid., 309.

15   **"Hardly a man takes a half-hour's nap . . . "** Ibid., 88.

17   **sleep of others** The phrase is taken from Kroker, The Sleep of Others. For Kroker, the phrase indicates the importance of turning sleep into an objective physiological state that can be observed and measured empirically rather than simply reported on subjectively by the individual who experiences it.

17   **"Done with the compass!"** Emily Dickinson, *Final Harvest: Poems* (Boston: Little, Brown, 1964), 38.

18   **"third state of brain activity"** Michel Jouvet, *The Paradox of Sleep: The Story of Dreaming*, trans. Laurence Garey (Cambridge, MA: MIT Press, 1999), 2.

18   **The philosopher Thomas Hobbes** Thomas Hobbes, *Leviathan; or, the Matter, Forme and Power of a Commonwealth Ecclesiasticall and Civil* (New York: Simon and Schuster, 2008), 100.

Notes to Chapter One

25   **Asabano believed** Roger Ivar Lohmann, "Sleeping Among the Asabano: Surprises in Intimacy and Sociality at the Margins of Consciousness," in *Sleep Around the World: Anthropological Perspectives*, eds. Katie Glaskin and Richard Chenhall (London: Palgrave Macmillan, 2013), 21–44.

25   **In the homes of the Cook Islanders** Kalissa Alexeyeff, "Sleeping Safe: Perceptions of Risk and Value in Western and Pacific Infant Co-Sleeping," in ibid., 122.

25   **Maori ancestral meetinghouses** Toon van Meijl, "Maori Collective Sleeping as Cultural Resistance," in ibid., 13–50.

25   **the introduction of electricity** Worthman and Brown, "Companionable Sleep," 124–135.

25   **the idea of a "bedroom"** Handley, *Sleep in Early Modern England*, 115.

26   **"If you share a bed with a comrade . . . "** Quoted in Elias, *The History of Manners*, 1:161.

26   **Samuel Pepys noted his preferences** Quoted in Sasha Handley, "Sociable Sleeping in Early Modern England, 1660–1760," *History & Health* 49 (2013): 102.

26   **"I s'pose you are goin' a whalin' . . . "; "No man prefers to sleep two in a bed . . . "; "affectionately throwing his brown tattooed legs"** Herman Melville, *Moby-Dick; or, the Whale* (New York: Penguin, 2001), 15, 17, 59.

27   **"new forms of sociability"** Handley, *Sleep in Early Modern England*, 150.

27   **"more intimate and private"** Elias, *The History of Manners*, 1:164, 168.

27   **" . . . all sorts of pernicious Excrements . . . "** Thomas Tryon, *A Treatise of Cleanness in Meats and Drinks, of the Preparation of Food, the Excellency of Good Airs, and the Benefits of Clean Sweet Beds, Also of the Generation of Bugs, and Their Cure* (London: Printed for the author, 1682), 5.

28   **The English parliament** Marcus Rediker, *The Slave Ship: A Human History* (New York: Viking, 2007), Kindle edition, loc. 4170.

28   **The Dolben Act** Ibid., loc. 4024.

28   **"so crowded . . . keeping others awake"** Quoted in ibid., loc. 1970.

28   **His widely publicized 1842 *Report*** Edwin Chadwick, *Report on the Sanitary Condition of the Labouring Population of Great Britain* (Edinburgh: Edinburgh University Press, 1965), 178.

29   **"The breathing at night . . . "** Ibid., 180.

29   **theory that was later debunked** Steven Johnson, *The Ghost Map: The Story of London's Most Terrifying Epidemic—and How It Changed Science, Cities, and the Modern World* (New York: Riverhead Books, 2006).

29   **Common Houses Lodging Act** See Simon J. Williams, *Sleep and Society: Sociological Ventures into the (Un)Known* (London: Routledge, 2005), 52–55.

29   **"the system of having beds . . . breathed breath"** Quoted in Hilary Hinds, "Together and Apart: Twin Beds, Domestic Hygiene and Modern Marriage, 1890–1945," *Journal of Design History* 23, no. 3 (2010): 275–304. Quoted material is on pp. 280–281.

29   **American doctor estimated** Bill Bryson, *At Home: A Short History of Private Life* (New York: Doubleday, 2010), 321.

30   **Jacob Riis's influential 1890 study** Jacob A. Riis, *How the Other Half Lives* (New York: Penguin, 1997), 20, 69.

30   **disabled people, who often lived quarantined** The disability studies scholar Tobin Siebers made the point that disabled people who were institutionalized tended to lack access to the private spaces that allow for the development of a "normal" sex life; the same holds true of their access to private sleep. See Tobin Siebers, "A Sexual Culture for Disabled People," in *Sex and Disability*, eds. Robert McRuer and Anna Mollow (Durham, NC: Duke University Press, 2012), 37–53.

30   **American physician William Whitty Hall** William Whitty Hall, *Sleep*, 3rd ed. (New York: W. W. Hall, 1863), 47.

30   **"a single sleeper . . . requires a chamber . . . "** Ibid., 51.

30   **"Calcutta Black Hole"** Ibid., 9–11.

30   **"crowd together . . . by Choice"** Quoted in Rediker, *Slave Ship*, loc. 5605.

31   **"the vilest, and the filthiest . . . as men improve in their condition . . . "** Hall, *Sleep*, 21–22.

31   **"The savages all sleep promiscuously together . . . "** François Le Vaillant, *Travels into the Interior Parts of Africa*, vol. 2 (London: G. G. and J. Robinson, 1796), 113.

31   **missionaries among the Asabano** Lohmann, "Sleeping Among the Asabano," 22; Toon van Meijl, "Maori Collective Sleeping," 133–149.

31   **to be "English" or "European" or "white"** On the ways in which the policing of behavior in colonial locales affected the policing of the lower classes in Europe, see Ann Laura Stoler, "Tense and Tender Ties: The Politics of Comparison in North American History and (Post) Colonial Studies," *Journal of American History* 88, no. 3 (2001): 829–865.

31   **a new sense of shame** Elias, *The History of Manners*, 1:160–168.

31   **"as nations advance . . . "** William Alexander Hammond, *Sleep and Its Derangements* (Philadelphia: J. B. Lippincott, 1873), 223.

32   **Sleep loss even became modish** Handley, *Sleep in Early Modern England*, 181–210.

33   **These two sleeps** Ekirch, *At Day's Close*; A. Roger Ekirch, "Sleep We Have Lost: Pre-Industrial Slumber in the British Isles," *American Historical Review* 106, no. 2 (2001): 343–386. The quotation is from *At Day's Close*, p. 300.

33   **Ekirch's subsequent work** Ekirch, "The Modernization of Western Sleep," 177–178.

33   **a newspaper advice column in 1911** Quoted in ibid., 166.

33   **we've disrupted our ancestral—perhaps our evolutionary—rhythms** Ibid., 149–192. Adding to the link between lighting and sleep patterns, anthropologist Carol Worthman found that in cultures that lack ubiquitous electricity, sleep patterns tend to be segmented—broken up into chunks rather than done all at once. See Worthman, "After Dark," 311.

34   **" . . . broadest and most enduring impact . . . "** Ekirch, "The Modernization of Western Sleep," 179.

34   **Wehr found that under these circumstances** Karen Fox, "Sleeping the Sleep of Our Ancestors," *Science* 262, no. 5137 (1993); Randall, *Dreamland*, 34–35.

34   **" . . . after the meate is digested . . . "** Quoted in Ekirch, *At Day's Close*, 310.

34 **"Many people wake up at night and panic"** Stephanie Hegarty, "The Myth of the Eight-Hour Sleep," *BBC News Magazine*, February 22, 2012, www.bbc.com/news/magazine-16964783.

35 **universal model of sleep** Handley, *Sleep in Early Modern England*, 9.

35 **Studying sleep patterns in three contemporary hunter-gatherer societies** Gandhi Yetish, Hillard Kaplan, Michael Gurven, Brian Wood, Herman Pontzer, Paul R. Manger, Charles Wilson, Ronald McGregor, and Jerome M. Siegel, "Natural Sleep and Its Seasonal Variations in Three Pre-Industrial Societies," *Current Biology* 25 (2015): 2862–2868.

35 **"all preindustrial peoples . . . "** A. Roger Ekirch, "Segmented Sleep in Preindustrial Societies," *Sleep* 39, no. 3 (2016): 715–716.

35 **a commentary on the Siegel group's article** Horacio O. de la Iglesia, Horacio O., Claudia Moreno, Arne Lowden, Fernando Louzada, Elaine Marqueze, Rosa Levandovski, Luisa K. Pilz, et al., "Ancestral Sleep," *Current Biology* 26, no. 7 (2016): R271–R272.

36 **question the notion** Gandhi Yetish, Hillard Kaplan, Michael Gurven, Brian Wood, Herman Pontzer, Paul R. Manger, Charles Wilson, Ronald McGregor, and Jerome M. Siegel. "Response to De La Iglesia et al.," *Current Biology* 26, no. 7 (April 4, 2016): R273–R274.

36 **"living fossil"** Kristen L. Knutson, "Should I Sleep More or Should I Sleep Less?," *Huffington Post*, 2015, www.huffingtonpost.com/kristen -knutson/should-i-sleep-more-or-sh_b_8434240.html.

36 **Matthew Wolf-Meyer went further** Matthew Wolf-Meyer, "Can We Ever Know the Sleep of Our Ancestors?," *Sleep Health* 2, no. 1 (2016):1–2.

37 **Edison himself** See Derickson, *Dangerously Sleepy*, 4–11.

37 **colonize the night** The phrase "colonize the night" comes from the sociologist Murray Melbin. See his *Night as Frontier: Colonizing the World After Dark* (New York: Free Press, 1987).

38 **" . . . It reduces the sound sleep . . . "** Karl Marx, *Das Kapital*, vol. 1, *A Critique of Political Economy* (New York: Dover, 2011), 291.

38 **some workers had always had to stay up while others slept** Peter C. Baldwin, *In the Watches of the Night: Life in the Nocturnal City, 1820–1930* (Chicago: University of Chicago Press, 2012), 213–275; Craig Koslofsky, *Evening's Empire: A History of the Night in Early Modern Europe* (Cambridge: Cambridge University Press, 2011), 201–203; Ekirch, *At Day's Close*, 156–160.

38 **A fundamental shift** Wolfgang Schivelbusch, *Disenchanted Night: The Industrialization of Light in the Nineteenth Century* (Berkeley: University of California Press, 1995).

39 **A survey in 1927** Baldwin, *In the Watches of the Night*, loc. 2588.

39   the dreaded "long turn" Derickson, *Dangerously Sleepy*, 53–83.

39   it was mainly only aristocrats Handley, "Sociable Sleeping in Early Modern England, 1660–1760," 79.

40   "I will wait no longer for the factory bell . . . " Sarah Savage, "The Factory Girl (1814)," *Common-place*, www.common-place.org /justteachone/wp-content/uploads/2013/12/Factory-Girl-1814-by-Sarah-Savage.pdf.

40   " . . . every hour of the twenty-four is accountable . . . " Charles Rumford Walker, *Steel: The Diary of a Furnace Worker* (Boston: Atlantic Monthly Press, 1922), 154.

40   "The second twelve hours were like nothing else . . . " Quoted in Derickson, *Dangerously Sleepy*, 60.

40   patterns that were directly or indirectly tied to the new industrial economy For changes in the sense of time across the nineteenth and twentieth centuries, see E. P. Thompson, "Time, Work-Discipline, and Industrial Capitalism," *Past & Present* 38, no. 1 (1967): 56–97; Michael O'Malley, *Keeping Watch: A History of American Time* (New York: Viking Penguin, 1990).

41   synchronize social activities Paul Glennie and Nigel Thrift, *Shaping the Day: A History of Timekeeping in England and Wales, 1300–1800* (Oxford: Oxford University Press, 2009). Glennie and Thrift are critical of Thompson's influential argument for making too sweeping a claim about industry's role in the spread of clock time.

41   research into the physiology of rest Anson Rabinbach, *The Human Motor: Energy, Fatigue, and the Origins of Modernity* (Berkeley: University of California Press, 1992).

41   "Eight hours for work . . . " Roy Rosenzweig, *Eight Hours for What We Will: Workers and Leisure in an Industrialized City, 1870–1920* (Cambridge: Cambridge University Press, 1985).

41   The sixteenth-century English physician Thomas Cogan Thomas Cogan, *The Haven of Health* (London: Anne Griffin, for Roger Bale, 1636), 275.

42   consulted for at least half a century Handley, *Sleep in Early Modern England*, 18.

42   Historian Graham Robb Graham Robb, *The Discovery of France: A Historical Geography from the Revolution to the First World War* (New York: Norton, 2007), 74–76. All sources mentioned in this paragraph are discussed in Robb's book.

42   A 1900 report "Human Hibernation," *British Medical Journal* (June 23, 1900): 1554–1555.

43   "the rhythm of the elements" Farley Mowat, *People of the Deer* (New York: Carroll and Graf, 1951), Kindle ed., loc. 1016.

43   **"huge fires burned all day . . . "** Ibid., loc. 1621.

44   **"fat . . . being burned—within their bodies"** Ibid., loc. 1250.

44   **"song-feasts"** Ibid., loc. 1945. For a more thorough account of seasonal variation in Inuit social behaviors and physiological processes, see Richard G. Condon, *Inuit Behavior and Seasonal Change in the Canadian Arctic* (Ann Arbor, MI: UMI Research Press, 1983).

44   **cerebral ischemia, is fatal to humans** Kunjan R. Dave, Sherri L. Christian, Miguel A. Perez-Pinzon, and Kelly L. Drew, "Neuroprotection: Lessons from Hibernators," *Comparative Biochemistry and Physiology Part B: Biochemistry and Molecular Biology* 162, no. 1–3 (2012).

44   **Workers in Arctic and Antarctic regions** Josephine Arendt, "Biological Rhythms During Residence in Polar Regions," *Chronobiology International: The Journal of Biological & Medical Rhythm Research* 29, no. 4 (2012): 379–394.

44   **"Let there be an appointed time . . . "** Hall, *Sleep*, 116.

44   **"following a definite routine . . . "** Quoted in Derickson, *Dangerously Sleepy*, 44.

45   **"how much sleep you need"** William C. Dement and Christopher Vaughan, *The Promise of Sleep: The Scientific Connection Between Health, Happiness, and a Good Night's Sleep* (New York: Dell, 2000), 335, 42.

45   **one of the surest routes toward insomnia** Maria Konnikova, "Why Can't We Fall Asleep," *New Yorker*, July 7, 2015, www.newyorker .com/science/maria-konnikova/why-cant-we-fall-asleep.

45   **While Kleitman himself was unable to adapt** Kroker, *The Sleep of Others*, 232–233.

45   **Kleitman specifically forbade napping** Matthew Wolf-Meyer, "Where Have All Our Naps Gone? Or Nathaniel Kleitman, the Consolidation of Sleep, and the Historiography of Emergence," *Anthropology of Consciousness* 24, no. 2 (2013): 96–116.

46   **Kleitman, to his credit, pushed back** Cited in Derickson, *Dangerously Sleepy*, 44.

46   **His advice about invariant sleep routines** Ibid.

46   **Other scientific research** The account of Aschoff and the origins of chronobiology is found in Till Roenneberg, *Internal Time: Chronotypes, Social Jet Lag, and Why You're So Tired* (Cambridge, MA: Harvard University Press, 2012), 40–46.

48   **"complex machine"** William Alexander Hammond, *On Wakefulness* (Philadelphia: J. B. Lippincott, 1865), 11.

49   **the timing of sleep was more dependent on changes in temperature** Yetish et al., "Natural Sleep and Its Seasonal Variations."

50   **"sleeping and eating patterns . . . "** Mark Sisson, *The Primal Blueprint* (Malibu, CA: Primal Nutrition, 2012), Kindle ed., loc. 4051.

51   **"excessive artificial light and digital stimulation . . . "** Ibid., loc. 4130.

51   **John Durant** John Durant, *The Paleo Manifesto: Ancient Wisdom for Lifelong Health* (New York: Harmony Books, 2013), Kindle ed., loc. 3394–3609.

52   **self-help books, exercise classes, training manuals** Alex Williams, "The Paleo Lifestyle: Way, Way, Way Back," *New York Times*, September 21, 2014.

53   **"TORPOR & HIBERNATION"** European Space Agency, Advanced Team Biomimetics website, www.esa.int/gsp/ACT/bio /projects/Hibernation.html.

54   **enable humans . . . to make deep penetration into space** Eric Niller, "Human Hibernation May Not Be a Pipedream Forever," *Washington Post*, April 13, 2015.

54   **"behavioral torpor"** Charles Q. Choi, "Mock Mars Flight Reveals Big Sleep Concerns for Astronauts," *Space*, 2013, www.space .com/19168-mock-mars-flight-reveals-big-sleep-concerns-for-astro nauts.html.

54   **induce prolonged torpor** Michael Venables, "Space Travel's Efficient, Cheaper Future: Sleeping Your Way to Mars in a Stasis Habitat," *Forbes/Tech*, October 6, 2013, www.forbes.com/sites/michael venables/2013/10/06/space-travels-efficient-cheaper-future-sleep ing-your-way-to-mars-in-stasis-habitat; John E. Bradford and Douglass Talk, "Torpor Inducing Transfer Habitat for Human Stasis to Mars" (Atlanta: Space Works Enterprises, 2014).

54   **"drugs that stimulate this in squirrels"** Author interview with Kelly Drew, September 11, 2014.

55   **customized or individually optimized sleep** See Lennard J. Davis, *The End of Normal: Identity in a Biocultural Era* (Ann Arbor: University of Michigan Press, 2013), esp. chap. 1; Simon J. Williams, Catherine M. Coveney, and Jonathan Gabe, "Medicalisation or Customisation? Sleep, Enterprise and Enhancement in the 24/7 Society," *Social Science & Medicine* 79 (2013): 40–47.

Notes to Chapter Two

58   **how to be fully awake** The critic who comes closest to tracking this dimension is Jeffrey E. Simpson, "Thoreau 'Dreaming Awake and Asleep,'" *Modern Language Studies* 14, no. 3 (1984): 54–62.

58   **"To be awake is to be alive"** Thoreau, *Walden and Other Writings*, 85.

59   **"overcome with drowsiness"** Ibid., 85.

59   **up late, staring out the window** Michael Sims, *The Adventures of Henry Thoreau: A Young Man's Unlikely Path to Walden Pond* (New York: Bloomsbury, 2014), 11.

59   **family complaint** Thoreau, *Walden and Other Writings*, 214.

60   **"I am a diseased bundle of nerves"** Quoted in Robert D. Richardson, Jr., *Henry Thoreau: A Life of the Mind* (Berkeley: University of California Press, 1986), 120.

60   **Concord, Massachusetts, was undergoing a startling transformation** Details taken from "A Brief History of Concord," Concord Library, www.concordlibrary.org/scollect/bhc/bhc.html.

61   **Adding to the pressure to develop regular sleep schedules** Stearns et al., "Children's Sleep."

62   **"awakened by . . . Genius"** Thoreau, *Walden and Other Writings*, 85.

62   **"The labor of the southern female slave . . . "** See Philip S. Foner, ed., *The Factory Girls: A Collection of Writings on Life and Struggles in the New England Factories of the 1840s* (Chicago: University of Illinois Press, 1977), 217.

62   **Thoreau was given a cannonball** Sims, *Adventures of Henry Thoreau*, 27.

63   **advised not to give children beds that were too comfortable** This advice came from John Locke, *Some Thoughts Concerning Education and of the Conduct of the Understanding* (Indianapolis, IN: Hackett, 1996). For Locke's influence on childrearing, see Hugh Cunningham, *Children and Childhood in Western Society Since 1500* (London: Longman, 1995), 62–78. For a sense of the cultural shifts around managing children's routines and habits, see Peter N. Stearns, *Anxious Parents: A History of Modern Childrearing in America* (New York: New York University Press, 2003).

63   **charging for rooms** On the importance of boardinghouses in nineteenth-century American culture, see David Falflik, *Boarding Out: Inhabiting the American Urban Literary Imagination, 1840–1860* (Evanston, IL: Northwestern University Press, 2012).

63   **Typically, boarders shared bedrooms** Baldwin, *In the Watches of the Night*, loc. 1035.

63   **Thoreau's sister** Quoted in Walter Harding, *The Days of Henry Thoreau* (New York: Dover, 1962; repr. 1980), 22.

63   **"I think I had rather keep a batchelor's hall . . . "** Quoted in Falflik, *Boarding Out*, 151.

64   **"to see if I could see God"** Quoted in Sims, *Adventures of Henry Thoreau*, 11.

64   **each proposing to her** At least this is the cover story. Recent scholars have questioned Henry's sexuality. See, for instance, Walter

Harding, "Thoreau's Sexuality," *Journal of Homosexuality* 21, no. 3 (1991): 23–45; Michael Warner, "Walden's Erotic Economy," in *Comparative American Identities: Race, Sex, and Nationality in the Modern Text*, ed. Hortense J. Spillers (New York: Routledge, 1991), 157–174.

65   **"Whenever we awoke in the night . . . "** Henry David Thoreau, *A Week on the Concord and Merrimack Rivers* (New York: Penguin, 1998), 267.

65   **By the late nineteenth century** Stearns et al., "Children's Sleep," 345–366.

66   **"Perhaps at midnight one was awakened . . . "** Thoreau, *A Week*, 138.

66   **" . . . He hibernates in this world . . . "** Ibid., 80.

66   **listening to the river** Ibid., 166.

66   **"Man thinks faster . . . "** Quoted in Sims, *Adventures of Henry Thoreau*, 40.

67   **Because the cause was unknown** Quoted in Harding, *The Days of Henry Thoreau*, 45.

68   **"I must confess"** Quoted in Richardson, *Henry Thoreau*, 125.

69   **The rattan slats came from palm trees** See Concord Museum, "Henry David Thoreau Collection," http://www.concordmuseum .org/henry-david-thoreau-collection.php.

70   **"I hear the iron horse . . . "** Thoreau, *Walden and Other Writings*, 110–111.

71   **Even wheeled clocks** Gerhard Dohrn-van Rossum, *History of the Hour: Clocks and Modern Temporal Orders*, trans. Thomas Dunlap (Chicago: University of Chicago Press, 1996), 17–27, 47.

71   **railroads set their clocks** Wolfgang Schivelbusch, *The Railway Journey* (Leamington Spa, UK: Berg, 1986), 43.

71   **By the late nineteenth century** Stearns et al., "Children's Sleep," 345–366.

71   **time itself became a commodity** O'Malley, *Keeping Watch*, 90.

72   **"The startings and arrivals . . . Have not men improved somewhat . . . "** Thoreau, *Walden and Other Writings*, 111.

72   **frantic panorama** I have borrowed the phrase from Nancy Bentley, *Frantic Panoramas: American Literature and Mass Culture, 1870–1920* (Philadelphia: University of Pennsylvania Press, 2009). The title of her book refers to literary writers' confrontation with mass culture later in the nineteenth century. But one of the panoramas she chronicles is that of the train wreck, which was a frequent topic in both the sensational press and in more reflective novels like those of William Dean Howells.

72   **"Everything was unfixed . . . "** Nathaniel Hawthorne, *Collected Novels: Fanshawe, the Scarlet Letter, the House of the Seven Gables, the*

Blithedale Romance, the Marble Faun (New York: Library of America, 1983), 572.

73   **"We do not ride on the railroad . . . "** Thoreau, *Walden and Other Writings*, 87–88.

74   **"men have become tools . . . "** Ibid., 35.

74   **"It seems almost beyond belief . . . "** Quoted in Derickson, *Dangerously Sleepy*, 27.

74   **"a danger to the general public . . . "** Stanley Coren, *Sleep Thieves: An Eye-Opening Exploration into the Science and Mysteries of Sleep* (New York: Free Press, 1996), 286.

74   **high-profile industrial and transportation accidents** Williams, *Sleep and Society*, 105.

74   **"Like many of my contemporaries"** Thoreau, *Walden and Other Writings*, 202.

75   **"Think of dashing the hopes of a morning"** Ibid., 204.

75   **"Gorrappit . . . "** Ibid., 138.

75   **"Ah, how low I fall . . . "** Ibid., 204.

75   **The Sufis of today's Yemen** Catherine M. Tucker, *Coffee Culture: Local Experiences, Global Connections* (New York: Routledge, 2011), 36.

75   **From there it spread through the Arab world** Wolfgang Schivelbusch, *Tastes of Paradise: A Social History of Spices, Stimulants, and Intoxicants*, trans. David Jacobson (New York: Random House, 1992), 17.

75   **By 1700 . . . dominant gathering places** See Roger Schmidt, "Caffeine and the Coming of the Enlightenment," *Raritan* 23, no. 1 (2003): 129–149.

76   **Richard Steele, editor of *The Tattler*** Schivelbusch, *Tastes of Paradise*, 51.

76   **Alexander Pope's "The Rape of the Lock"** Schmidt, "Caffeine and the Coming of the Enlightenment," 129–149.

76   **"I do not know if coffee and sugar . . . "** Quoted in Mark Pendergrast, *Uncommon Grounds: The History of Coffee and How It Transformed Our World* (New York: Basic Books, 1999), 18.

77   **"nobody tasted blood in it . . . "** Ralph Waldo Emerson, *Essays & Poems* (New York: Library of America, 1996), 980.

77   **Commentators were complaining** Schivelbusch, *Tastes of Paradise*, 43–48; Hammond, *On Wakefulness*, 79; Justine S. Murison, *The Politics of Anxiety in Nineteenth-Century American Culture* (Cambridge: Cambridge University Press, 2011), 25.

77   **"finely pulverized, dense coffee"; "sparks shoot all the way to the brain"** Honoré de Balzac, "The Pleasures and Pains of Coffee," *Michigan Quarterly Review* 25, no. 2 (1996): 275–276.

78   **a test online** See *Caffeine Informer: Accurate Caffeine Information Available to All*, www.caffeineinformer.com/death-by-caffeine.

78   **"I did not use tea, nor coffee"; "You'd better go now, John"** Thoreau, *Walden and Other Writings*, 193–194.

79   **Neural jolts became pleasurable** For an interesting theory of how the search for neural stimulation drives historical change, see Daniel Lord Smail, *On Deep History and the Brain* (Berkeley: University of California Press, 2008).

79   **"Hardly a man takes a half-hour's nap . . . "** Thoreau, *Walden and Other Writings*, 88–89.

80   **Telegraph transmission** See Yoshiaki Furui, "Networked Solitude: American Literature in the Age of Modern Communications, 1831–1898" (Dissertation, Emory University, 2015), chap. 1.

80   **"the practical annihilation of time and space . . . "** Quoted in Scrivner, *Becoming Insomniac*, 18.

80   **"a herd of highly excited newsboys"** Quoted in Baldwin, *In the Watches of the Night*, loc. 2360.

81   **"like rabbits in their burrows . . . "** Riis, *How the Other Half Lives*, 149.

81   **"a city resident who began the day . . . "** Baldwin, *In the Watches of the Night*, loc. 2374.

81   **The female factory operatives in the famous mills** Thomas M. Allen, *A Republic in Time: Temporality and Social Imagination in Nineteenth-Century America* (Chapel Hill: University of North Carolina Press, 2008), 133.

81   **"Consider the girls in the factory . . . "** Thoreau, *Walden and Other Writings*, 129.

82   **" . . . standing for nature . . . "** Lawrence Buell, *The Environmental Imagination: Thoreau, Nature Writing, and the Formation of American Culture* (Cambridge, MA: Belknap Press of Harvard University Press, 1995), 2.

82   **followed the work of modern naturalists** See Laura Dassow Walls, *Seeing New Worlds: Henry David Thoreau and Nineteenth-Century Natural Science* (Madison: University of Wisconsin Press, 1995).

82   **"Thoreau was a climate change scientist . . . "** Richard B. Primack, *Walden Warming: Climate Change Comes to Thoreau's Woods* (Chicago: University of Chicago Press, 2014), x, 30.

83   **layers of time** On Thoreau's sense of the multiplicity of time frames, see Thomas M. Allen, "Clockwork Nation: Modern Time, Moral Perfectionism and American Identity in Catharine Beecher and Henry Thoreau," *Journal of American Studies* 39, no. 1 (2005): 65–86.

83   "How we eat, drink, sleep . . . " Henry David Thoreau, *The Journal: 1837–1861* (New York: New York Review of Books, 2009), 18.

83   "I hear, just as the night sets in . . . " Ibid., 56.

83   "What is the earliest sign of spring? . . . " Ibid., 179.

83   "My soul and body have tottered along . . . " Ibid., 22.

83   "Methinks my seasons revolve more slowly . . . " Ibid., 62.

83   "I feel as if I could go to sleep under a hedge . . . " Ibid., 129.

84   "Health is a sound relation . . . " Ibid., 269.

84   "visceral sense of belonging . . . " Donald Worster, *Nature's Economy: A History of Ecological Ideas* (Cambridge: Cambridge University Press, 1994), 78.

84   submitting his body to the natural rhythms Christopher Sellers, "Thoreau's Body: Towards an Embodied Environmental History," *Environmental History* 4, no. 4 (1999): 486–515.

84   "The vials of summer . . . " Quoted in Ronald A. Bosco, ed., *Nature's Panorama: Thoreau on the Seasons* (Amherst: University of Massachusetts Press, 2005), 47.

84   health as a matter of being attuned See Stacy Alaimo, *Bodily Natures: Science, Environment, and the Material Self* (Bloomington: Indiana University Press, 2010).

84   "The morning, which is the most memorable season . . . " Thoreau, *Walden and Other Writings*, 84–85.

85   "Little is to be expected of that day . . . " Ibid., 85.

85   His fascination with natural rhythms William Stowe, "Linnaean Poetics: Emerson, Cooper, Thoreau, and the Names of Plants," *Isle: Interdisciplinary Studies in Literature and Environment* 17, no. 3 (2010): 563–583; Richardson, *Henry Thoreau*, 283.

85   "Not solicitous for the means of gratification . . . " Henry David Thoreau, "The Laws of Menu," *Dial* 43 (1843): 331.

86   "While lying thus on our oars . . . " Thoreau, *A Week*, 101.

86   "Sometimes, after coming home thus late . . . " Thoreau, *Walden and Other Writings*, 160.

86   "I believe that men are generally still a little afraid . . . " Ibid., 123.

86   "a slight insanity in my mood" Ibid., 124.

86   "ghouls and idiots and insane howlings" Ibid., 118.

87   "sluggish by constitution and by habit" Henry David Thoreau, *Collected Essays and Poems* (New York: Library of America, 2001), 404.

87   "We aspire to be something more . . . " Ibid., 401.

87   "It seems as if no man had ever died . . . " Ibid., 414.

Notes to Chapter Three

91   "more needs she the divine . . . " William Shakespeare, *Macbeth*, Act V, scene 1, 39, 82.

91   **"our great-grandmother Nature's universal, vegetable, botanic medicines"** Thoreau, *Walden and Other Writings*, 150.

92   **medicinal remedies** Karl H. Dannenfeldt, "Sleep: Theory and Practice in the Late Renaissance," *Journal of the History of Medicine and Allied Sciences* 41, no. 4 (October 1986): 436–437.

92   **The sixteenth-century French physician André du Laurens** Ibid., 436.

93   **the extraordinary staying power of Aristotle** David Gallop, ed. *Aristotle: On Sleep and Dreams* (Warminster, UK: Aris and Phillips, 1996); Dannenfeldt, "Sleep," 418; Kroker, *The Sleep of Others*, 29–34.

93   **dissipate excess heat** Handley, *Sleep in Early Modern England*, 64.

94   **"rational powers of intellect"** Garrett A. Sullivan Jr., *Sleep, Romance and Human Embodiment: Vitality from Spenser to Milton* (Cambridge: Cambridge University Press, 2012), 1.

94   **Medical theories of sleep** Michael J. Thorpy, "History of Sleep and Man," in *The Encyclopedia of Sleep and Sleep Disorders*, eds. Michael J. Thorpy and Jan Yager (New York: Facts on File, 1991).

94   **role of blood flow to the brain** Handley, *Sleep in Early Modern England*, 33–35.

94   **Fresh air** Ibid., 40–44.

94   **"devoted Christian"; attacks by the devil** Ibid., 69, 71.

95   **"And Paul went down and fell on him . . . "** Acts 20:9–10.

95   **"by sleeping at sermons . . . "** Increase Mather, *Practical Truths Tending to Promote the Power of Godliness* (Boston: Samuel Green, 1682), 192.

95   **"men are more naturally inclined to sleep"; "If thou dost find thyself inclined to sleep . . . "** Ibid., 220.

96   **Sleeping in church was a favorite topic** Koslofsky, *Evening's Empire*, 214.

96   **"Is it possible! . . . "; "with his *Energy* to make us *Drowsy* . . . "** Cotton Mather, *Vigilius; or, the Awakener* (Boston: J. Franklin, 1719), 1, 5–6.

96   **"Sinners, there's no sleeping in Hell . . . "** Azariah Mather, *Wo to Sleepy Sinners; or, a Discourse Upon Amos VI.1.* (Timothy Green, printer, 1720), 3, 27.

96   **"take his Word away from them"** Mather, *Practical Truths*, 205.

96   **"Sinful Sleep . . . "** Mather, *Vigilius*, 6; Robert S. Cox, "The Suburbs of Eternity: On Visionaries and Miraculous Sleepers," in *Worlds of Sleep*, eds. Lodewijk Brunt and Brigitte Steger (Berlin: Frank and Timme, 2008), 61.

97   **"We must not be afraid of *offending* our Neighbour . . . "** Mather, *Vigilius*, 7.

97   **Donald Trump mocked Jeb Bush** Colin Campbell, "Donald Trump Just Trolled Jeb Bush with a Video Touting Him as a Cure for Insomnia," *Business Insider,* September 8, 2015, www.businessinsider.com/donald-trump-jeb-bush-can-help-you-sleep-2015-9.

97   **exhaustion was sometimes taken as a sign** Koslofsky, *Evening's Empire,* 214.

98   **the grim necessity of policing the night** Gregory S. Jackson, *The Word and Its Witness: The Spiritualization of American Realism* (Chicago: University of Chicago Press, 2009), 45–65.

98   **"The world is in a deep sleep"; "sweat[ing] so much . . . "** Frank Lambert, *Inventing the "Great Awakening"* (Princeton, NJ: Princeton University Press, 1999); Joanne van der Woude, "The Great Awakening," in *A New Literary History of America,* eds. Greil Marcus and Werner Sollors (Cambridge, MA: Harvard University Press, 2009), 79–84.

98   **"It sows the seeds of foolish and hurtful Desires . . . "** John Wesley, "The Duty and Advantage of Early Rising" (Cambridge, Eng.: J. Archdeacon, Printer to the University, 1785), 11.

99   **"What if an Holy GOD should punish your drowsiness . . . "** Mather, *Vigilius,* 8.

99   **"cause me to *Awake unto Righteousness* . . . "; "oil of Roses . . . "** *The Angel of Bethesda* (1724), ed. Gordon W. Jones (Barre, MA: American Antiquarian Society and Barre Publishers, 1972), 150.

99   **the role of the brain in producing or disrupting sleep** Handley, *Sleep in Early Modern England,* 181–188.

100   **Rachel Baker rose from her bed** See John H. Douglass, *Devotional Somnium; or, a Collection of Prayers and Exhortations Uttered by Miss Rachel Baker, in the City of New-York, in the Winter of 1815, During Her Abstracted and Unconscious State* (New York: Van Winkle and Riley, 1815). Baker's story is detailed in Robert S. Cox, *Body and Soul: A Sympathetic History of American Spiritualism* (Charlottesville: University of Virginia Press, 2003), 53–68; Kristen Anne Keerma Friedman, "Soul Sleepers: A History of Somnambulism in the United States, 1740–1840" (Dissertation, Harvard University, 2014). Medical interest in the case began in 1814, but Douglass—who compiled the first published records of her case—makes clear that the episodes began in 1811 and the public became interested a year later.

100   **"the thoughts of God and eternity . . . "; far from possessing very quick perceptions . . . "** Douglass, *Devotional Somnium,* 15.

100   **"sighing and groaning . . . "; "like one somewhat deranged . . . "** Ibid., 17.

100   **"plump, hale country lass . . . "; "unsteady, wild and capricious"** Charles Mais, *The Surprising Case of Rachel Baker, Who Prays and Preaches in Her Sleep* (New York: S. Marks, 1814), 32.

101 "that God would give them a sense of her danger . . . "; "She would beg them not to give sleep to their eyes . . . " Douglass, *Devotional Somnium*, 23.

101 "Soon after she went to bed . . . " Ibid., 17.

101 "the shuddering terrors . . . "; "colourless as the dead" Quoted in Friedman, "Soul Sleepers," 89–90.

101 "[did] not appear to be possessed of a clear mind . . . " Douglass, *Devotional Somnium*, 19–20.

102 an alternating consciousness Ann Taves, *Fits, Trances, & Visions: Experiencing Religion and Explaining Experience from Wesley to James* (Princeton, NJ: Princeton University Press, 1999), 1–9.

102 "It is no longer I who live . . . " Quoted in ibid, 8.

102 " . . . in the body or out of the body" Quoted in ibid, 9.

102 Evidence of witchcraft . . . prostitution Friedman, "Soul Sleepers," 26–28.

102 The clash of scientific and theological explanations See Roy Porter, *Madness: A Brief History* (Oxford: Oxford University Press, 2002), 10–33; Alberto Toscano, *Fanaticism: On the Uses of an Idea* (London: Verso, 2010), xiii.

103 As much as a century later This account of the French prophets comes from Taves, *Fits, Trances, & Visions*, 15–19.

103 "the Weakness of their Nerves . . . " Quoted in ibid., 23, 28–29.

103 "People struck with somnambulism . . . " John Bell, *An Essay on Somnambulism, or Sleep-Walking, Produced by Animal Electricity and Magnetism, as Well as by Sympathy, &C.* (Dublin: Printed for the author, 1788), 23.

103 other notable examples Handley, *Sleep in Early Modern England*, 190–193.

104 associated with genius Ibid., 190.

104 "draught of porter . . . "; " . . . taste and correctness" Benjamin Rush, *Medical Inquiries and Observations upon the Diseases of the Mind*, 5th ed. (Philadephia: Grigg and Elliott, 1835), 302.

104 Novelist Charles Brockden Brown Charles Brocken Brown, *Edgar Huntly; or, Memoirs of a Sleepwalker* (New York: Penguin, 1988); Karen Halttunen, *Murder Most Foul: The Killer and the American Gothic Imagination* (Cambridge, MA: Harvard University Press, 1998), 217–230.

104 A Rhode Island woman Cox, *Body and Soul*, 40–42.

104 A German woman *Journeys into the Moon, Several Planets, and the Sun: History of a Female Somnambulist, of Wilhelm on the Teck, in the Kingdom of Wuehtemberg, in the Years 1832 and 1833* (Philadelphia: Vollmer and Hagenmacher, 1837).

104 A Scottish sleepwalker Cox, *Body and Soul*, 42

105   **"continual weeping and lamentation"** Quoted in Friedman, "Soul Sleepers," 72–76.

106   **historian of medicine Kristen Keerma Friedman** Ibid., 3.

106   **"It is a strange thing . . . "** Ibid., 140.

106   **Samuel Latham Mitchill, a professor at the College** On Mitchill's life, see Courtney Robert Hall, *A Scientist of the Early Republic: Samuel Latham Mitchill, 1764–1831* (New York: Russell and Russell, 1967); Alan David Aberbach, *In Search of an American Identity: Samuel Latham Mitchill, Jeffersonian Naturalist* (New York: Peter Lang, 1988).

106   **"some cunning . . . "; " . . . the result of devotional somnium"** Douglass, *Devotional Somnium*, 40.

106   **"a period when the female frame acquires additional sensibilities . . . "** Quoted in Cox, *Body and Soul*, 61.

106   **triggered by menstruation** Handley, *Sleep in Early Modern England*, 195.

107   **"the case is indeed interesting to the physician . . . "** Douglass, *Devotional Somnium*, 12. On Douglass's career, see Friedman, "Soul Sleepers," 125.

107   **In the spring of 1833, Jane C. Rider** Details are taken from "Interesting Case of Somnambulism," *Springfield Republican*, October 30, 1833; "Somnambulism," *Springfield Republican*, November 13, 1833. Many details below come from L. W. Belden, *An Account of Jane C. Rider, the Somnambulist* (Springfield, MA: G. and C. Merriam, 1834); Alexandre Jacques François Brierre de Boismont, *Hallucinations; or, the Rational History of Apparitions, Visions, Dreams, Ecstasy, Magnetism, and Somnambulism*, 1st American ed. (Philadelphia: Lindsay and Blakiston, 1853). The case has also been discussed in Friedman, "Soul Sleepers," chap. 6; and I draw on my own previous article, Benjamin Reiss, "The Springfield Somnambulist; or, the End of the Enlightenment in America," *Common-place* 4, no. 2 (2004), www .common-place.org/vol-04/no-02/reiss.

108   **"the fervor of her praying . . . "** E. Griffith, "Another Sleeping Preacher," *Springfield Republican*, October 3, 1833.

108   **He originally diagnosed her with chorea** Details from this paragraph and the next are taken from Belden, *An Account of Jane C. Rider, the Somnambulist*.

109   **"who made no bustle in his business . . . "** Quoted in Friedman, "Soul Sleepers," 250.

109   **struck by the stagey appearance** Friedman, in "Soul Sleepers," responded to my suggestion of staging in an earlier article published on this episode by defending both Rider and Belden from charges of chicanery: "There was no evidence whatsoever that Rider and

Belden were involved in some sort of scheme" (ibid.). Yet it seems manifestly implausible that Rider could read and write letters in her sleep, while blindfolded. My interpretation is not one of a straight scam, but of what disability studies scholars call a "masquerade": an exaggeration of a genuine experience of impairment that might not be legible to the public unless it is amplified in a visible way. See Tobin Siebers, "Disability as Masquerade," *Literature and Medicine* 23, no. 4 (2004): 1–22. See also Jeffrey A. Brune and Daniel J. Wilson, eds., *Disability and Passing* (Philadelphia: Temple University Press, 2013); Ellen Samuels, "Passing," in *Keywords for Disability Studies*, eds. Rachel Adams, Benjamin Reiss, and David Serlin (New York: New York University Press, 2015), 135–137.

110 **Schenck was inclined to give some credence** Carlos Schenck, personal communication, November 11, 2010.

110 **"She complained . . . that she was locked up . . . "** Belden, *An Account of Jane C. Rider, the Somnambulist*, 66.

111 **first state-run asylum** Gerald N. Grob, *The State and the Mentally Ill: A History of Worcester State Hospital in Massachusetts* (Chapel Hill: University of North Carolina Press, 1966), 46–50.

111 **The "moral treatment"** See David Rothman, *The Discovery of the Asylum: Social Order and Disorder in the New Republic* (Boston: Little, Brown, 1971); Benjamin Reiss, *Theaters of Madness: Insane Asylums and Nineteenth-Century American Culture* (Chicago: University of Chicago Press, 2008).

111 **The asylum offered a humane way** On such economic explanations for the rise of asylum care, see Andrew Scull, *The Most Solitary of Afflictions: Madness and Society in Britain, 1700–1900* (New Haven, CT: Yale University Press, 1993).

112 **The soreness in Rider's head** Woodward's views are included in Belden, *An Account of Jane C. Rider, the Somnambulist*, 77–94.

112 **"she actually *saw*"; " . . . even a confused image of the object"** Ibid., 99.

113 **"this she was permitted to continue"; "My head, my head, do cut it open!"** L. W. Belden, "An Account of Jane C. Rider, the Springfield Somnambulist," *Boston Medical and Surgical Journal* 11, no. 4 (September 10, 1834): 4–74.

113 **Given Rider's clear desire** All details in this paragraph are taken from Belden, *An Account of Jane C. Rider, the Somnambulist*, 91–94.

115 **"no return" of the affliction** "The Nervous System," *New Englander and Yale Review* 4, no. 15 (July 1846): 438.

115 **"total institutions"** Erving Goffman, *Asylums: Essays on the Social Situation of Mental Patients and Other Inmates* (New York: Anchor Books, 1961), 5.

116   **"If they sleep well"** Amariah Brigham, "Annual Report of the Managers of the State Lunatic Asylum" (Albany, NY: Carroll and Cook, 1844), 31.

116   **controlling the sleep routines** Ellen Dwyer, *Homes for the Mad: Life Inside Two Nineteenth-Century Asylums* (New Brunswick, NJ: Rutgers University Press, 1987), 15; Rothman, *The Discovery of the Asylum*, 145.

116   **"Utica crib"** Mary Elene Wood, *The Writing on the Wall: Women's Autobiography and the Asylum* (Urbana: University of Illinois Press, 1994), 74.

116   **Patients who would not get out of bed** Nancy Tomes, *A Generous Confidence: Thomas Story Kirkbride and the Art of Asylum-Keeping, 1840–1883* (Cambridge: Cambridge University Press, 1984), 206.

116   **those who overslept** Elizabeth Parsons Ware Packard, *The Prisoners' Hidden Life; or, Insane Asylums Unveiled* (Chicago: Published by the author, 1868), 225–227.

117   **a critic of the Worcester asylum** "The Worcester Asylum for the Insane," *Vermont Chronicle*, April 22, 1846.

117   **Particularly disturbed patients' rooms** Kathleen Brian, "'The Weight of Perhaps Ten or a Dozen Lives': Suicide, Accountability, and the Life-Saving Technologies of the Asylum," *Bulletin of the History of Medicine* 90, no. 4 (2016).

117   **Over seventy sleep disorders** *International Classification of Sleep Disorders*, 3rd ed. (Darien, IL: American Academy of Sleep Medicine, 2014).

117   **Forty million Americans . . . ; More than 2,500 accredited treatment centers** "Sleep Centers Increase to Highest Number Ever," *Huffington Post*, January 3, 2013, www.huffingtonpost .com/2013/01/03/sleep-centers-highest-number-american-academy -of-sleep-medicine_n_2366719.html.

118   **Critics claim this is driven** Kroker, *The Sleep of Others*, 395–428; Wolf-Meyer, *Slumbering Masses*, 27–50.

118   **a host of new technologies** Molly Wood, "Bedtime Technology for a Better Night's Sleep," *New York Times*, December 24, 2014, www .nytimes.com/2014/12/25/technology/personaltech/bedroom -technology-for-a-better-nights-sleep.html.

Notes to Chapter Four

119   **"sleep debt . . . is the contemporary complaint . . . "** Horne, *Sleep-faring*, 188.

120   **You Can't Sleep Here** Edward Newhouse, *You Can't Sleep Here* (New York: Macaulay, 1934).

120 **George Orwell decided to cross over** George Orwell, *Down and Out in Paris and London* (Orlando, FL: Harcourt, 1961).

121 **"Without a doubt, sleep is the biggest issue . . . "; " . . . 5 a.m. every single morning."** Quoted in Hannah Brooks Olsen, "Homelessness and the Impossibility of a Good Night's Sleep," *The Atlantic*, August 14, 2014, www.theatlantic.com/health/archive/2014/08/homelessness-and-the-impossibility-of-a-good-nights-sleep/375671.

121 **The poetically haunting Indian documentary film** See "Cities of Sleep (Official Trailer), YouTube, posted September 4, 2015, https://www.youtube.com/watch?v=rXzElV75x08.

122 **"inconsiderate masters"; "overcome with weariness . . . "** Thomas Tryon, *Friendly Advice to the Gentlemen-Planters of the East and West Indies* (London: Andrew Sowle, 1684), 89.

123 **"We rise early, and lie down late . . . "** Ibid., 122.

123 **"a thing worthy to be considered . . . "** Ibid., 96.

123 **most of the southern slaves** See Eugene D. Genovese, *Roll, Jordan, Roll: The World the Slaves Made* (New York: Vintage Books, 1976), 285–293.

123 **"the difference between . . . rising at six and at eight . . . "** Mark M. Smith, *Mastered by the Clock: Time, Slavery, and Freedom in the American South* (Chapel Hill: University of North Carolina Press, 1997), 103.

124 **" . . . The foreman calls the roll . . . "** Ibid., 112.

124 **" . . . in winter at 8, in summer at 9 . . . "** Ibid., 115.

124 **"With a prayer that he may be on his feet . . . "** Solomon Northup, *Twelve Years a Slave: Narrative of Solomon Northup* (Buffalo, NY: Derby, Orton and Mulligan, 1853), 16.

124 **"no regular periods of rest"** Ibid., 194.

124 **"Oh, don't, sir! . . . "** Quoted in Walter Johnson, *River of Dark Dreams: Slavery and Empire in the Cotton Kingdom* (Cambridge, MA: Belknap Press of Harvard University Press, 2013), 172.

125 **"seem to require less sleep . . . "** Thomas Jefferson, *Notes on the State of Virginia* (London: Printed for John Stockdale, 1787), 231.

125 **certain mental afflictions** Handley, *Sleep in Early Modern England*, 181–182.

126 **" . . . More slaves are whipped . . . "** Frederick Douglass, *Autobiographies* (New York: Library of America, 1994), 187.

126 **"Sunday was my only leisure time . . . "** Ibid., 268.

127 **tactics of enforced sleep deprivation** Johnson, *River of Dark Dreams*, 173.

127 **violation of the Geneva Convention** Simon J. Williams, *The Politics of Sleep: Governing (Un)Consciousness in the Late Modern Age* (Houndsmills, UK: Palgrave Macmillan, 2011), 68–70.

127   **a matter of security** See Ekirch, *At Day's Close*, 256–258.

127   **" . . . he may be expected anytime"** Quoted in Smith, *Mastered by the Clock*, 146.

128   **an ability that . . . many whites assumed** See Daylanne K. English, *Each Hour Redeem: Time and Justice in African American Literature* (Minneapolis: University of Minnesota Press, 2013), chap. 1.

128   **"about two hours in the night"** Kenneth S. Greenberg, ed. *The Confessions of Nat Turner and Related Documents* (Boston: Bedford Books of St. Martin's Press, 1996), 48.

128   **" . . . than rouse a sleeping Negro"** "The Narrative of Gregory Gamble, Esq.," *New-York Mirror*, 1835, 337.

128   **"he can sleep anywhere . . . "** Caroline Lee Hentz, *The Planter's Northern Bride*, vol. 1 (Philadelphia: Carey and Hart, 1854), 224.

129   **" . . . that sleep was not slow in its approaches . . . "** William Gilmore Simms, *The Yemassee: A Romance of Carolina* (Fayetteville: University of Arkansas Press, 1994), 311.

129   **"like most negroes suddenly awaking . . . "** Ibid., 320.

129   **" . . . want of natural *Sleep*"** George Cheyne, *The English Malady; or, a Treatise of Nervous Diseases of All Kinds* (London: G. Strahan, 1735), 208.

130   **members of "advanced" civilizations** Hammond, *On Wakefulness*, 39–40.

130   **less blood was drawn into the brain** Bonnie Ellen Blustein, *Preserve Your Love for Science: Life of William A. Hammond, American Neurologist* (New York: Cambridge University Press, 1991), 145–149.

130   **insomnia was particularly prevalent** Hammond, *On Wakefulness*, 46, 56.

130   **The southern physician Samuel Adolphus Cartwright** On Cartwright and his place in southern medicine and the slavery debate, see George M. Fredrickson, *The Black Image in the White Mind: The Debate on Afro-American Character and Destiny, 1817–1914* (New York: Harper and Row, 1971), 87–88; Todd L. Savitt, *Medicine and Slavery: The Diseases and Health Care of Blacks in Antebellum Virginia* (Urbana: University of Illinois Press, 1978), 8–16; Harriet A. Washington, *Medical Apartheid* (New York: Anchor Books, 2006), 35–39; Steven M. Stowe, *Doctoring the South: Southern Physicians and Everyday Medicine in the Mid-Nineteenth Century* (Chapel Hill: University of North Carolina Press, 2003), 215–218.

130   **" . . . direct and practical bearing . . . "** Samuel Cartwright, "Diseases and Peculiarities of the Negro Race," *Debow's Review of the Southern and Western States* 11, new ser. 4 (1851): 64.

130   **"a deficiency of red blood . . . "** Ibid., 66.

131   **"hebetude . . . of intellect . . . "; " . . . or they will run into excess"** Ibid., 67.

132   **" . . . sleeps in perfect security among them"** Ibid., 68.

132   **not completely innate** Steven Stowe makes the point about Cartwright's openness to environmental explanations for racial difference. See Stowe, *Doctoring the South*, 217–218.

132   **prolonged exposure to cold air** See Evelleen Richards, "The 'Moral Anatomy' of Robert Knox: The Interplay Between Biological and Social Thought in Victorian Scientific Naturalism," *Journal of the History of Biology* 22 (1989): 373–436.

132   **"Dysaesthesia Aethiopica . . . "** Cartwright, "Diseases and Peculiarities of the Negro Race," 333.

133   **"break, waste and destroy everything . . . "** Ibid., 334.

134   **"parasite"** Orlando Patterson, *Slavery and Social Death: A Comparative Study* (Cambridge, MA: Harvard University Press, 1982).

134   **" . . . society is asleep"; "man seems idle"** Alexis de Tocqueville, *Democracy in America: Historical-Critical Edition of De La Démocratie en Amérique*, trans. James T. Schleifer (Indianapolis, IN: Liberty Fund, 2010), 556.

134   **"There was no end of her various complaints . . . "** Harriet Beecher Stowe, *Uncle Tom's Cabin; or, Life Among the Lowly* (New York: Penguin, 1981), 243.

135   **Pullman Company began to run** Details of the Pullman porters' story are drawn from Derickson, *Dangerously Sleepy*, 84–107.

136   **the effects of sleep deprivation** Ibid., 84–85.

136   **"an abundance of life stressors . . . "** Lauren Hale and D. Phuong Do, "Racial Differences in Self-Reports of Sleep Duration in a Population-Based Study," *Sleep* 30, no. 9 (2009): 1096–1103.

136   **African Americans experienced significantly less slow-wave sleep** Uma Rao, Russell E. Poland, Preetam Lutchmansingh, Geoffrey E. Ott, James T. McCracken, and Keh-Ming Lin, "Relationship Between Ethnicity and Sleep Patterns in Normal Controls: Implications for Psychopathology and Treatment," *Journal of Psychiatric Research* 33, no. 5 (1999).

137   **such differences as anything but innate** See Natasha J. Williams, Michael A. Grandner, Shedra A. Snipes, April Rogers, Olajide Williams, Collins Airhihenbuwa, and Jean-Louis Girardin, "Racial/Ethnic Disparities in Sleep Health and Healthcare: Importance of the Sociocultural Context," *Sleep Health* 1, no. 1 (2015). For a good overview of the issues, see Brian Resnick, "The Black-White Sleep Gap," *National Journal*, October 23, 2015, www.nationaljournal .com/s/91261/black-white-sleep-gap.

137   **anything that occurs in the waking world** Benjamin Hale and Lauren Hale, "Is Justice Good for Your Sleep (and Therefore, Good for Your Health)?" *Social Theory and Health* 7, no. 4 (2009): 354–370.

137   **the founder of the Slave Dwelling Project** Jennifer Schuessler, "Confronting Slavery at Long Island's Oldest Estates," *New York Times*, August 12, 2015, www.nytimes.com/2015/08/14/arts /confronting-slavery-at-long-islands-oldest-estates.html.

138   **"This was the life of a slave"** Joseph McGill, "The Slave Dwelling Project," http://slavedwellingproject.org.

Notes to Chapter Five

141   **more parents seek pediatric advice** Cited in Randall, *Dreamland*, 71.

141   **runaway best-selling mock-bedtime book** Adam Mansbach, *Go the F**k to Sleep* (New York: Akashic Books, 2011).

142   **timed differently** Salome Kurth, Peter Acherman, Thomas Ruster-holz, and Monique K. LeBourgeois, "Development of Brain EEG Connectivity Across Early Childhood: Does Sleep Play a Role?," *Brain Sciences* 3, no. 4 (2013): 1445–1460.

142   **brisk market for baby sleep gizmos** Pamela Paul, *Parenting, Inc.: How the Billion-Dollar Baby Business Has Changed the Way We Raise Our Children* (New York: Henry Holt, 2008), 235–241.

143   **"We must make haste . . . "** Mary Collier, *The Woman's Labour: An Epistle to Mr. Stephen Duck; in Answer to His Late Poem, Called the Thresher's Labour* (London: Printed for the author, 1739), 7.

144   **"the most arduous and prolonged work . . . "** Thompson, "Time, Work-Discipline, and Industrial Capitalism," 79.

145   **"To get a living . . . "** Collier, *Woman's Labour*, 10.

147   **"Nothing is more to be indulg'd children . . . "** Locke, *Some Thoughts Concerning Education*, 20.

147   **"the great cordial of nature"** Ibid., 22.

147   **antagonist in theories of childhood** On the influence of these two thinkers on childrearing practices over the centuries, see Cunningham, *Children and Childhood*, 61–77; Ann Hulbert, *Raising America: Experts, Parents, and a Century of Advice to Children* (New York: Alfred A. Knopf, 2003), 23–24.

149   **Several eighteenth-century physicians** Walter Harris, *A Full View of All the Diseases Incident to Children* (London: A. Millar, 1742), 16; *Directions and Observations Relative to Food, Exercise, and Sleep* (London: S. Bladon, 1772), 22.

149   **"Supposing the Mother go to Bed at ten . . . "** James Nelson, *An Essay on the Government of Children, Under Three General Heads, Viz. Health, Manners, and Education* (London: R. and J. Dodsley, 1763), 63.

149   " . . . a gentle Puke" George Armstrong, *An Account of the Diseases, Most Incident to Children, from the Birth Till the Age of Puberty* (London: T. Cadell, 1783), 17.

149   bones may become damaged . . . nightmares Handley, *Sleep in Early Modern England*, 27.

149   " . . . white Poppie seeds with milk . . . " Cogan, *The Haven of Health*, 95.

149   "Doses of Meconium, or Syrup of white Poppies . . . " Thomas Apperley, *Observations in Physick, Both Rational and Practical* (London: W. Innys, 1731), 163.

150   " . . . Many children have by this means been killed . . . " Nelson, *Essay on the Government of Children*, 91.

150   " . . . an accident that scarcely happens . . . " William Moss, *An Essay on the Management and Nursing of Children in the Earlier Period of Infancy* (London: J. Johnson, 1781), 47.

150   " . . . a custom it may hereafter be difficult to break him of . . . " Ibid., 48.

150   "one of the strongest indications of health" "Time for Sleep," *Journal of Health* 1 (1830): 75.

150   "marked success in life" "Early Rising," *Children's Missionary Record of the Free Church of Scotland* 5 (1849): 235; Ekirch, "The Modernization of Western Sleep," 167–175.

150   "Get up the moment you wake . . . " Quoted in "The Modernization of Western Sleep," 168.

151   "a relay of guards should be so employed . . . " Luther Bell, *An Hour's Conference with Fathers and Sons, in Relation to a Common and Fatal Indulgence* (Boston: Whipple and Damrell, 1840), 86.

151   erection alarms, penis cases, sleeping mitts Thomas W. Laqueur, *Solitary Sex: A Cultural History of Masturbation* (New York: Zone Books, 2003), 46.

152   " . . . the dark underbelly . . . " Ibid., 249.

152   "To lay on the bed in the day time . . . " Bell, *An Hour's Conference*, 51.

152   " . . . children dead as a result of masturbation" Quoted in Laqueur, *Solitary Sex*, 200.

152   co-sleeping with each other Hall, *Sleep*, 140.

153   "waste away the vigor and flesh . . . " Ibid., 141.

153   "your neighbor may be as pure and blameless . . . " Ibid., 146.

153   " . . . unbridled indulgence" Ibid., 146.

153   " . . . sometimes persons become deranged by it . . . " Ibid., 147.

153   Freud's lurid 1918 case study Sigmund Freud, "From the History of an Infantile Neurosis ('Wolf-Man')," in *The Freud Reader*, ed. Peter Gay (New York: W. W. Norton, 1989), 400–428.

154   "Spock babies" Hulbert, *Raising America*, 12.

154   a latter-day Rousseau Ibid., 260.

154   "As long as a baby is satisfied . . . " Benjamin Spock, *The Common Sense Book of Baby and Child Care* (New York: Duell, Sloan and Pearce, 1957), 162.

154   "The young child may be upset . . . " Ibid., 165.

154   "cut in half and the two pieces sewed together . . . " Ibid., 352.

154   "closed compartment about as spacious as a standard crib" B. F. Skinner, "Baby in a Box: The Mechanical Baby-Tender," *Ladies' Home Journal* 62 (1945): 30–31.

155   " . . . a routine acceptable to the baby . . . " Ibid., 130.

156   " . . . a morbid fear of anything sexual . . . " Spock, *Common Sense Book of Baby and Child Care*, 371.

157   "responsible, lone sleeper" Wolf-Meyer, *Slumbering Masses*, 137.

157   private sleeping rooms are the exception Eyal Ben-Ari, "'It's Bedtime' in the World's Urban Middle Classes: Children, Families and Sleep," in *Worlds of Sleep*, eds. Lodewijk Brunt and Brigitte Steger (Berlin: Frank and Timme, 2008), 175–191; Brigitte Steger and Lodewijk Brunt, "Introduction: Into the Night and the World of Sleep," in *Night-Time and Sleep in Asia and the West*, eds. Brigitte Steger and Lodewijk Brunt (London: Routledge, 2003), 1–23; Worthman and Brown, "Companionable Sleep," 124–135.

157   No ethnographic research has found James J. McKenna and Thomas McDade, "Why Babies Should Never Sleep Alone: A Review of the Co-Sleeping Controversy in Relation to SIDS, Bedsharing, and Breast Feeding," *Pediatric Respiratory Reviews* 6 (2005): 142.

157   " . . . having children sleep in the beds of their parents" Philippe Ariès, "The Sentimental Revolution," *Wilson Quarterly* 6, no. 4 (1982): 49. For Ariès's fuller view, see *Centuries of Childhood: A Social History of Family Life*, trans. Robert Baldick (New York: Alfred A. Knopf, 1962).

157   A health manual published in 1781 Handley, *Sleep in Early Modern England*, 47.

158   Most early modern European homes Ibid., 111.

158   nineteenth and twentieth centuries as the crucial period Ben-Ari, "'It's Bedtime,'" 175–191; Stearns et al., "Children's Sleep," 345–366.

158   By the 1890s Stearns et al., "Children's Sleep," 345–366.

158   "Do you sleep in a bed all by yourself? . . . " Quoted in ibid., 359.

159   "Sleep was a new issue . . . " Ibid., 350.

159   " . . . they soon had me packed into bed" Roger C. Lewis, ed. *The Collected Poems of Robert Louis Stevenson* (Edinburgh: Edinburgh University Press, 2003), 35.

159   **"Must we to bed indeed? . . . "** Ibid., 46. This poem is also cited in Mary Galbraith, "'Goodnight Nobody' Revisited: Using an Attachment Perspective to Study Picture Books About Bedtime," *Children's Literature Association Quarterly* 23, no. 4 (1998): 172.

160   **"Long before the time when I should have to go to bed . . . "** Marcel Proust, *Remembrance of Things Past*, vol. 1, *Swann's Way; Within a Budding Grove*, trans. C. K. Scott Moncrief and Kevin Kilmartin (New York: Random House, 1982), 9.

160   **"so as to prolong the time of respite . . . "** Ibid., 14.

160   **"Leave your mother alone . . . "** Ibid., 29.

160   **" . . . We mustn't let the child get into the habit . . . "** Ibid., 39.

161   **"I ought to have been happy . . . "** Ibid., 41.

161   **in Proust's own life** Michael Wood, "Proust's Mother," *London Review of Books* 34, no. 6 (2012).

163   **"it was never our policy . . . "** Alexandra Rutherford, *Beyond the Box: B. F. Skinner's Technology of Behavior from Laboratory to Life, 1950s–1970s* (Toronto: University of Toronto Press, 2009), 23.

163   **"simple, straightforward measures"** Richard Ferber, *Solve Your Child's Sleep Problems* (New York: Simon and Schuster, 1985), 10.

163   **rigidly enforced schedules** Ibid., 36–37.

163   **"Bedtime means separation"** Ibid., 37.

164   **"to see himself as an independent individual"; "separating the two of you"** Ibid., 39.

165   **" . . . your child will certainly resent being displaced . . . "** Ibid.

165   **" . . . your whole family, will suffer"** Ibid., 40.

165   **" . . . whatever you feel comfortable doing . . . "** Quoted in Martha Brant and Anna Kuchment, "The Little One Said 'Roll Over,'" *Newsweek* 147, no. 22 (2006): 54–55.

165   **. . . sleep on its own by six months** Richard Ferber, *Solve Your Child's Sleep Problems: New, Revised, and Expanded Edition* (New York: Fireside, 2006).

165   **no evidence that people living in societies** Worthman, "After Dark," 291–313; McKenna and McDade, "Why Babies Should Never Sleep Alone," 134–152.

165   **family structures tend to be tighter** Worthman and Brown, "Companionable Sleep," 124.

165   **"in Laos, a baby was never apart . . . "** Anne Fadiman, *The Spirit Catches You and You Fall Down: A Hmong Child, Her American Doctors, and the Collision of Two Cultures* (New York: Farrar, Straus and Giroux, 1997; repr. 2012), 22.

166   **"mutual recognition"** Worthman and Brown, "Companionable Sleep," 125.

166 "You know it's an Inuit tradition . . . " "Physicians Call for End of an Inuit Sleep Tradition," *CBCNews*, November 8, 2005, www.cbc.ca/news/technology/physicians-call-for-end-of-an-inuit-sleep-tradition-1.551990.

166 **45 percent of all parents** Brant and Kuchment, "The Little One Said 'Roll Over,'" 44–45.

166 **"detachment parenting"** William Sears, *Nighttime Parenting: How to Get Your Baby and Child to Sleep* (New York: Plume, 1999), 7.

166 **"a simplistic and harsh way to treat another human being"** Elizabeth Pantley, *The No-Cry Sleep Solution* (New York: McGraw-Hill, 2002), 6.

167 **"attachment parenting"** Katha Pollitt, "Attachment Parenting: More Guilt for Mother," *The Nation*, June 4, 2012, 9; Elisabeth Badinter, *The Conflict: How Modern Motherhood Undermines the Status of Women*, trans. Adriana Hunter (New York: Metropolitan Books, 2012).

167 **" . . . economically and socially 'primitive'"** Ferber, *Solve Your Child's Sleep Problems: New, Revised, and Expanded Edition*, 42.

167 **unexpected sudden death** Ibid., 45–46.

167 **SIDS and other nocturnal catastrophes** McKenna and McDade, "Why Babies Should Never Sleep Alone," 136.

167 **immigrant and racial minority families** Betsy Lozoff, Abraham W. Wolf, and Nancy S. Davis, "Cosleeping in Urban Families with Young Children in the United States," *Pediatrics* 74, no. 2 (1984): 171–182.

168 **"Goodnight moon . . . goodnight air . . . "** Margaret Wise Brown and Clement Hurd, *Goodnight Moon* (New York: Harper and Collins, 1947).

168 **"how to behave and what to feel . . . "** Galbraith, "'Goodnight Nobody' Revisited, 174. Several of the bedtime books discussed below are also analyzed in Galbraith's illuminating study.

168 **Bettelheim castigated Sendak** Quoted in Margalit Fox, "Maurice Sendak, 1928–2012: A Conjurer of Luminous Worlds, Both Beautiful and Terrifying," *New York Times*, May 9, 2012.

170 **" . . . children might be heedlessly bossed about"** Stearns et al., "Children's Sleep," 363.

170 **homes with separate master bedrooms** Tracie Rozhon, "To Have, Hold, and Cherish, Until Bedtime," *New York Times*, March 11, 2007.

Notes to Chapter Six

172 **in the midst of a "sleep crisis"** Arianna Huffington, *The Sleep Revolution: Transforming Your Life, One Night at a Time* (New York: Harmony Books, 2016), 17–45.

172   **"sleep wish list"** Ibid, 280.

172   **organic cotton sheets** Bob Morris, "Arianna Huffington's Sleep Revolution Begins at Home," *New York Times*, April 28, 2016, www.nytimes
.com/2016/05/01/realestate/arianna-huffingtons-sleep-revolution
-starts-at-home.html. The Huffington line can be found at Coco-
Mat, www.coco-mat.com/store/us_en/kalipso-beige-stripe-6374.

173   **"optimal sleep and recuperation in everyday life"** Bich Phoung
Nguyen, Elbrich Postma, David Ekkers, Fabian Degener, and
Thomas Meijer, "Bad Kissingen: A Blueprint for Future Urban
Design" (Groningen, Netherlands, 2013), 5, http://docplayer
.net/19477784-Bad-kissingen-bad-kissingen-a-blueprint-for
-future-urban-design.html.

173   **"modern 24/7 lifestyle . . . "; " . . . chronobiology technologies"**
Ibid., 24.

174   **"to wrap work around humans . . . "** Thomas Kantermann, email
to the author, August 18, 2015.

175   **"the great lazy gang of priests"; " . . . each man's individual
discretion"** Sir Thomas More, *Utopia* (New York: W. W. Norton,
1975), 41–42.

175   **The Shakers** All details about Ann Lee and the Shakers are taken
from Chris Jennings, *Paradise Now: The Story of American Utopianism*
(New York: Random House, 2016), 3–77.

176   **The most famous such community, at Brook Farm** See ibid.,
193–236. The detail about the sleepless visitor is on p. 222.

177   **bachelor's hall in hell** Harding, *The Days of Henry Thoreau*, 125.

177   **Charlotte's troubles with sleep** I am using her first name when
referring to the early part of her biography because her last name
changed from Perkins to Stetson to Gilman during this story.

177   **"pretend to fall asleep . . . "** Helen Lefkowitz Horowitz, *Wild
Unrest: Charlotte Perkins Gilman and the Making of "The Yellow
Wall-Paper"* (Oxford: Oxford University Press, 2010), 8. Unless oth-
erwise noted, details from Gilman's life are taken from this book.

178   **"corsets, tea, coffee . . . "** Quoted in ibid., 113.

178   **"Isn't catalepsy something like this? . . . "** Quoted in ibid., 71.

178   **"She is more sensitive and easily fatigued . . . "** Quoted in ibid., 93.

178   **a remedy for insomnia** Kroker, *The Sleep of Others*, 354.

179   **"Get hysterical in the evening . . . "** Quoted in Horowitz, *Wild
Unrest*, 106.

179   **"constant self supervision and restraint"** Quoted in ibid., 114.

179   **"People tire me frightfully"** Quoted in ibid., 116.

179   **the foremost authority** Michael Blackie, "Reading the Rest Cure,"
Arizona Quarterly 60 (2004): 58.

179   "the woman's desire to be on a level . . . " Quoted in Elaine Showalter, *Hystories: Hysterical Epidemics and Modern Culture* (New York: Columbia University Press, 1997), 50.

179   "tired by much marching . . . " S. Weir Mitchell, "The Evolution of the Rest Treatment," *Journal of Nervous & Mental Disease* 31, no. 6 (1904): 368.

180   the most modish of all diagnoses Edward Shorter, *From Paralysis to Fatigue: A History of Psychosomatic Illness in the Modern Era* (New York: Free Press, 1992), 220–232.

180   "a diagnostic wastebasket" Quoted in ibid., 222.

180   featured fatigue and sleep disturbance Megan Barke, Rebecca Fribush, and Peter N. Stearns, "Nervous Breakdown in 20th-Century American Culture," *Journal of Social History* 33, no. 3 (2000): 567.

180   "a natural and legitimate result of lawful use" S. Weir Mitchell, *Wear and Tear; or, Hints for the Overworked* (Philadelphia: J. B. Lippincott, 1871), 6–7.

180   "the overeducation and overstraining of our young people" Ibid., 9.

180   " . . . he has taxed it enough" Ibid., 12.

180   " . . . renders them remarkably sensitive" Ibid., 27.

180   "if the mothers of a people . . . " Ibid., 23.

180   a diagnosis for Emily Dickinson John F. McDermott, "Emily Dickinson's 'Nervous Prostration' and Its Possible Relationship to Her Work," *Emily Dickinson Journal* 9, no. 1 (2000): 72.

181   gynecological surgery Blackie, "Reading the Rest Cure," 68.

181   bed rest as a sort of vacation Carroll Smith-Rosenberg, *Disorderly Conduct: Visions of Gender in Victorian America* (New York: Knopf, 1985), 197–216.

182   "work, with excitement and change . . . " Charlotte Perkins Gilman, *The Yellow Wallpaper: A Bedford Cultural Edition*, ed. Dale M. Bauer (Boston: Bedford Books of St. Martin's Press, 1998), 42.

182   "smouldering unclean yellow"; "like a woman stooping down . . . " Ibid., 46, 47, 50.

182   "tiresome and perplexing" Ibid., 52, 54.

182   "Now why should that man have fainted?" Ibid., 58.

183   "live as domestic a life as far as possible" Ibid., 348.

183   Contemporary scholars question See Blackie, "Reading the Rest Cure"; Horowitz, *Wild Unrest*.

183   "I cast the noted specialist's advice . . . " Gilman, *The Yellow Wallpaper*, 349.

183   " . . . it was enough to drive anyone mad . . . " Ibid., 348–349.

183   **"foremost feminist theorist . . . "** Clare Virginia Eby, *Until Choice Do Us Part: Marriage Reform in the Progressive Era* (Chicago: University of Chicago Press, 2014), chap. 2.

184   **"There was no reason . . . "** Charlotte Perkins Gilman, *Concerning Children* (Boston: Small, Maynard, 1900), 189.

184   **"awake nearly all night . . . "** Charlotte Perkins Gilman, *Herland, the Yellow Wall-Paper, and Selected Writings* (New York: Penguin, 1999), 239.

184   **"a form of torture"** Ibid., 240.

184   **"Sleep—Sleep—Sleep . . . "** Ibid., 242.

184   **" . . . not what it's cracked up to be"** Ibid., 243.

185   **"This being married and bringing up children . . . "** Ibid., 246.

186   **" . . . feminine regime"; " . . . dependence upon man . . . "** Edward Bellamy, *Looking Backward* (New York: Viking Penguin, 1982), 185.

186   **lectures sounded Nationalist themes** Mark W. Van Wienen, "A Rose by Any Other Name: Charlotte Perkins Stetson (Gilman) and the Case for American Reform Socialism," *American Quarterly* 55, no. 4 (2003): 603–634.

186   **"We have given them a world of their own"** Bellamy, *Looking Backward*, 182.

186   **"The youngest ones . . . "** Gilman, *Herland*, 103, 108.

188   **"The women wouldn't hear of giving up their share . . . "** Quoted in Bruno Bettelheim, *The Children of the Dream* (London: Collier-Macmillan, 1969), 19.

188   **"the going-to-bed scene . . . "** Yael Darr, "Discontent from Within: Hidden Dissent Against Communal Upbringing in Kibbutz Children's Literature of the 1940s & 1950s," *Israel Studies* 16, no. 2 (2011): 127–150. The quotation is from p. 134.

188   **largest utopian experiment** Melford E. Spiro, "Utopia and Its Discontents: The Kibbutz and Its Historical Vicissitudes," *American Anthropologist* 106, no. 3 (2004): 556–568.

189   **"family sleeping"** Ibid., 561–562.

192   **"never know what it's like to be rested . . . "** B. F. Skinner, *Walden Two* (Indianapolis: Hackett, 1948; repr. 1976), 165.

192   **"a sort of second Thoreau"** Ibid., 7.

192   **"any group of people . . . "** Ibid., 10.

193   **"they have no reason to wait . . . "** Ibid., 34.

193   **"pathological aberrations"** Ibid., 122.

193   **"Living in a separate room . . . "** Ibid., 129.

194   **Critics on the left** Rutherford, *Beyond the Box*, 19–40.

194   **"automated mass society"** Ibid., 30.

194   **" . . . manipulate it for their own benefit"** Quoted in ibid., 127.

195　**"We go in for father love, too . . ."** Skinner, *Walden Two*, 98.

195　**collective arrangements were discontinued** Hilke Kuhlmann, *Living Walden Two: B. F. Skinner's Behaviorist Utopia and Experimental Communities* (Urbana: University of Illinois Press, 2005), 102–106.

195　**still run as a collective** See Twin Oaks Community website, www .twinoaks.org.

Notes to Chapter Seven

200　**increasingly becoming global norms** See Wolf-Meyer, *Slumbering Masses*, 182.

200　**physicians warned** Ernest Freeberg, *The Age of Edison: Electric Light and the Invention of Modern America* (New York: Penguin, 2013), 7.

200　**historians and anthropologists** Ekirch, "Sleep We Have Lost"; Worthman, "After Dark."

200　**Yemen in the 1970s** Cited in Dan Falk, *In Search of Time: Journeys Along a Curious Dimension* (Toronto: McClelland and Stewart, 2008), 90.

200　**"insomnia squad"** Derickson, *Dangerously Sleepy*, 7.

201　**"sleep mafia"** Ellen Barry, "Desperate for Slumber in Delhi, Homeless Encounter a 'Sleep Mafia,'" *New York Times*, January 18, 2016, www.nytimes.com/2016/01/19/world/asia/delhi-sleep-economy.html.

201　**"global weirding"** Thomas L. Friedman, "Global Weirding Is Here," *New York Times*, February 17, 2010. On the connections between altered sleep and environmental catastrophe, see Crary, *24/7*. This work is discussed in greater detail below.

201　**eradicate napping** Steger and Brunt, "Introduction: Into the Night and the World of Sleep," 18; Williams, *Sleep and Society*, 109.

201　**"We need a more efficient culture"** Quoted in Jim Yardley, "Spain, Land of 10 p.m. Dinners, Asks If It's Time to Reset the Clock," *New York Times*, February 18, 2014.

201　**government offices in Spain** Wolf-Meyer, *Slumbering Masses*, 183.

202　**after we've turned them off** Lauren Hale and Stanford Guan, "Screen Time and Sleep Among School-Aged Children and Adolescents: A Systematic Literature Review," *Sleep Medicine Reviews* 21 (2015): 50–58.

202　**one of the fastest-growing areas of sleep research** Van den Bulck, Jan. "Television Viewing, Computer Game Playing, and Internet Use and Self-Reported Time to Bed and Time Out of Bed in Secondary School Children," *Sleep* 27, no. 1 (2004): 101–104

204　**"Since my sleep in the daytime was not very good . . ."** "Chinese Labor Workers Exploited by U.S.-Owned iPhone Supplier: An Investigation of Labor Conditions at Jabil Green Point in Wuxi,

China," *China Labor Watch*, 2013, 21, www.chinalaborwatch.org /upfile/Jabil_Green_Point.final.pdf.

204 **creating an efficient workforce** See Rabinbach, *The Human Motor*.

205 **computer animators and software developers in the Philippines** Jingky P. Lozano-Kühne, Maria Eliza R. Aguila, Gayline F. Manalang Jr., Richard Bryann Chua, Roselyn S. Gabud, and Eduardo R. Mendoza, "Shift Work Research in the Philippines: Current State and Future Directions," *Philippine Science Letters* 5, no. 1 (2012): 17–29.

205 **radiologists in India and Australia** Kevin Birth, "Time and the Biological Consequences of Globalization," *Current Anthropology* 48, no. 2 (2007): 216.

205 **sleep labs themselves** Theresa Shumard, "Tapping into Outsourcing," *Sleep Review: The Journal for Sleep Specialists*, July 5, 2007, www .sleepreviewmag.com/2007/07/tapping-into-outsourcing.

205 **serious health consequences** Jeyapal Dinesh Raja and Sanjiv Kumar Bhasin, "Health Issues Amongst Call Center Employees, an Emerging Occupational Group in India," *Indian Journal of Community Medicine: Official Publication of Indian Association of Preventive & Social Medicine* 39, no. 3 (2014): 175–177.

205 **"conflicts between global and local schedules . . . "** Birth, "Time and the Biological Consequences of Globalization," 216. Birth cites the detail about global outsourcing of CAT scan reading from Thomas Friedman's book *The World Is Flat* (New York: Farrar, Straus and Giroux, 2005).

205 **outfit your phone to produce highly detailed records** Elicia Toon, Margot J. Davey, Samantha L. Hollis, Gillian M. Nixon, Rosemary S. C. Horne, and Sarah N. Bigg, "Comparison of Commercial Wrist-Based and Smartphone Accelerometers, Actigraphy, and PSG in a Clinical Cohort of Children and Adolescents," *Journal of Clinical Sleep Medicine* 12, no. 3 (March 2016): 343–350.

206 **the most economically advantaged** Birth, "Time and the Biological Consequences," 225.

206 **telegraph as a metaphor** Paul Gilmore, *Aesthetic Materialism: Electricity and American Romanticism* (Stanford, CA: Stanford University Press, 2009), 187.

206 **"the battery of the brain . . . "** Quoted in Scrivner, *Becoming Insomniac*, 47.

206 **electrified sleep gadgetry** Ibid., 28–29.

206 **Sleep Shepherd Biofeedback Sleep Hat** Patricia Marx, "In Search of Forty Winks: Gizmos for a Good Night's Sleep," *New Yorker*, February 8 and 15, 2016, www.newyorker.com/magazine/2016/02/08 /in-search-of-forty-winks.

207   **other kinds of neural stimulation** Smail, *On Deep History and the Brain*, 157–189.

207   **newest wonder drug** Arlene Weintraub, "Merck's Quest to Revive the Market for Insomnia Drugs," *Forbes*, June 14, 2015, www .forbes.com/sites/arleneweintraub/2015/06/04/mercks-quest-to -revive-the-market-for-insomnia-drugs; Ian Parker, "The Big Sleep," *The New Yorker*, December 9, 2013, www.newyorker.com /magazine/2013/12/09/the-big-sleep-2.

208   **Armed forces have long sought to gain a competitive edge** For a detailed history of such uses, see Lukasz Kamienski, *Shooting Up: A Short History of Drugs and War* (New York: Oxford University Press, 2016).

208   **" . . . a 21st century revolution in military affairs"** Randall, *Dreamland*, 135.

208   **Military Energy Gum** See Military Energy Gum, www.military energygum.com/clinical-studies.

208   **Other DARPA projects** See Patricia Morrisroe, *Wide Awake: A Memoir of Insomnia* (New York: Spiegel and Grau, 2010), 137–141.

209   **"If there is a war in Europe . . . "** "Sleepless Pill," *British Medical Journal* 298, no. 6687 (1989): 1543–1544.

209   **tends to promote overconfidence** See Dimitris Repantis, Peter Schlattmann, Oona Laisney, and Isabella Heuser, "Modafinil and Methylphenidate for Neuroenhancement in Healthy Individuals: A Systematic Review," *Pharmacological Research* 62, no. 3 (2010): 187– 206; Will Saletan, "The War on Sleep," *Slate*, May 29, 2013, www .slate.com/articles/health_and_science/superman/2013/05/sleep _deprivation_in_the_military_modafinil_and_the_arms_race_for _soldiers.html.

209   **Somneo Sleep Trainer** Jessa Gamble, "The End of Sleep," *Aeon*, 2015, https://aeon.co/essays/technology-to-cut-down-on-sleep -is-just-around-the-corner.

209   **a whopping $1.4 billion** See "Modafinil: A Chronology of Three Decades," H.M. Pharma Consultancy Blog, *http://hmpharmacon .blogspot.com/2012/04/modafinil-chronology-of-three-decades.html*; "Modafinil Sales Data," Drugs, *www.drugs.com/stats/modafinil*.

210   **The drug's developer** "Sleepless Pill," 1543–1544.

210   **a 2009 poll** Margaret Talbot, "Brain Gain: The Underground World of Brain-Enhancing Drugs," *New Yorker*, April 27, 2009, www.new yorker.com/magazine/2009/04/27/brain-gain.

210   **attempts to optimize cognitive functioning** See Paul Root Wolpe, "Treatment, Enhancement, and the Ethics of Neurotherapeutics," *Brain & Cognition* 50 (2002): 387–395; Williams, *Politics of Sleep*, 137–140.

210   **"If you're a fifty-five-year-old . . . "** Quoted in Talbot, "Brain Gain."

210   **So where is sleep heading?** "What Is the Future of Sleep?" *Test-Tube Plus!* YouTube, May 24, 2015, https://www.youtube.com /watch?v=M-bQzqdwUk0; Dominic Basulto, "7 Reasons Why the Future of Sleep Could Be Wilder Than Your Wildest Dreams," *Washington Post*, May 20, 2014, www.washingtonpost.com/news /innovations/wp/2014/05/20/7-reasons-why-the-future-of-sleep -could-be-wilder-than-your-wildest-dreams.

211   **According to these would-be oracles** Williams, *The Politics of Sleep*, 146–155; Wolf-Meyer, *Slumbering Masses*, 243–261. The quotation is on p. 21.

212   **"sleeping on the job"** See "Policy and Procedures: Policy 4.62, Standards of Conduct," Emory University, http://policies.emory .edu/4.62.

212   **"customization" of sleep** Williams et al., "Medicalisation or Customisation," 40–47.

212   **" . . . the end of capitalism"** Fredric Jameson, "Future City," *New Left Review* 21 (2003): 76.

212   **Thatcher boasted of her ability** Williams, *Sleep and Society*, 140.

212   **a 1997 satirical novel** Jonathan Coe, *The House of Sleep* (New York: Vintage Contemporaries, 1997; repr. 1999).

213   **conquered the final frontier** Crary, *24/7*.

213   **a future in which sleep has literally become impossible** Karen Russell, *Sleep Donation: A Novella* (New York: Atavist Books, 2014).

214   **detached from individual bodies** See Nikolas Rose, *The Politics of Life Itself: Biomedicine, Power, and Subjectivity in the Twenty-First Century* (Princeton, NJ: Princeton University Press, 2007), 14–15.

215   **"end of nature"** Bill McKibben, *The End of Nature* (New York: Random House, 1989).

216   **"Humans have never been 'natural'"** Rose, *The Politics of Life Itself*, 80.

216   **fastidious vegetarian diet** Michelle C. Neely, "Embodied Politics: Antebellum Vegetarianism and the Dietary Economy of *Walden*," *American Literature* 85, no. 1 (2013): 34–60.

216   **sleeping and getting a cold . . . ; positions might lead to nightmares** Roni Caryn Rabin, "Ask Well: More Sleep, Fewer Colds?" *New York Times*, January 29, 2016, www.well.blogs.nytimes .com/2016/01/29/ask-well-sleep-and-colds; Maya Dangerfield, "Scientists May Have Discovered What Sleeping Position Gives You Nightmares," *Tech Insider*, January 19, 2016, www.techinsider.io /sleep-positions-affect-dreams-2016-1.

216 **new fascination in literature** See Michael Greaney, "'Observed, Measured, Contained': Contemporary Fiction and the Science of Sleep," *Contemporary Literature* 56, no. 1 (2015): 56–80.

217 **popular disability memoirs** See G. Thomas Couser, *Signifying Bodies: Disability in Contemporary Life Writing* (Ann Arbor: University of Michigan Press, 2009).

217 **some severe sleep disorders are classified as disabilities** Benjamin Reiss, "Sleeping While Disabled, Disabled While Sleeping," *Sleep Health* 2, no. 3 (2016): 187–190.

218 **reallocation of funds** Gayle Greene, *Insomniac* (Berkeley: University of California Press, 2008). See esp. chap. 12.

218 **"Panels of color . . ."; "Often the clog . . ."** Blake Butler, *Nothing: A Portrait of Insomnia* (New York: Harper Perennial, 2011). The quotations are from pp. 109, 110, 118, 34, 61, 38, and 263.

219 **"I fall inside myself . . ."** Jean-Luc Nancy, *The Fall of Sleep*, trans. Charlotte Mandell (New York: Fordham University Press, 2009), 5.

219 **Andy Warhol's famous 1963 film *Sleep*** For an account of the film's first screening and audience reaction, see "Sleep (1963)," www.warholstars.org/sleep.html.

219 **"I fell asleep 25 minutes into it . . ."** Austin Sweetwater, "Lena Dunham to Remake Andy Warhol's *Sleep*," *News Examiner*, 2015, http://newsexaminer.net/movies/lena-dunham-to-remake-andy-warhols-sleep.

219 **co-sleeping with her parents** Meghan Daum, "Lena Dunham Is Not Done Confessing," *New York Times Magazine*, September 10, 2014, www.nytimes.com/2014/09/14/magazine/lena-dunham.html.

220 **Kanye West's notorious video "Famous"** Kanye West, "Famous" YouTube, June 28, 2016, https://www.youtube.com/watch?v=wCg1_IKXmQc.

220 **"I am Warhol . . ."** See "I Am Warhol," YouTube, December 5, 2013, https://www.youtube.com/watch?v=bINO64iDaeY.

220 **Trump's . . . erratic public behavior** Krithika Varagur, "Can Sleep Deprivation Explain Donald Trump's Behavior?" *Huffington Post*, March 6, 2016, www.huffingtonpost.com/entry/donald-trump-sleep-deprivation_us_56d5d020e4b03260bf78343a; Timothy Egan, "A Unified Theory of Trump," *New York Times*, February 26, 2015, www.nytimes.com/2016/02/26/opinion/a-unified-theory-of-trump.html.

221 **"They want to be in the bed"** Dirk Standen, "Exclusive: Kanye West on His 'Famous' Video, Which Might Be His Most Thought-Provoking Work Yet," *Vanity Fair*, June 24, 2016, www.vanityfair.com/culture/2016/06/kanye-famous-video-interview.

221 " . . . slumbering idiots"; " . . . spark of empathy . . . " Rachel Martin, "A Chat with the Painter Whose Work Inspired Kanye West's 'Famous,'" National Public Radio, Weekend Edition, July 23, 2016, www.npr.org/2016/07/03/484402517/a-chat-with-the-painter -whose-work-inspired-kanye-wests-famous.

221 **"the stuff of snuff films"** Lena Dunham, June 27, 2016, https:// www.facebook.com/lenadunham/posts/1756770211270449:0.

222 **how Taylor Swift felt** Amber Belus, "Taylor Swift's Retaliation to Kanye West's 'Famous' Video Revealed! (Exclusive)," *InTouch*, June 27, 2016. www.intouchweekly.com/posts/taylor-swift-kanye -west-famous-106399.

Notes to Epilogue

227 **aversion to steady work** Jimmy Carter, *An Outdoor Journal* (New York: Bantam Books, 1988), 10.

227 **"the poor man's wealth . . . "** Philip Sidney, "Come, Sleep!," in *Poems of Sleep and Dreams*, ed. Peter Washington (New York: Alfred A. Knopf, 2004), 33.

228 **" . . . with kings and counselors"** Herman Melville, *Great Short Works* (New York: Harper Perennial, 2004), 73.

228 **"I swear they are averaged now . . . "** Walt Whitman, *Leaves of Grass and Other Writings*, 2nd ed., ed. Michael Moon (New York: W. W. Norton, 2002).

BIBLIOGRAPHY

Aberbach, Alan David. *In Search of an American Identity: Samuel Latham Mitchill, Jeffersonian Naturalist*. New York: Peter Lang, 1988.

Ahlheim, Hannah, ed. *Die Geschichte des Schlafs in der Moderne*. Frankfurt: Campus Verlag, 2014.

Alaimo, Stacy. *Bodily Natures: Science, Environment, and the Material Self*. Bloomington: Indiana University Press, 2010.

Alexeyeff, Kalissa. "Sleeping Safe: Perceptions of Risk and Value in Western and Pacific Infant Co-Sleeping." In *Sleep Around the World: Anthropological Perspectives*, edited by Katie Glaskin and Richard Chenhall, 113–131. London: Palgrave Macmillan, 2013.

Allen, Thomas M. "Clockwork Nation: Modern Time, Moral Perfectionism and American Identity in Catharine Beecher and Henry Thoreau." *Journal of American Studies* 39, no. 1 (2005): 65–86.

———. *A Republic in Time: Temporality and Social Imagination in Nineteenth-Century America*. Chapel Hill: University of North Carolina Press, 2008.

Apperley, Thomas. *Observations in Physick, Both Rational and Practical*. London: W. Innys, 1731.

Arendt, Josephine. "Biological Rhythms During Residence in Polar Regions." *Chronobiology International: The Journal of Biological & Medical Rhythm Research* 29, no. 4 (2012): 379–394.

Ariès, Philippe. *Centuries of Childhood: A Social History of Family Life*. Translated by Robert Baldick. New York: Alfred A. Knopf, 1962.

———. "The Sentimental Revolution." *Wilson Quarterly* 6, no. 4 (1982): 47–53.

Armstrong, George. *An Account of the Diseases, Most Incident to Children, from Their Birth Till the Age of Puberty*. London: T. Cadell, 1783.

Badinter, Elisabeth. *The Conflict: How Modern Motherhood Undermines the Status of Women*. Translated by Adriana Hunter. New York: Metropolitan Books, 2012.

Baldwin, Peter C. *In the Watches of the Night: Life in the Nocturnal City, 1820–1930*. Chicago: University of Chicago Press, 2012.

Balzac, Honoré de. "The Pleasures and Pains of Coffee." *Michigan Quarterly Review* 25, no. 2 (Spring 1996): 273–277.

"Barbara Bush Calls Evacuees Better Off." *New York Times*, September 7, 2005.

Barke, Megan, Rebecca Fribush, and Peter N. Stearns. "Nervous Breakdown in 20th-Century American Culture." *Journal of Social History* 33, no. 3 (2000): 565–584.

Barry, Ellen. "Desperate for Slumber in Delhi, Homeless Encounter a 'Sleep Mafia.'" *New York Times*, January 18, 2016, www.nytimes.com/2016/01/19 /world/asia/delhi-sleep-economy.html.

Basulto, Dominic. "7 Reasons Why the Future of Sleep Could Be Wilder Than Your Wildest Dreams." *Washington Post*, May 20, 2014, www.wash ingtonpost.com/news/innovations/wp/2014/05/20/7-reasons-why-the -future-of-sleep-could-be-wilder-than-your-wildest-dreams.

Beard, George, and Alphonso David Rockwell. *A Practical Treatise on the Medical and Surgical Uses of Electricity*. New York: William Wood, 1878.

Belden, L. W. *An Account of Jane C. Rider, the Somnambulist*. Springfield, MA: G. and C. Merriam, 1834.

———. "An Account of Jane C. Rider, the Springfield Somnambulist." *Boston Medical and Surgical Journal* 11, no. 4 (September 10, 1834): 4–84.

Bell, John. *An Essay on Somnambulism; or, Sleep-Walking, Produced by Animal Electricity and Magnetism, as Well as by Sympathy, &C.* Dublin: Printed for the author, 1788.

Bell, Luther. *An Hour's Conference with Fathers and Sons, in Relation to a Common and Fatal Indulgence*. Boston: Whipple and Damrell, 1840.

Bellamy, Edward. *Looking Backward*. New York: Viking Penguin, 1982.

Belus, Amber. "Taylor Swift's Retaliation to Kanye West's 'Famous' Video Revealed! (Exclusive)." *In Touch*, June 27, 2016, www.intouchweekly.com /posts/taylor-swift-kanye-west-famous-106399.

Ben-Ari, Eyal. "'It's Bedtime' in the World's Urban Middle Classes: Children, Families and Sleep." In *Worlds of Sleep*, edited by Lodewijk Brunt and Brigitte Steger, 175–191. Berlin: Frank and Timme, 2008.

Bentley, Nancy. *Frantic Panoramas: American Literature and Mass Culture, 1870–1920*. Philadelphia: University of Pennsylvania Press, 2009.

Bettelheim, Bruno. *The Children of the Dream*. London: Collier-Macmillan, 1969.

Bin, Yu Su, Nathaniel S. Marshall, and Nick Glozier. "Secular Trends in Adult Sleep Duration: A Systematic Review." *Sleep Medicine Reviews* 16 (2012): 223–230.

Birth, Kevin. "Time and the Biological Consequences of Globalization." *Current Anthropology* 48, no. 2 (2007): 215–236.

Blackie, Michael. "Reading the Rest Cure." *Arizona Quarterly* 60 (Spring 2004): 57–85.

Blustein, Bonnie Ellen. *Preserve Your Love for Science: Life of William A. Hammond, American Neurologist*. New York: Cambridge University Press, 1991.

Bosco, Ronald A., ed. *Nature's Panorama: Thoreau on the Seasons*. Amherst: University of Massachusetts Press, 2005.

Bradford, John E., and Douglass Talk. "Torpor Inducing Transfer Habitat for Human Stasis to Mars." Atlanta: Space Works Enterprises, 2014, https://www.nasa.gov/content/torpor-inducing-transfer-habitat-for-human-stasis-to-mars.

Brant, Martha, and Anna Kuchment. "The Little One Said 'Roll Over.'" *Newsweek* 147, no. 22 (2006): 54–55.

Brian, Kathleen. "'The Weight of Perhaps Ten or a Dozen Lives': Suicide, Accountability, and the Life-Saving Technologies of the Asylum." *Bulletin of the History of Medicine* 90, no. 4 (Winter 2016).

"A Brief History of Concord." Concord Library, www.concordlibrary.org/scollect/bhc/bhc.html.

Brierre de Boismont, Alexandre Jacques François. *Hallucinations; or, the Rational History of Apparitions, Visions, Dreams, Ecstasy, Magnetism, and Somnambulism*. 1st American ed. Philadelphia: Lindsay and Blakiston, 1853.

Brigham, Amariah. "Annual Report of the Managers of the State Lunatic Asylum." Albany, NY: Carroll and Cook, 1844.

Brown, Charles Brocken. *Edgar Huntly; or, Memoirs of a Sleepwalker*. New York: Penguin, 1988.

Brown, Margaret Wise, and Clement Hurd. *Goodnight Moon*. New York: Harper and Collins, 1947.

Brune, Jeffrey A., and Daniel J. Wilson, eds. *Disability and Passing*. Philadelphia: Temple University Press, 2013.

Brunt, Lodewijk, and Brigitte Steger, eds. *Worlds of Sleep*. Leipzig, Germany: Frank and Timme, 2008.

Bryson, Bill. *At Home: A Short History of Private Life*. New York: Doubleday, 2010.

Buell, Lawrence. *The Environmental Imagination: Thoreau, Nature Writing, and the Formation of American Culture*. Cambridge, MA: Belknap Press of Harvard University Press, 1995.

Butler, Blake. *Nothing: A Portrait of Insomnia*. New York: Harper Perennial, 2011.

Caffeine Informer: Accurate Caffeine Information Available to All, www.caffeineinformer.com/death-by-caffeine.

Campbell, Colin. "Donald Trump Just Trolled Jeb Bush with a Video Touting Him as a Cure for Insomnia." *Business Insider*, September 8, 2015, www.businessinsider.com/donald-trump-jeb-bush-can-help-you-sleep-2015-9.

Carter, Jimmy. *An Outdoor Journal*. New York: Bantam Books, 1988.

Cartwright, Samuel. "Diseases and Peculiarities of the Negro Race." *Debow's Review of the Southern and Western States* 11, new ser. 4 (1851): 64–69, 209–213, 331–336.

Chadwick, Edwin. *Report on the Sanitary Condition of the Labouring Population of Great Britain*. Edinburgh: Edinburgh University Press, 1965.

Cheyne, George. *The English Malady; or, a Treatise of Nervous Diseases of All Kinds*. London: G. Strahan, 1735.

"Chinese Labor Workers Exploited by U.S.-Owned iPhone Supplier: An Investigation of Labor Conditions at Jabil Green Point in Wuxi, China." China Labor Watch, 2013, www.chinalaborwatch.org/upfile/Jabil_Green _Point.final.pdf.

Choi, Charles Q. "Mock Mars Flight Reveals Big Sleep Concerns for Astronauts." Space, January 8, 2013, www.space.com/19168-mock-mars-flight -reveals-big-sleep-concerns-for-astronauts.html.

Clurman, Carol. "In Bed with Arianna Huffington: Tips for Getting More (and Better) Sleep." *Parade*, July 16, 2015, http://parade.com/411133/parade /go-to-sleep-with-arianna-tips-for-getting-more-zzzs/2.

Coe, Jonathan. *The House of Sleep*. New York: Vintage Contemporaries, 1997 (repr. 1999).

Cogan, Thomas. *The Haven of Health*. London: Anne Griffin, for Roger Bale, 1636.

Collier, Mary. *The Woman's Labour: An Epistle to Mr. Stephen Duck; in Answer to His Late Poem, Called the Thresher's Labour*. London: Printed for the author, 1739.

Collins, Anne. *In the Sleep Room: The Story of the CIA Brainwashing Experiments in Canada*. Toronto: Lester and Orpen Dennys, 1988.

Concord Museum, "Henry David Thoreau Collection," http://www.concord museum.org/henry-david-thoreau-collection.php.

Condon, Richard G. *Inuit Behavior and Seasonal Change in the Canadian Arctic*. Ann Arbor, MI: UMI Research Press, 1983.

Coren, Stanley. *Sleep Thieves: An Eye-Opening Exploration into the Science and Mysteries of Sleep*. New York: Free Press, 1996.

Couser, G. Thomas. *Signifying Bodies: Disability in Contemporary Life Writing*. Ann Arbor: University of Michigan Press, 2009.

Cox, Robert S. *Body and Soul: A Sympathetic History of American Spiritualism*. Charlottesville: University of Virginia Press, 2003.

———. "The Suburbs of Eternity: On Visionaries and Miraculous Sleepers." In *Worlds of Sleep*, edited by Lodewijk Brunt and Brigitte Steger, 53–73. Berlin: Frank and Timme, 2008.

Crary, Jonathan. *24/7: Late Capitalism and the Ends of Sleep*. London: Verso, 2013.

Cunningham, Hugh. *Children and Childhood in Western Society Since 1500*. London: Longman, 1995.

Dangerfield, Maya. "Scientists May Have Discovered What Sleeping Position Gives You Nightmares," *Tech Insider*, January 19, 2016, www.tech insider.io/sleep-positions-affect-dreams-2016-1.

Dannenfeldt, Karl H. "Sleep: Theory and Practice in the Late Renaissance." *Journal of the History of Medicine and Allied Sciences* 41, no. 4 (October 1986): 415–441.

Darr, Yael. "Discontent from Within: Hidden Dissent Against Communal Upbringing in Kibbutz Children's Literature of the 1940s & 1950s." *Israel Studies* 16, no. 2 (Summer 2011): 127–150.

Daum, Meghan. "Lena Dunham Is Not Done Confessing." *New York Times Magazine*, September 10, 2014, www.nytimes.com/2014/09/14/magazine /lena-dunham.html.

Dave, Kunjan R., Sherri L. Christian, Miguel A. Perez-Pinzon, and Kelly L. Drew. "Neuroprotection: Lessons from Hibernators." *Comparative Biochemistry and Physiology Part B: Biochemistry and Molecular Biology* 162, no. 1–3 (May 2012): 1–9.

Davis, Lennard J. *The End of Normal: Identity in a Biocultural Era*. Ann Arbor: University of Michigan Press, 2013.

De la Iglesia, Horacio O., Claudia Moreno, Arne Lowden, Fernando Louzada, Elaine Marqueze, Rosa Levandovski, Luisa K. Pilz, *et al.* "Ancestral Sleep." *Current Biology* 26, no. 7 (April 4, 2016): R271–R272.

Dement, William C., and Christopher Vaughan. *The Promise of Sleep: The Scientific Connection Between Health, Happiness, and a Good Night's Sleep*. New York: Dell, 2000.

Derickson, Alan. *Dangerously Sleepy: Overworked Americans and the Cult of Manly Wakefulness*. Philadelphia: University of Pennsylvania Press, 2014.

Dickinson, Emily. *Final Harvest: Poems*. Boston: Little, Brown, 1964.

Directions and Observations Relative to Food, Exercise, and Sleep. London: S. Bladon, 1772.

Dohrn-van Rossum, Gerhard. *History of the Hour: Clocks and Modern Temporal Orders*. Translated by Thomas Dunlap. Chicago: University of Chicago Press, 1996.

Douglass, Frederick. *Autobiographies*. New York: Library of America, 1994.

Douglass, John H. *Devotional Somnium; or, a Collection of Prayers and Exhortations Uttered by Miss Rachel Baker, in the City of New-York, in the Winter of 1815, During Her Abstracted and Unconscious State*. New York: Van Winkle and Riley, 1815.

Durant, John. *The Paleo Manifesto: Ancient Wisdom for Lifelong Health*. New York: Harmony Books, 2013.

Dwyer, Ellen. *Homes for the Mad: Life Inside Two Nineteenth-Century Asylums*. New Brunswick, NJ: Rutgers University Press, 1987.

"Early Rising." *Children's Missionary Record of the Free Church of Scotland* 5 (February 1849): 235.

Eby, Clare Virginia. *Until Choice Do Us Part: Marriage Reform in the Progressive Era*. Chicago: University of Chicago Press, 2014.

Egan, Timothy. "A Unified Theory of Trump." *New York Times*, February 26, 2016, www.nytimes.com/2016/02/26/opinion/a-unified-theory-of-trump.html.

Ekirch, A. Roger. *At Day's Close: Night in Times Past*. New York: W. W. Norton, 2005.

———. "The Modernization of Western Sleep; or, Does Insomnia Have a History?" *Past & Present* 226, no. 1 (February 1, 2015): 149–192.

———. "Segmented Sleep in Preindustrial Societies." *Sleep* 39, no. 3 (2016): 715–716.

———. "Sleep We Have Lost: Pre-Industrial Slumber in the British Isles." *American Historical Review* 106, no. 2 (2001): 343–386.

Elias, Norbert. *The History of Manners*. Vol. 1, *The Civilizing Process*. Translated by Edmund Jephcott. New York: Pantheon, 1978.

Emerson, Ralph Waldo. *Essays & Poems*. New York: Library of America, 1996.

English, Daylanne K. *Each Hour Redeem: Time and Justice in African American Literature*. Minneapolis: University of Minnesota Press, 2013.

European Space Agency, Advanced Team Biomimetics website, www.esa.int/gsp/ACT/bio/projects/Hibernation.html.

Fadiman, Anne. *The Spirit Catches You and You Fall Down: A Hmong Child, Her American Doctors, and the Collision of Two Cultures*. New York: Farrar, Straus and Giroux, 1997 (repr. 2012).

Falflik, David. *Boarding Out: Inhabiting the American Urban Literary Imagination, 1840–1860*. Evanston, IL: Northwestern University Press, 2012.

Falk, Dan. *In Search of Time: Journeys Along a Curious Dimension*. Toronto: McClelland and Stewart, 2008.

Ferber, Richard. *Solve Your Child's Sleep Problems*. New York: Simon and Schuster, 1985.

———. *Solve Your Child's Sleep Problems: New, Revised, and Expanded Edition*. New York: Fireside, 2006.

Foner, Philip S., ed. *The Factory Girls: A Collection of Writings on Life and Struggles in the New England Factories of the 1840s*. Chicago: University of Illinois Press, 1977.

Fox, Karen. "Sleeping the Sleep of Our Ancestors." *Science* 262, no. 5137 (November 19, 1993): 1297.

Fox, Margalit. "Maurice Sendak, 1928–2012: A Conjurer of Luminous Worlds, Both Beautiful and Terrifying." *New York Times*, May 9, 2012.

Fredrickson, George M. *The Black Image in the White Mind: The Debate on Afro-American Character and Destiny, 1817–1914*. New York: Harper and Row, 1971.

Freeberg, Ernest. *The Age of Edison: Electric Light and the Invention of Modern America*. New York: Penguin, 2013.

Freud, Sigmund. "From the History of an Infantile Neurosis ('Wolf-Man')." In *The Freud Reader*, edited by Peter Gay, 400–428. New York: W. W. Norton, 1989.

Friedman, Kristen Anne Keerma. "Soul Sleepers: A History of Somnambulism in the United States, 1740–1840." Dissertation, Harvard University, 2014.

Friedman, Thomas L. "Global Weirding Is Here." *New York Times*, February 17, 2010.

Furui, Yoshiaki. "Networked Solitude: American Literature in the Age of Modern Communications, 1831–1898." Dissertation, Emory University, 2015.

Galbraith, Mary. "'Goodnight Nobody' Revisited: Using an Attachment Perspective to Study Picture Books About Bedtime." *Children's Literature Association Quarterly* 23, no. 4 (1998): 172–180.

Gallop, David, ed. *Aristotle: On Sleep and Dreams*. Warminster, UK: Aris and Phillips, 1996.

Gamble, Jessa. "The End of Sleep." *Aeon*, 2015, https://aeon.co/essays/technology-to-cut-down-on-sleep-is-just-around-the-corner.

Genovese, Eugene D. *Roll, Jordan, Roll: The World the Slaves Made*. New York: Vintage Books, 1976.

Gilman, Charlotte Perkins. *Concerning Children*. Boston: Small, Maynard, 1900.

———. *Herland, the Yellow Wall-Paper, and Selected Writings*. New York: Penguin, 1999.

———. *The Yellow Wallpaper: A Bedford Cultural Edition*. Edited by Dale M. Bauer. Boston: Bedford Books of St. Martin's Press, 1998.

Gilmore, Paul. *Aesthetic Materialism: Electricity and American Romanticism*. Stanford, CA: Stanford University Press, 2009.

Glaskin, Katie, and Richard Chenhall, eds. *Sleep Around the World: Anthropological Perspectives*. London: Palgrave Macmillan, 2013.

Glennie, Paul, and Nigel Thrift. *Shaping the Day: A History of Timekeeping in England and Wales, 1300–1800*. Oxford: Oxford University Press, 2009.

Goffman, Erving. *Asylums: Essays on the Social Situation of Mental Patients and Other Inmates*. New York: Anchor Books, 1961.

Greaney, Michael. "'Observed, Measured, Contained': Contemporary Fiction and the Science of Sleep." *Contemporary Literature* 56, no. 1 (2015): 56–80.

Greenberg, Kenneth S., ed. *The Confessions of Nat Turner and Related Documents*. Boston: Bedford Books of St. Martin's Press, 1996.

Greene, Gayle. *Insomniac*. Berkeley: University of California Press, 2008.

Griffith, E. "Another Sleeping Preacher." *Springfield Republican*, October 3, 1833.

Grob, Gerald N. *The State and the Mentally Ill: A History of Worcester State Hospital in Massachusetts*. Chapel Hill: University of North Carolina Press, 1966.

Hale, Benjamin, and Lauren Hale. "Is Justice Good for Your Sleep (and Therefore, Good for Your Health)?" *Social Theory and Health* 7, no. 4 (2009): 354–370.

Hale, Lauren, and D. Phuoung Do. "Racial Differences in Self-Reports of Sleep Duration in a Population-Based Study." *Sleep* 30, no. 9 (2009): 1096–1103.

Hale, Lauren, and Stanford Guan. "Screen Time and Sleep Among School-Aged Children and Adolescents: A Systematic Literature Review." *Sleep Medicine Reviews* 21 (June 2015): 50–58.

Hall, Courtney Robert. *A Scientist of the Early Republic: Samuel Latham Mitchill, 1764–1831*. New York: Russell and Russell, 1967.

Hall, William Whitty. *Sleep*, 3rd ed. New York: W. W. Hall, 1863.

Halttunen, Karen. *Murder Most Foul: The Killer and the American Gothic Imagination*. Cambridge, MA: Harvard University Press, 1998.

Hammond, William Alexander. *On Wakefulness*. Philadelphia: J. B. Lippincott, 1865.

———. *Sleep and Its Derangements*. Philadelphia: J. B. Lippincott, 1873.

Handley, Sasha. *Sleep in Early Modern England*. New Haven, CT: Yale University Press, 2016.

———. "Sociable Sleeping in Early Modern England, 1660–1760." *History & Health* 49 (2013): 79–104.

Harding, Walter. *The Days of Henry Thoreau*. New York: Dover, 1962 (repr. 1980).

———. "Thoreau's Sexuality." *Journal of Homosexuality* 21, no. 3 (1991): 23–45.

Harris, Walter. *A Full View of All the Diseases Incident to Children*. London: A. Millar, 1742.

Hawthorne, Nathaniel. *Collected Novels: Fanshawe, the Scarlet Letter, the House of the Seven Gables, the Blithedale Romance, the Marble Faun*. New York: Library of America, 1983.

Hegarty, Stephanie. "The Myth of the Eight-Hour Sleep." *BBC News Magazine*, February 22, 2012, www.bbc.com/news/magazine-16964783.

Hentz, Caroline Lee. *The Planter's Northern Bride*, vol. 1. Philadelphia: Carey and Hart, 1854.

Hinds, Hilary. "Together and Apart: Twin Beds, Domestic Hygiene and Modern Marriage, 1890–1945." *Journal of Design History* 23, no. 3 (September 1, 2010): 275–304.

Hobbes, Thomas. *Leviathan; or, the Matter, Forme and Power of a Commonwealth Ecclesiasticall and Civil*. New York: Simon and Schuster, 2008.

Horne, Jim. *Sleepfaring: A Journey Through the Science of Sleep*. Oxford: Oxford University Press, 2006.

Horowitz, Helen Lefkowitz. *Wild Unrest: Charlotte Perkins Gilman and the Making of "The Yellow Wall-Paper."* Oxford: Oxford University Press, 2010.

Huffington, Arianna. *The Sleep Revolution: Transforming Your Life, One Night at a Time*. New York: Harmony Books, 2016.

Hulbert, Ann. *Raising America: Experts, Parents, and a Century of Advice to Children*. New York: Alfred A. Knopf, 2003.

"Human Hibernation." *British Medical Journal* (June 23, 1900): 1554–1555.

"Interesting Case of Somnambulism." *Springfield Republican*, October 30, 1833.

International Classification of Sleep Disorders, 3rd ed. Darien, IL: American Academy of Sleep Medicine, 2014.

Jackson, Gregory S. *The Word and Its Witness: The Spiritualization of American Realism*. Chicago: University of Chicago Press, 2009.

Jameson, Fredric. "Future City." *New Left Review* 21 (May-June 2003): 65–79.

Jefferson, Thomas. *Notes on the State of Virginia*. London: Printed for John Stockdale, 1787.

Jennings, Chris. *Paradise Now: The Story of American Utopianism*. New York: Random House, 2016.

Johnson, Steven. *The Ghost Map: The Story of London's Most Terrifying Epidemic— and How It Changed Science, Cities, and the Modern World*. New York: Riverhead Books, 2006.

Johnson, Walter. *River of Dark Dreams: Slavery and Empire in the Cotton Kingdom*. Cambridge, MA: Belknap Press of Harvard University Press, 2013.

Journeys into the Moon, Several Planets, and the Sun: History of a Female Somnambulist, of Wilhelm on the Teck, in the Kingdom of Wuehtemberg, in the Years 1832 and 1833. Philadelphia: Vollmer and Hagenmacher, 1837.

Jouvet, Michel. *The Paradox of Sleep: The Story of Dreaming*. Translated by Laurence Garey. Cambridge, MA: MIT Press, 1999.

Kamienski, Lukasz. *Shooting Up: A Short History of Drugs and War*. New York: Oxford University Press, 2016.

Knutson, Kristen L. "Should I Sleep More or Should I Sleep Less?" *Huffington Post*, November 13. 2015, www.huffingtonpost.com/kristen-knutson /should-i-sleep-more-or-sh_b_8434240.html.

Knutson, Kristen L., Eve Van Cauter, Paul J. Rathouz, Thomas DeLeire, and Diane S. Lauderdale. "Trends in the Prevalence of Short Sleepers in the USA: 1975–2006." *Sleep* 33, no. 1 (2010): 37–45.

Konnikova, Maria. "Why Can't We Fall Asleep?" *New Yorker*, July 7, 2015, www.newyorker.com/science/maria-konnikova/why-cant-we-fall-asleep.

Koslofsky, Craig. *Evening's Empire: A History of the Night in Early Modern Europe*. Cambridge: Cambridge University Press, 2011.

Kroker, Kenton. *The Sleep of Others and the Transformation of Sleep Research*. Toronto: University of Toronto Press, 2007.

Kuhlmann, Hilke. *Living Walden Two: B. F. Skinner's Behaviorist Utopia and Experimental Communities*. Urbana: University of Illinois Press, 2005.

Kurth, Salome, Peter Acherman, Thomas Rusterholz, and Monique K. LeBourgeois. "Development of Brain EEG Connectivity Across Early Childhood: Does Sleep Play a Role?" *Brain Sciences* 3, no. 4 (December 2013): 1445–1460.

Lambert, Frank. *Inventing the "Great Awakening."* Princeton, NJ: Princeton University Press, 1999.

Laqueur, Thomas W. *Solitary Sex: A Cultural History of Masturbation*. New York: Zone Books, 2003.

Le Vaillant, François. *Travels into the Interior Parts of Africa*, vol. 2. London: G. G. and J. Robinson, 1796.

Lewis, Roger C., ed. *The Collected Poems of Robert Louis Stevenson*. Edinburgh: Edinburgh University Press, 2003.

Locke, John. *Some Thoughts Concerning Education and of the Conduct of the Understanding*. Indianapolis, IN: Hackett, 1996.

Lohmann, Roger Ivar. "Sleeping Among the Asabano: Surprises in Intimacy and Sociality at the Margins of Consciousness." In *Sleep Around the World: Anthropological Perspectives*, edited by Katie Glaskin and Richard Chenhall, 21–44. London: Palgrave Macmillan, 2013.

Lozano-Kühne, Jingky P., Maria Eliza R. Aguila, Gayline F. Manalang, Jr., Richard Bryann Chua P., Roselyn S. Gabud, and Eduardo R. Mendoza. "Shift Work Research in the Philippines: Current State and Future Directions." *Philippine Science Letters* 5, no. 1 (2012): 17–29.

Lozoff, Betsy, Abraham W. Wolf, and Nancy S. Davis. "Cosleeping in Urban Families with Young Children in the United States." *Pediatrics* 74, no. 2 (1984): 171–182.

Mais, Charles. *The Surprising Case of Rachel Baker, Who Prays and Preaches in Her Sleep*. New York: S. Marks, 1814.

Mansbach, Adam. *Go the F**k to Sleep*. New York: Akashic Books, 2011.

Martin, Rachel. "A Chat with the Painter Whose Work Inspired Kanye West's 'Famous.'" National Public Radio, Weekend Edition, July 23, 2016. www.npr.org/2016/07/03/484402517/a-chat-with-the-painter-whose-work-inspired-kanye-wests-famous.

Marx, Karl. *Das Kapital*. Vol. 1, *A Critique of Political Economy*. New York: Dover, 2011.

Marx, Patricia. "In Search of Forty Winks: Gizmos for a Good Night's Sleep." *New Yorker*, February 8 and 15, 2016, www.newyorker.com/magazine/2016/02/08/in-search-of-forty-winks.

Mather, Azariah. *Wo to Sleepy Sinners; or, a Discourse upon Amos VI.1.* Timothy Green, printer, 1720.

Mather, Cotton. *The Angel of Bethesda (1724).* Edited by Gordon W. Jones. Barre, MA: American Antiquarian Society and Barre Publishers, 1972.

———. *Vigilius; or, the Awakener.* Boston: J. Franklin, 1719.

Mather, Increase. *Practical Truths Tending to Promote the Power of Godliness.* Boston: Samuel Green, 1682.

McDermott, John F. "Emily Dickinson's 'Nervous Prostration' and Its Possible Relationship to Her Work." *Emily Dickinson Journal* 9, no. 1 (2000): 71–86.

McGill, Joseph. "The Slave Dwelling Project," http://slavedwellingproject.org.

McKenna, James J., and Thomas McDade. "Why Babies Should Never Sleep Alone: A Review of the Co-Sleeping Controversy in Relation to SIDS, Bedsharing, and Breast Feeding." *Pediatric Respiratory Reviews* 6 (2005): 134–152.

McKibben, Bill. *The End of Nature.* New York: Random House, 1989.

Melbin, Murray. *Night as Frontier: Colonizing the World After Dark.* New York: Free Press, 1987.

Melville, Herman. *Great Short Works.* New York: Harper Perennial, 2004.

———. *Moby-Dick; or, the Whale.* New York: Penguin, 2001.

Mitchell, S. Weir. "The Evolution of the Rest Treatment." *Journal of Nervous & Mental Disease* 31, no. 6 (1904): 368–373.

———. *Wear and Tear; or, Hints for the Overworked.* Philadelphia: J. B. Lippincott, 1871.

Mooallem, Jon. "The Sleep-Industrial Complex." *New York Times Magazine,* November 18, 2007, www.nytimes.com/2007/11/18/magazine/18sleep -t.html.

More, Sir Thomas. *Utopia.* New York: W. W. Norton, 1975.

Morris, Bob. "Arianna Huffington's Sleep Revolution Begins at Home." *New York Times,* April 28, 2016, www.nytimes.com/2016/05/01/realestate/arianna -huffingtons-sleep-revolution-starts-at-home.html.

Morrisroe, Patricia. *Wide Awake: A Memoir of Insomnia.* New York: Spiegel and Grau, 2010.

Moss, William. *An Essay on the Management and Nursing of Children in the Earlier Period of Infancy.* London: J. Johnson, 1781.

Mowat, Farley. *People of the Deer.* New York: Carroll and Graf, 1951.

Murison, Justine S. *The Politics of Anxiety in Nineteenth-Century American Culture.* Cambridge: Cambridge University Press, 2011.

Nancy, Jean-Luc. *The Fall of Sleep.* Translated by Charlotte Mandell. New York: Fordham University Press, 2009.

"The Narrative of Gregory Gamble, Esq." *New-York Mirror,* 1835, 337–338.

National Sleep Foundation. "2009 Sleep in America Poll: Highlights and Key Findings," 2009. https://sleepfoundation.org/sites/default/files/2009%20 POLL%20HIGHLIGHTS.pdf.

Neely, Michelle C. "Embodied Politics: Antebellum Vegetarianism and the Dietary Economy of *Walden*." *American Literature* 85, no. 1 (March 2013): 34–60.

Nelson, James. *An Essay on the Government of Children, Under Three General Heads, Viz. Health, Manners, and Education*. London: R. and J. Dodsley, 1763.

"The Nervous System." *New Englander and Yale Review* 4, no. 15 (July 1846): 433–447.

Newhouse, Edward. *You Can't Sleep Here*. New York: Macaulay, 1934.

Nguyen, Bich Phoung, Elbrich Postma, David Ekkers, Fabian Degener, and Thomas Meijer. "Bad Kissingen: A Blueprint for Future Urban Design." Groningen, Netherlands, 2013, http://docplayer.net/19477784-Bad -kissingen-bad-kissingen-a-blueprint-for-future-urban-design.html.

Niller, Eric. "Human Hibernation May Not Be a Pipedream Forever." *Washington Post*, April 13 2015.

Northup, Solomon. *Twelve Years a Slave: Narrative of Solomon Northup*. Buffalo, NY: Derby, Orton and Mulligan, 1853.

Olsen, Hannah Brooks. "Homelessness and the Impossibility of a Good Night's Sleep." *The Atlantic*, August 14, 2014, www.theatlantic.com /health/archive/2014/08/homelessness-and-the-impossibility-of-a -good-nights-sleep/375671.

O'Malley, Michael. *Keeping Watch: A History of American Time*. New York: Viking Penguin, 1990.

Orwell, George. *Down and Out in Paris and London*. Orlando, FL: Harcourt, 1961.

Packard, Elizabeth Parsons Ware. *The Prisoners' Hidden Life; or, Insane Asylums Unveiled*. Chicago: Published by the author, 1868.

Pantley, Elizabeth. *The No-Cry Sleep Solution*. New York: McGraw-Hill, 2002.

Parker, Ian. "The Big Sleep." *The New Yorker*, December 9, 2013, www .newyorker.com/magazine/2013/12/09/the-big-sleep-2.

Patterson, Orlando. *Slavery and Social Death: A Comparative Study*. Cambridge, MA: Harvard University Press, 1982.

Paul, Pamela. *Parenting, Inc.: How the Billion-Dollar Baby Business Has Changed the Way We Raise Our Children*. New York: Henry Holt, 2008.

Pendergrast, Mark. *Uncommon Grounds: The History of Coffee and How It Transformed Our World*. New York: Basic Books, 1999.

"Physicians Call for End of an Inuit Sleep Tradition." *CBCNews*, November 8, 2005, www.cbc.ca/news/technology/physicians-call-for-end-of-an -inuit-sleep-tradition-1.551990.

Pollitt, Katha. "Attachment Parenting: More Guilt for Mother." *The Nation* (June 4, 2012): 9.

Porter, Roy. *Madness: A Brief History*. Oxford: Oxford University Press, 2002.

Primack, Richard B. *Walden Warming: Climate Change Comes to Thoreau's Woods*. Chicago: University of Chicago Press, 2014.

Proust, Marcel. *Remembrance of Things Past*. Translated by C. K. Scott Moncrief and Kevin Kilmartin. Vol. 1, *Swann's Way; Within a Budding Grove*. New York: Random House, 1982.

Rabin, Roni Caryn. "Ask Well: More Sleep, Fewer Colds?" *New York Times*, January 29, 2016, www.well.blogs.nytimes.com/2016/01/29/ask-well-sleep-and-colds.

Rabinbach, Anson. *The Human Motor: Energy, Fatigue, and the Origins of Modernity*. Berkeley: University of California Press, 1992.

Raja, Jeyapal Dinesh, and Sanjiv Kumar Bhasin. "Health Issues Amongst Call Center Employees, an Emerging Occupational Group in India." *Indian Journal of Community Medicine: Official Publication of Indian Association of Preventive & Social Medicine* 39, no. 3 (2014): 175–177.

Randall, David K. *Dreamland: Adventures in the Strange Science of Sleep*. New York: W. W. Norton, 2012.

Rao, Uma, Russell E. Poland, Preetam Lutchmansingh, Geoffrey E. Ott, James T. McCracken, and Keh-Ming Lin. "Relationship Between Ethnicity and Sleep Patterns in Normal Controls: Implications for Psychopathology and Treatment." *Journal of Psychiatric Research* 33, no. 5 (September 1999): 419–426.

Rediker, Marcus. *The Slave Ship: A Human History*. New York: Viking, 2007.

Reiss, Benjamin. "Sleeping While Disabled, Disabled While Sleeping." *Sleep Health* 2, no. 3 (2016): 187–190.

———. "Sleep's Hidden Histories." *Los Angeles Review of Books*, February 15, 2014, https://lareviewofbooks.org/review/sleeps-hidden-histories.

———. "The Springfield Somnambulist; or, the End of the Enlightenment in America." *Common-place* 4, no. 2 (2004), www.common-place.org/vol-04/no-02/reiss.

———. *Theaters of Madness: Insane Asylums and Nineteenth-Century American Culture*. Chicago: University of Chicago Press, 2008.

Repantis, Dimitris, Peter Schlattmann, Oona Laisney, and Isabella Heuser. "Modafinil and Methylphenidate for Neuroenhancement in Healthy Individuals: A Systematic Review." *Pharmacological Research* 62, no. 3 (September 2010): 187–206.

Resnick, Brian. "The Black-White Sleep Gap." *National Journal*, October 23, 2015, www.nationaljournal.com/s/91261/black-white-sleep-gap.

Richards, Evelleen. "The 'Moral Anatomy' of Robert Knox: The Interplay Between Biological and Social Thought in Victorian Scientific Naturalism." *Journal of the History of Biology* 22 (1989): 373–426.

Richardson, Robert D., Jr. *Henry Thoreau: A Life of the Mind*. Berkeley: University of California Press, 1986.

Riis, Jacob A. *How the Other Half Lives*. New York: Penguin, 1997.

Robb, Graham. *The Discovery of France: A Historical Geography from the Revolution to the First World War*. New York: Norton, 2007.

Roenneberg, Till. *Internal Time: Chronotypes, Social Jet Lag, and Why You're So Tired*. Cambridge, MA: Harvard University Press, 2012.

Rose, Nikolas. *The Politics of Life Itself: Biomedicine, Power, and Subjectivity in the Twenty-First Century*. Princeton, NJ: Princeton University Press, 2007.

Rosenzweig, Roy. *Eight Hours for What We Will: Workers and Leisure in an Industrialized City, 1870–1920*. Cambridge: Cambridge University Press, 1985.

Rothman, David. *The Discovery of the Asylum: Social Order and Disorder in the New Republic*. Boston: Little, Brown, 1971.

Rozhon, Tracie. "To Have, Hold, and Cherish, Until Bedtime." *New York Times*, March 11, 2007.

Rush, Benjamin. *Medical Inquiries and Observations upon the Diseases of the Mind*, 5th ed. Philadelphia: Grigg and Elliott, 1835.

Russell, Karen. *Sleep Donation: A Novella*. New York: Atavist Books, 2014.

Rutherford, Alexandra. *Beyond the Box: B. F. Skinner's Technology of Behavior from Laboratory to Life, 1950s–1970s*. Toronto: University of Toronto Press, 2009.

Saletan, Will. "The War on Sleep." *Slate*, May 29, 2013, www.slate.com/articles /health_and_science/superman/2013/05/sleep_deprivation_in_the _military_modafinil_and_the_arms_race_for_soldiers.html.

Samuels, Ellen. "Passing." In *Keywords for Disability Studies*, edited by Rachel Adams, Benjamin Reiss, and David Serlin, 135–137. New York: New York University Press, 2015.

Savage, Sarah. "The Factory Girl (1814)." *Common-place*, www.common-place .org/justteachone/wp-content/uploads/2013/12/Factory-Girl-1814-by -Sarah-Savage.pdf.

Savitt, Todd L. *Medicine and Slavery: The Diseases and Health Care of Blacks in Antebellum Virginia*. Urbana: University of Illinois Press, 1978.

Schivelbusch, Wolfgang. *Disenchanted Night: The Industrialization of Light in the Nineteenth Century*. Berkeley: University of California Press, 1995.

———. *The Railway Journey*. Leamington Spa, UK: Berg, 1986.

———. *Tastes of Paradise: A Social History of Spices, Stimulants, and Intoxicants*. Translated by David Jacobson. New York: Random House, 1992.

Schmidt, Roger. "Caffeine and the Coming of the Enlightenment." *Raritan* 23, no. 1 (Summer 2003): 129–149.

Schuessler, Jennifer. "Confronting Slavery at Long Island's Oldest Estates." *New York Times*, August 12, 2015, www.nytimes.com/2015/08/14/arts/con fronting-slavery-at-long-islands-oldest-estates.html.

Scrivner, Lee. *Becoming Insomniac: How Sleeplessness Alarmed Modernity*. New York: Palgrave Macmillan, 2014.

Scull, Andrew. *The Most Solitary of Afflictions: Madness and Society in Britain, 1700–1900*. New Haven, CT: Yale University Press, 1993.

Sears, William. *Nighttime Parenting: How to Get Your Baby and Child to Sleep*. New York: Plume, 1999.

Sellers, Christopher. "Thoreau's Body: Towards an Embodied Environmental History." *Environmental History* 4, no. 4 (1999): 486–514.

Shorter, Edward. *From Paralysis to Fatigue: A History of Psychosomatic Illness in the Modern Era*. New York: Free Press, 1992.

Showalter, Elaine. *Hystories: Hysterical Epidemics and Modern Culture*. New York: Columbia University Press, 1997.

Shumard, Theresa. "Tapping into Outsourcing." *Sleep Review: The Journal for Sleep Specialists*, July 5, 2007, www.sleepreviewmag.com/2007/07 /tapping-into-outsourcing.

Sidney, Sir Philip. "Come, Sleep!" In *Poems of Sleep and Dreams*, edited by Peter Washington. New York: Alfred A. Knopf, 2004.

Siebers, Tobin. "Disability as Masquerade." *Literature and Medicine* 23, no. 4 (2004): 1–22.

———. "A Sexual Culture for Disabled People." In *Sex and Disability*, edited by Robert McRuer and Anna Mollow, 37–53. Durham, NC: Duke University Press, 2012.

Simms, William Gilmore. *The Yemassee: A Romance of Carolina*. Fayetteville: University of Arkansas Press, 1994.

Simpson, Jeffrey E. "Thoreau 'Dreaming Awake and Asleep.'" *Modern Language Studies* 14, no. 3 (1984): 54–62.

Sims, Michael. *The Adventures of Henry Thoreau: A Young Man's Unlikely Path to Walden Pond*. New York: Bloomsbury, 2014.

Sisson, Mark. *The Primal Blueprint*. Malibu, CA: Primal Nutrition, 2012.

Skinner, B. F. "Baby in a Box: The Mechanical Baby-Tender." *Ladies' Home Journal* 62 (October 1945): 30–31, 135–136, 138.

———. *Walden Two*. Indianapolis: Hackett, 1948 (repr. 1976).

"Sleep Centers Increase to Highest Number Ever." *Huffington Post*, January 3, 2013, www.huffingtonpost.com/2013/01/03/sleep-centers-highest -number-american-academy-of-sleep-medicine_n_2366719.html.

"Sleepless Pill." *British Medical Journal* 298, no. 6687 (June 10, 1989): 1543–1544.

Smail, Daniel Lord. *On Deep History and the Brain*. Berkeley: University of California Press, 2008.

Smith, Mark M. *Mastered by the Clock : Time, Slavery, and Freedom in the American South*. Chapel Hill: University of North Carolina Press, 1997.

Smith-Rosenberg, Carroll. *Disorderly Conduct: Visions of Gender in Victorian America*. New York: Alfred A. Knopf, 1985.

"Somnambulism." *Springfield Republican*, November 13, 1833.

Spiro, Melford E. "Utopia and Its Discontents: The Kibbutz and Its Historical Vicissitudes." *American Anthropologist* 106, no. 3 (2004): 556–568.

Spock, Benjamin. *The Common Sense Book of Baby and Child Care*. New York: Duell, Sloan and Pearce, 1957.

Standen, Dirk. "Exclusive: Kanye West on His 'Famous' Video, Which Might Be His Most Thought-Provoking Work Yet." *Vanity Fair*, June 24, 2016, www.vanityfair.com/culture/2016/06/kanye-famous-video-interview.

Stearns, Peter N. *Anxious Parents: A History of Modern Childrearing in America*. New York: New York University Press, 2003.

Stearns, Peter N., Perrin Rowland, and Lori Giarnella. "Children's Sleep: Sketching Historical Change." *Journal of Social History* 30, no. 2 (1996): 345–366.

Steger, Brigitte, and Lodewijk Brunt. "Introduction: Into the Night and the World of Sleep." In *Night-Time and Sleep in Asia and the West*, edited by Brigitte Steger and Lodewijk Brunt, 1–23. London: Routledge, 2003.

Stoler, Ann Laura. "Tense and Tender Ties: The Politics of Comparison in North American History and (Post) Colonial Studies." *Journal of American History* 88, no. 3 (2001): 829–865.

Stowe, Harriet Beecher. *Uncle Tom's Cabin; or, Life Among the Lowly*. New York: Penguin, 1981.

Stowe, Steven M. *Doctoring the South: Southern Physicians and Everyday Medicine in the Mid-Nineteenth Century*. Chapel Hill: University of North Carolina Press, 2003.

Stowe, William. "Linnaean Poetics: Emerson, Cooper, Thoreau, and the Names of Plants." *Isle: Interdisciplinary Studies in Literature and Environment* 17, no. 3 (2010): 567–583.

Sullivan, Garrett A., Jr. *Sleep, Romance and Human Embodiment: Vitality from Spenser to Milton*. Cambridge: Cambridge University Press, 2012.

Sweetwater, Austin. "Lena Dunham to Remake Andy Warhol's *Sleep*." *News Examiner*, 2015, http://newsexaminer.net/movies/lena-dunham-to-remake-andy-warhols-sleep.

Talbot, Margaret. "Brain Gain: The Underground World of Brain-Enhancing Drugs." *New Yorker*, April 27, 2009, www.newyorker.com/magazine/2009/04/27/brain-gain.

Taves, Ann. *Fits, Trances, & Visions: Experiencing Religion and Explaining Experience from Wesley to James*. Princeton, NJ: Princeton University Press, 1999.

Thompson, E. P. "Time, Work-Discipline, and Industrial Capitalism." *Past & Present* 38, no. 1 (1967): 56–97.

Thoreau, Henry David. *Collected Essays and Poems*. New York: Library of America, 2001.

———. *The Journal: 1837–1861*. New York: New York Review of Books, 2009.

———. "The Laws of Menu." *Dial* 43 (January 1843): 331–340.

———. *Walden and Other Writings*. New York: Random House, 1992.

———. *A Week on the Concord and Merrimack Rivers*. New York: Penguin, 1998.

Thorpy, Michael J. "History of Sleep and Man." In *The Encyclopedia of Sleep and Sleep Disorders*, edited by Michael J. Thorpy and Jan Yager, ix–xxxiii. New York: Facts on File, 1991.

"Time for Sleep." *Journal of Health* 1 (1830): 73–76.

Tocqueville, Alexis de. *Democracy in America: Historical-Critical Edition of De La Démocratie en Amérique*. Translated by James T. Schleifer. Indianapolis, IN: Liberty Fund, 2010.

Tomes, Nancy. *A Generous Confidence: Thomas Story Kirkbride and the Art of Asylum-Keeping, 1840–1883*. Cambridge: Cambridge University Press, 1984.

Toon, Elicia, Margot J. Davey, Samantha L. Hollis, Gillian M. Nixon, Rosemary S. C. Horne, and Sarah N. Bigg. "Comparison of Commercial Wrist-Based and Smartphone Accelerometers, Actigraphy, and PSG in a Clinical Cohort of Children and Adolescents." *Journal of Clinical Sleep Medicine* 12, no. 3 (March 2016): 343–350.

Toscano, Alberto. *Fanaticism: On the Uses of an Idea*. London: Verso, 2010.

Tripp, C. A. *The Intimate World of Abraham Lincoln*. New York: Basic Books, 2005.

Tryon, Thomas. *Friendly Advice to the Gentlemen-Planters of the East and West Indies*. London: Andrew Sowle, 1684.

———. *A Treatise of Cleanness in Meats and Drinks, of the Preparation of Food, the Excellency of Good Airs, and the Benefits of Clean Sweet Beds, Also of the Generation of Bugs, and Their Cure*. London: Printed for the author, 1682.

Tucker, Catherine M. *Coffee Culture: Local Experiences, Global Connections*. New York: Routledge, 2011.

Van den Bulck, Jan. "Television Viewing, Computer Game Playing, and Internet Use and Self-Reported Time to Bed and Time Out of Bed in Secondary-School Children." *Sleep* 27, no. 1 (2004): 101–104.

Van der Woude, Joanne. "The Great Awakening." In *A New Literary History of America*, edited by Greil Marcus and Werner Sollors, 79–84. Cambridge, MA: Harvard University Press, 2009.

Van Meijl, Toon. "Maori Collective Sleeping as Cultural Resistance." In *Sleep Around the World: Anthropological Perspectives*, edited by Katie Glaskin and Richard Chenhall, 133–150. London: Palgrave Macmillan, 2013.

Van Wienen, Mark W. "A Rose by Any Other Name: Charlotte Perkins Stetson (Gilman) and the Case for American Reform Socialism." *American Quarterly* 55, no. 4 (2003): 603–634.

Varagur, Krithika. "Can Sleep Deprivation Explain Donald Trump's Behavior?" *Huffington Post*, March 6, 2016, www.huffingtonpost.com/entry/donald-trump-sleep-deprivation_us_56d5d020e4b03260bf78343a.

Venables, Michael. "Space Travel's Efficient, Cheaper Future: Sleeping Your Way to Mars in a Stasis Habitat." *Forbes/Tech*, October 6, 2013, www.forbes.com/sites/michaelvenables/2013/10/06/space-travels-efficient-cheaper-future-sleeping-your-way-to-mars-in-stasis-habitat.

Walker, Charles Rumford. *Steel: The Diary of a Furnace Worker*. Boston: Atlantic Monthly Press, 1922.

Walls, Laura Dassow. *Seeing New Worlds: Henry David Thoreau and Nineteenth-Century Natural Science*. Madison: University of Wisconsin Press, 1995.

Warner, Michael. "Walden's Erotic Economy." In *Comparative American Identities: Race, Sex, and Nationality in the Modern Text*, edited by Hortense J. Spillers, 157–174. New York: Routledge, 1991.

Washington, Harriet A. *Medical Apartheid*. New York: Anchor Books, 2006.

Washington, Peter, ed. *Poems of Sleep and Dreams*. New York: Alfred A. Knopf, 2004.

Weintraub, Arlene. "Merck's Quest to Revive the Market for Insomnia Drugs." *Forbes*, June 14, 2015, www.forbes.com/sites/arleneweintraub/2015/06/04/mercks-quest-to-revive-the-market-for-insomnia-drugs.

Weissbluth, M., J. Poncher, G. Given, J. Schwab, R. Mervis, and M. Rosenberg. "Sleep Duration and Television Viewing." *Journal of Pediatrics* 99, no. 3 (1981): 486–488.

Wesley, John. "The Duty and Advantage of Early Rising." Cambridge, Eng: J. Archdeacon, Printer to the University, 1785.

West, Kanye. "Famous." YouTube, June 28, 2016, https://www.youtube.com/watch?v=wCg1_IKXmQc.

"What Is the Future of Sleep?" *Test-Tube Plus!* YouTube, May 24, 2015, www.youtube.com/watch?v=M-bQzqdwUk0.

Whitman, Walt. *Leaves of Grass and Other Writings*, 2nd ed. Edited by Michael Moon. New York: W. W. Norton, 2002.

Williams, Alex. "The Paleo Lifestyle: Way, Way, Way Back." *New York Times*, September 21, 2014, ST1.

Williams, Natasha J., Michael A. Grandner, Shedra A. Snipes, April Rogers, Olajide Williams, Collins Airhihenbuwa, and Jean-Louis Girardin. "Racial/Ethnic Disparities in Sleep Health and Healthcare: Importance of the Sociocultural Context." *Sleep Health* 1, no. 1 (2015): 28–35.

Williams, Simon J. *The Politics of Sleep: Governing (Un)Consciousness in the Late Modern Age*. Houndsmills, UK: Palgrave Macmillan, 2011.

———. *Sleep and Society: Sociological Ventures into the (Un)Known*. London: Routledge, 2005.

Williams, Simon J., Catherine M. Coveney, and Jonathan Gabe. "Medicalisation or Customisation? Sleep, Enterprise and Enhancement in the 24/7 Society." *Social Science & Medicine* 79 (2013): 40–47.

Wolf-Meyer, Matthew. "Can We Ever Know the Sleep of Our Ancestors?" *Sleep Health* 2, no. 1 (2016): 1–2.

———. *The Slumbering Masses: Sleep, Medicine, and Modern American Life*. Minneapolis: University of Minnesota Press, 2012.

———. "Where Have All Our Naps Gone? Or Nathaniel Kleitman, the Consolidation of Sleep, and the Historiography of Emergence." *Anthropology of Consciousness* 24, no. 2 (2013): 96–116.

Wolpe, Paul Root. "Treatment, Enhancement, and the Ethics of Neurotherapeutics." *Brain & Cognition* 50 (2002): 387–395.

Wood, Mary Elene. *The Writing on the Wall: Women's Autobiography and the Asylum*. Urbana: University of Illinois Press, 1994.

Wood, Michael. "Proust's Mother." *London Review of Books* 34, no. 6 (2012): 5–10.

Wood, Molly. "Bedtime Technology for a Better Night's Sleep." *New York Times*, December 24, 2014, www.nytimes.com/2014/12/25/technology /personaltech/bedroom-technology-for-a-better-nights-sleep.html.

"The Worcester Asylum for the Insane." *Vermont Chronicle*, April 22, 1846.

Worster, Donald. *Nature's Economy: A History of Ecological Ideas*. Cambridge: Cambridge University Press, 1994.

Worthman, Carol M. "After Dark: The Evolutionary Ecology of Human Sleep." In *Evolutionary Medicine and Health*, edited by Wenda R. Trevathan, E. O. Smith, and James J. McKenna, 291–313. Oxford: Oxford University Press, 2008.

Worthman, Carol M., and Ryan A. Brown. "Companionable Sleep: Social Regulation of Sleep and Cosleeping in Egyptian Families." *Journal of Family Psychology* 21, no. 1 (2007): 124–135.

Yardley, Jim. "Spain, Land of 10 p.m. Dinners, Asks If It's Time to Reset the Clock." *New York Times*, February 18, 2014, A1.

Yetish, Gandhi, Hillard Kaplan, Michael Gurven, Brian Wood, Herman Pontzer, Paul R. Manger, Charles Wilson, Ronald McGregor, and Jerome M. Siegel. "Natural Sleep and Its Seasonal Variations in Three Pre-Industrial Societies." *Current Biology* 25 (November 2, 2015): 2862–2868.

———. "Response to De La Iglesia et al." *Current Biology* 26, no. 7 (April 4, 2016): R273–R274.

INDEX

abolitionist writing, 124
Abu Ghraib, 127
adenosine/adenosine A1, 54
agribusiness, 49
agricultural revolution, 207
altered states of consciousness, 102
Ambien, 118, 207
American Business, 46
Americans with Disabilities Act, 217
amphetamines, 208
Angel of Bethesda, The (C. Mather), 99
anthropology, 24, 36, 45, 51, 200, 205, 206
anxiety, 5, 14, 23, 36, 143, 145, 150, 151, 156, 160, 168, 179, 215
Apperley, Thomas, 149
Apple's iPhone 5c, 203
Arctic/Antarctic regions, 44
Ariès, Philippe, 157
Aristotle, 93–94, 106
artificial lighting, 9–10, 33–34, 35, 37, 38, 48, 119, 159, 173, 174, 200
    experiments in deprivation of, 34
    gas light, 9, 10, 38, 62–63, 119
Art of Nursing, The, 149
Asabano people, 24–25, 31
Aschoff, Jürgen, 46
Aserinsky, Eugene, 46

asylums. *See* insane asylums
At Day's Close: Night in Times Past (Ekirch), 33
attachment parenting, 167
Australia, 205

Baby and Child Care (Spock), 154
Bach, Johann Sebastian, 76
Bad Kissingen, Germany, 173
Baker, Rachel, 100–102, 105, 106
    death of, 107
Baldwin, Peter, 81
Balzac, Honoré de, 77
Barbieux, Kevin, 121
"Bartleby, the Scrivener" (Melville), 228
Beard, George, 179
Bedtime for Frances (Hoban), 168–169f
behavioral psychology/engineering, 148, 192. *See also* Skinner, B. F.
Belden, Lemuel, 108–110, 112, 113, 114
Bell, John, 103
Bell, Luther, 151, 152
Bell, Thomas, 40
Bellamy, Edward, 185–-186
Belsomra, 207–208
Bettelheim, Bruno, 168, 187–188
Birth, Kevin, 205, 206

birth control, 159
Blithedale Romance, The
        (Hawthorne), 177
Blumenbach, Johann, 130, 131
boarders, 63, 81
bodily contact, 144–145
Book of Job, 227
Boston Medical and Surgical Journal,
        113
brain chemistry, 207
breastfeeding, 149
Brigham, Amariah, 116
British Medical Journal, 42
bromides, 69, 84, 178
Brook Farm (Massachusetts),
        176–177
Brotherhood of Sleeping Car
        Porters, 135
Brown, Charles Brockden, 104
Brown, John, 87
Brown, Margaret Wise, 16, 168
Brown, Ryan, 165
Brown, William Wells, 124
bruxism, 117
Buell, Lawrence, 82
Buqueras y Bach, Ignacio, 201
Burgundian day laborers, 42
Bush, Barbara, 5
Bush, Jeb, 97
Butler, Blake, 218–219

caffeine, 12, 14, 58, 69, 74, 75, 77, 80,
        207
    caffeinated gum, 208
    See also coffee
Calcutta Black Hole, 30
Canada, 43–44, 166
capitalism, 34, 38, 143, 210, 212
Carter, Jimmy, 226–227
Cartwright, Samuel Adolphus,
        130–133, 134, 136–137
castoreum, 92

catastrophic layovers, 150
Centers for Disease Control and
        Prevention, 172
Chadwick, Edwin, 28–29, 120
Challenger space shuttle, 74
Chauncy, Charles, 103
Chernobyl, 74
Cheyne, George, 129
children, 17, 63, 131, 139, 141–170,
        183, 195, 228
    baby-in-a-box system, 154–155,
        161, 163, 191, 193
    books for bedtime stories,
        167–169, 188
    books for parents concerning,
        161–162
    brain development of, 142
    co-sleeping of children and
        parents, 144, 157, 165–167,
        184, 219
    cradles vs. beds for, 149–150
    cry-it-out vs. no-cry methods
        concerning, 162–164
    and digital age, 202
    economic dimensions of
        children's sleep, 142
    infants' sleep routines, 154
    parents rolling over on, 158,
        166, 167
    psychological independence of,
        164
    raised collectively, 176, 186–187,
        189–190, 192–193, 195
        (*see also* Israeli kibbutz
        movement)
    seeing parents' intercourse, 154,
        156, 169
    sleeping separately in own
        rooms, 2, 4, 10–11, 15, 24,
        31, 61, 65, 120, 141, 154,
        157–158, 163, 167, 187, 188
    sleepovers, 153

Children of the Dream, The
    (Bettelheim), 187–188
Child's Garden of Verses, A
    (Stevenson), 159–160
China, 157, 201, 204–205
cholera, 29
chorea, 108
Christianity, 86, 94, 95–100. *See*
    also sleepwalking: female
    sleepwalkers
chronobiology, 46, 48, 85, 173–174
Chrono City, 173–174
circadian rhythms, 4, 6, 46, 52–53,
    85, 171, 173, 200, 204, 205,
    206, 210
Cities of Sleep (film), 121
civil disobedience, 87
class divides, 212
climate change, 82, 174, 201, 206
climate control, 48, 49, 51
clocks, 40–41, 69, 71, 85, 128, 145,
    173. *See also* time
coal, 62
cocaine, 178–179, 207
codeine, 93, 183
Coe, Jonathan, 212
coffee, 74–78. *See also* caffeine
coffeehouses, 75–76
Cogan, Thomas, 34, 41–42, 51, 149
cognitive issues, 136–137, 208, 210
Collier, Mary, 143–144, 145, 159
colonialism, 76
Concerning Children (Gilman), 184
Concord, Massachusetts, 60–63, 68
consumerism, 16, 79, 81, 82, 155,
    193, 194, 201
continuous positive airway pressure
    machines (CPAPs), 118
Cook Islanders, 25
Coren, Stanley, 74
counterculture, 194
Crary, Jonathan, 213, 214, 215

DARPA. See Defense Advanced
    Research Projects Agency
Darr, Yael, 188
Darwin, Charles, 82
Darwin, Erasmus, 106
Das Kapital (Marx), 38
Defense Advanced Research Projects
    Agency (DARPA), 208
Defense Department, 208
Delhi, 200–201
Dement, William, 45
Derickson, Alan, 136
Desiderio, Vincent, 220, 221
De somno et vigilia (Aristotle), 93
Devotional Somnium (Mitchill and
    Rathbone), 17
Dial, The (journal), 85
Dickinson, Emily, 16–17, 180
diet, 50, 112, 113, 179, 216
digestion, 93, 94, 106, 109, 112
digital age, 55, 202, 222
Dinges, David, 54
disabilities, 217
disease, 28, 29, 94, 112
    categories pertaining only to
        slaves, 132–133
    See also medical issues;
        tuberculosis
diurnal sleep-wake rhythm, 45, 200,
    206
Doctor and Patient (Mitchell), 179
dolphins, 3
Douglass, Frederick, 16, 89
    on sleep deprivation, 126, 133,
        136
Douglass, John, 106–107
Down and Out in Paris and London
    (Orwell), 120
dreaming, 18, 46, 104, 211, 214
Drew, Kelly, 54
ducks, 3
du Laurens, André, 92

Dunbar, Charles, 61
Dunham, Lena, 219, 221
Durant, John, 51, 52
dystopian views, 212–215, 216

early rising movement, 150–151
Eby, Clare, 183
economic issues, 7, 8, 13, 15, 34, 43,
        61, 64, 70, 81, 125, 136, 150,
        180, 183, 186, 192, 215
    business process outsourcing
        industry, 205
    and controlling sleep, 216
    economic dimensions of
        children's sleep, 142
    global economy/workforce, 199,
        202, 203, 212, 214
*Edgar Huntly; or, Memoirs of a
    Sleepwalker* (C. Brown), 104
Edison, Thomas, 37, 200
education, 61, 146, 176, 179, 180,
        191, 202, 203
Egypt, 157
Ekirch, Roger, 9, 33–34, 35, 37, 51
electrification, 9–10, 25, 35, 37
electroencephalographic (EEG)
        readouts, 118
Elias, Norbert, 11, 12, 122
Emerson, Ralph Waldo, 67, 68, 69,
        77, 176
emetics, 109, 118
Émile, or On Education (Rousseau),
        147
Emory University, 17, 226
England, 25, 28–29, 42, 103
    Common Houses Lodging Act,
        29
    Conservative Party, 212
    Dolben Act of 1788, 28
    London, 75–76
English, Daylanne, 128
English Malady, The (Cheyne), 129

Enlightenment era, 76, 151
entertainment, 10, 11, 15, 191
Equiano, Olaudah, 28
Erasmus, 26
"Escape at Bedtime" (Stevenson),
        159
*Essay Concerning Human
    Understanding, An* (Locke),
        146
Europe/Europeans, 12, 25, 28, 31,
        32, 33, 75, 92, 93, 94, 102,
        105, 157, 158
European Space Agency (ESA), 53,
        54
Eutychus, 95–96
evolution, 33, 34–35, 35–36, 36–37,
        48, 50, 51
exhaustion. *See* fatigue/exhaustion
Exxon Valdez oil spill, 74

Factory Girl, The (Savage), 40
Fadiman, Anne, 165–166
Fall of Sleep, The (Nancy), 219
Famous (video), 220–222
fatigue/exhaustion, 15, 40, 58, 60,
        69, 74, 97, 122, 123, 125–
        126, 127, 135, 143, 144, 178,
        179, 180, 184, 185, 190, 205,
        206
    treating, 210
feminism, 166–167, 177, 181, 183,
        186
Ferber, Richard, 163–165, 167
Ficino, Marcelo, 92–93
Field, John, 78–79
Fielding, Henry, 76
food issues, 42, 43, 44, 50, 52, 93
Forerunner, The (magazine), 182
Foster, Russell, 34
Fourier, Charles, 176
Franklin, Benjamin, 150
French Ministry of Defense, 209

French Pyrenees, 42
Freud, Sigmund, 153, 154, 158, 161, 180
Friedman, Kristen Keerma, 105–106
Friendly Advice to the Gentlemen-Planters of the East and West Indies (Tryon), 122–123
Fuller, Henry, 74

Galbraith, Mary, 168
gender issues, 142, 175, 179, 186, 187
Giarnella, Lori, 158, 170
Gibson, William, 50, 197
Gilman, Charlotte Perkins, 16, 139, 177–179, 181–187
Giorno, John, 219
Goffman, Erving, 115–116
Goodnight Gorilla (Rathmann), 169
Goodnight Moon (M. Brown), 168
*Go the F**k to Sleep* (Mansbach), 16, 139, 141, 145, 169
Grand Dictionnaire (Larousse), 152
Great Awakening movement, 98, 100
Great Depression, 120
Greeks, ancient, 68, 93, 208
Greene, Gayle, 217–218
Grob, Gerald, 111
guilt feelings, 161

habit, 46, 87, 147, 148, 161, 163
Hale, Lauren, 136–137
Hall, William Whitty, 30, 31, 44, 152
Hammond, William Alexander, 31–32, 48, 129–130, 131
Handley, Sasha, 25, 27, 35, 94
Hawthorne, Nathaniel, 73, 177
heat, 42, 43–44
   body heat, 61, 93
   warming pans for beds, 62
Hentz, Caroline Lee, 128, 134

Herland (Gilman), 186–187
hibernation, 41, 42, 43, 45, 52, 66, 211
   and blood flow to the brain, 44, 54
   safe suspension of human consciousness, 53–54
historical issues, 7, 24, 27–32, 36, 37, 44, 51, 58, 112, 122, 137, 142, 188, 204
   and children's sleep, 143–150, 158, 165
   history of sleep remedies, 92–93
   and segmented sleep, 9–10, 32–37
   seventeenth/eighteenth centuries, 8, 10, 11, 25, 26, 32, 38, 39, 75, 76, 93, 94, 95, 96, 99, 102, 103, 106, 125, 148–149, 157, 158, 175, 207
   sleep's hidden history, 18, 19
   suppression of premodern sleep customs, 17
   Victorian era, 29, 206, 208
   See also premodern societies; slavery
Hmong people, 165–166
Hoban, Russell, 168
Hobbes, Thomas, 18
homeless people, 121, 201
homework, 203
Horne, Jim, 119
Horowitz, Helen Lefkowitz, 177
Hottentots, 31
House of Seven Gables, The (Hawthorne), 72
House of Sleep, The (Coe), 212
How the Other Half Lives (Riis), 30
Huffington, Arianna, 172–173, 201, 211
Hurd, Clement, 168
Hurricane Katrina, 3–4, 5

Ihalmiut people, 43–44
Inca warriors, 208
Inception (film), 214, 215, 222
India, 157, 205. *See also* Delhi
individualism, 58, 63, 170
Indonesia, 157
industrialization, 6, 8–9, 10, 12, 13, 25, 28, 30, 38, 48, 49, 51, 60, 62, 82, 83, 176, 199
    children's sleep in preindustrial period, 148
    and commercialism, 152
    continuous-process industries, 39
    industrial capitalism, 34, 38
    industrial revolution, 7, 38, 41, 55, 143, 144
    industrial time, 14, 71
    steel industry, 39, 40, 204
    and taming sleep, 16
    See also workers
information flow, 80
information overload, 10, 215
insanity, 103, 104, 111, 116, 151
    insane asylums, 69, 104, 110–111, 115–116, 228
insomnia, 31–32, 45, 59, 69, 80, 97, 99, 117, 170, 178, 200, 208, 213, 224
    vs. ancestral sleep rhythms, 37, 92
    and racial theory, 129–130
    memoirs concerning, 217–219
    middle-of-the-night insomnia, 33 (*see also* sleep; segmented)
    and technology, 206
    See also under Thoreau, Henry David
Insomniac (Greene), 217–218
intergenerational bedtime struggles, 203

International Classification of Sleep Disorders, 117
Internet, 10, 80, 216, 222
Interstellar (film), 53
In the Night Kitchen (Sendak), 168
intifada, 190
Inuit people, 45, 166
Iraq War, 209
Israeli kibbutz movement, 187–191

Jameson, Fredric, 212
Jefferson, Thomas, 125–126, 128, 130, 133, 134
Johnson, Walter, 127
Jordan, Hamilton, 227
journalism, 76. *See also* newspapers
Jouvet, Michel, 210

Kantermann, Thomas, 173, 174
Kardashian West, Kim, 220, 221
Kleitman, Nathaniel, 44–45
    Mammoth Cave experiment of, 45–46, 55
Knutson, Kristen, 36
Koslofsky, Craig, 97

labor, 42, 81, 82, 123, 133, 144, 174, 183, 191
    democratization of, 175, 176
    flexible patterns of work, 211–212
    labor laws, 214–215
    and life of the mind, 193
    rationalizing, 192
    variable labor credit system, 194–195
    See also slavery; workers
La Comédie Humaine (Balzac), 77
Laos, 166
Laqueur, Thomas, 151–152
Larousse, Pierre, 152
Laws of Menu, The, 85

Lee, Ann, 175, 176
leeches, 92, 93, 114, 118
Linnaeus, Carolus, 85, 93
"Little Boxes" (Seeger), 194
Locke, John, 146–148, 170
Lohmann, Roger, 24–25
Looking Backward: 2000–1887
        (Bellamy), 185–186
lotska, 42–43
love, 195

Macbeth (Shakespeare), 91, 99
McDade, Thomas, 167
McGill, Joseph, 137–138
McKenna, James, 165, 167
McKibben, Bill, 215
McLean Asylum for the Insane,
        Massachusetts, 151
Mais, Charles, 106
"Making a Change" (Gilman),
        184–185, 186
Mansbach, Adam, 16, 139, 145,
        169
Maori people, 25
MARS 500, 54
Marx, Karl, 38
masturbation, 151–153, 156
Mather, Azariah, 96
Mather, Cotton, 96, 97–98, 98–99
Mather, Increase, 95–96, 96–97
media, 7, 14, 80, 210–211. *See also*
        newspapers; social media
medical issues, 2, 6, 9, 23, 35, 41, 49,
        93, 115, 120, 129, 164, 200,
        205, 210, 216, 226
    arousal disorders, 110
    blood flow to the brain, 44, 54,
        130, 131, 132
    and children's sleep, 149
    and fatigue, 205, 206, 210
    health as sound relation to
        nature, 84

health risks of sociable sleeping,
        27–30
    and masturbation, 152
    medications, 92
    medicine vs. religion, 92, 100,
        102–103, 111
    neurasthenia, 179–181
    optimal times for healing, 173
    pediatric sleep hygiene books,
        162
    self-diagnosis, 118
    sleepwalking as disease of the
        brain, 104, 108
    and factory work, 62
    See also disease; sleep: sleep
        disorders
melatonin, 202, 203
Melville, Herman, 16, 21, 26,
        227–228
*Memoirs of the Year Two Thousand
        Five Hundred* (Mercier),
        53
menstruation, 106, 114
Mercier, Louis-Sébastien, 53
miasma, 29, 94
migraine, 110
military, 9, 209
misogyny, 181
missionaries, 25, 31
Mitchell, Silas Weir, 179–181, 182,
        183
Mitchill, Samuel Latham, 106, 107
Moby-Dick (Melville), 26–27
modafinil, 207, 209–210
More, Sir Thomas, 174–175, 177
morphine, 178–179
Moss, William, 150
Mowat, Farley, 43

Nancy, Jean-Luc, 219
naps, 8, 35, 41, 45, 50, 51, 61, 79, 171,
        172, 190, 224

naps *(continued)*
  napping in the workplace, 201, 211, 212
NASA, 52, 53, 54
National Association of Homebuilders, 170
National Institutes of Health, 166
Nationalism movement, 185, 186
National Sleep Foundation, 6
Nature, 210
Nelson, James, 150
neural enhancement, 210
neurasthenia, 179–181, 183
neuroscientists, 98
Newhouse, Edward, 120
news, 15, 76, 79, 80
newsboys, 81
newspapers, 33, 62, 70, 80
Newsweek, 165
New Yorker, 45
New Zealand, 31
nightmares, 99, 149, 216
Nolan, Christopher, 214, 222
Northup, Solomon, 124, 136
"Northwest Passage" (Stevenson), 159–160
Notes on the State of Virginia (Jefferson), 125
Nothing: A Portrait of Insomnia (Butler), 218–219
novels, 76
nuclear families, 31, 185, 187, 214

obsessive compulsive disorder, 118
Oedipus complex, 154, 156, 158, 161
Olmsted, Frederick Law, 124
O'Malley, Michael, 71
Onania, or the Heinous Sin of Self-Pollution, and Its Frightful Consequences in Both Sexes, Considered, 151

opium, 92, 93, 99, 104, 113, 116, 118, 151, 178, 207, 208
  as sleep aid for children, 149
orexin, 98, 208
Oromo people, 75
Orwell, George, 16, 120, 194
Outdoor Journal, An (Carter), 227
Out of This Furnace (Bell), 40
outsourcing, 190, 204, 205

Paleo Manifesto, The (Durant), 51
Paleo movement/diet, 50–51, 52, 55
Pantley, Elizabeth, 166
Papua New Guinea, 24–25
parrot fish, 3
Patterson, Orlando, 134
Pauktuutit Inuit Women of Canada, 166
Paul (apostle), 102
peasants, 43, 45, 49
Pepys, Samuel, 26
Philippines, 205
phrenology, 109, 112
"Plea for Captain John Brown" (Thoreau), 87–88
Pope, Alexander, 76
poverty, 30, 120, 133, 195
  poor women, 143
premodern societies, 15, 24–25, 33, 35, 49
Primack, Richard, 82
Primal Blueprint, The (Sisson), 50–51
privacy, 4, 11, 29, 30, 49, 64, 120, 122, 146, 151, 156, 190, 191, 222, 229
prolactin, 34
Promise of Sleep, The (Dement), 45
Proust, Marcel, 16, 57, 160–161, 164
Provigil, 209–210
psychiatry/psychoanalysis, 112, 115, 153. *See also* Freud, Sigmund
Pullman Company, 135

racial issues, 30–31, 32, 131–134, 195
   fantasy of black laziness, 122, 133–134
    theories of self-reflection, 125, 129
   theories of differential sleep requirements, 125–126, 128
   and normal sleep spectrum, 136
   racial superiority, 137
   and unionization, 135
   whites' insomnia, 129–130
railroads, 61, 63, 70–71, 72–73, 80, 180, 186, 206
   trains with sleeping berths, 135
Randolph, A. Philip, 135
"Rape of the Lock" (Pope), 76
Rathbone, David, 107
Rathmann, Peggy, 169
Reagan, Ronald, 133
reforms, 31, 32, 41, 122, 174, 186, 187
religious revivals, 108. *See also* Great Awakening movement
Remembrance of Things Past (Proust), 160–161, 164
REM (rapid eye movement) sleep, 18, 46
   REM behavior disorder, 117, 118
Renaissance, 92
Renard, Jules, 42
Report on the Sanitary Conditions of the Labouring Population of Great Britain (Chadwick), 28–29
rest cures, 179, 181
Richardson (Dr.), 29
Richardson, Bruce, 45
Richardson, Samuel, 76
Rider, Jane C., 107–115
Riis, Jacob, 30, 81, 120
Ripley, George, 176

Robb, Graham, 42
Rose, Nikolas, 216
Rousseau, Jean-Jacques, 147–148, 154, 161
Rowland, Perrin, 158, 170
Rush, Benjamin, 104
Russell, Karen, 213–214, 215
Rye, David, 17, 118, 157

Salem witch trials, 97–98, 102
San Domingo, 76
Savage, Sarah, 40
Schenck, Carlos, 110
Schmidt, Roger, 76
Scrivner, Lee, 206
Sears, William, 166
seasons, 45, 48, 51, 59, 60, 83, 84, 123. *See also* winter
Seeger, Pete, 194
Sellers, Christopher, 84
Sendak, Maurice, 16, 168
sensibility, 32
Sewall, Ellen, 74
sexuality, 29, 34, 146, 153, 161, 164–165, 175, 176, 193
   parents' intercourse, 154, 156, 164
   sexual morality, 157
   See also masturbation
Shakers, 175–176
sharing beds, 24–25, 26–27. *See also* sleep: social sleep
shelter, 3
Sidney, Sir Philip, 227
SIDS. *See* Sudden Infant Death Syndrome
Siegel, Jerome, 35, 36, 37, 51
siesta breaks, 202
Simms, William Gilmore, 129, 130, 134
single parents, 165
Sisson, Mark, 50–51, 52

Skinner, B. F., 154–156, 163, 191–195
slavery, 28, 30, 31, 58, 70, 76, 77, 79, 87, 89, 119–138, 175
and balance between rest and labor, 123, 172
supposed medical justification for, 130–133
nocturnal surveillance of slaves, 127
and oversleeping, 116, 124, 126, 128
Slave Dwelling Project, 137
sleeping conditions of slaves, 28, 137–138, 228
sleep
amount of, 5–6, 35, 41, 42, 45, 49, 61, 119, 135, 136, 142, 176–177, 215 (*see also* sleep: sleep deprivation *and* oversleeping)
arousal disorders, 117
brain's role in controlling, 130
buying, 213
challenges to regular, 2
co-sleeping of children and parents, 144, 157, 165–167, 184, 219
consolidated, 1, 11, 32, 33, 34, 35, 46, 120, 165, 170, 202 (*see also* sleep: eight-hour ideal concerning)
control of sleep environments, 48–49, 170
democratization of, 175
diversity of sleeping arrangements, 7–8
eight-hour ideal concerning, 9, 41, 51, 55 (*see also* sleep: consolidated)
flexibility of sleep-wake cycle, 54, 148, 211
future of, 199–222

health risks of sociable sleeping, 27–30
literary descriptions of, 217
natural, 7, 8, 35, 36–37, 46, 48, 49, 52, 55, 215
normal, 2, 4, 5, 12, 17, 23–24, 34, 55, 120, 121, 162, 199, 202, 212, 216
obsession with, 5, 6–7, 8, 170, 174
oversleeping, 89, 98, 116, 124, 126, 128
as psychosomatic enterprise, 6–7
regularizing/managing, 45, 61, 69, 94–95, 96, 116, 117, 122, 127, 145, 147, 196, 202, 224, 229
routines concerning, 44–45, 48, 49, 121, 172
rules concerning, 2, 4, 5, 7, 8, 11, 19, 24, 25, 36, 116, 121, 163, 171, 174, 191, 199, 202, 215, 216, 222, 228
segmented, 9–10, 33, 36, 51
in separate master bedrooms, 170
sleep apnea, 117, 118, 206, 210
sleep clinics/labs, 5, 6, 117, 205
sleep crises, 7, 172
sleep debt, 119
sleep deprivation, 6, 35, 73, 74, 80, 119, 124, 126, 127, 136, 145, 172, 184, 201, 208
sleep disorders, 6, 7, 37, 58, 59, 91, 93, 117–118, 170, 205 (*see also* insomnia; sleepwalking)
sleeping in church, 96, 98
sleeping pills, 6, 50, 118, 207–208, 211, 213
sleeping posture, 149
sleep memoirs (*see* insomnia: memoirs concerning)

sleep products, 172–173, 201,
    205–207
sleep research, 7, 9, 16, 35, 37,
    44, 46, 54, 93, 110, 119, 201,
    202, 208, 215, 216, 218
sleep revolution, 171, 172
sleep science, 9, 18
sleep stages, 18
slow-wave sleep, 136
and social inequities, 228
as social leveler, 227–228
social sleep, 4, 24–32, 42, 55,
    63, 64 (*see also* bed sharing;
    children: raised collectively)
as source of shared humanity,
    226
spiritual meanings of, 19
stressful sleep environments,
    136
vulnerability of, 3, 18, 221, 229
wake-up times, 150
See also insomnia; sleepwalking
Sleep (film), 219
Sleep (Hall), 152
Sleep (painting), 220
Sleep and Its Derangements
    (Hammond), 31–32
Sleep and *Sleep Medicine Reviews*
    journals, 6
Sleep and Wakefulness (Kleitman),
    46
Sleep Around the World, 24
Sleep Donation (Russell), 213–214
sleep-industrial complex, 5
"Sleep in Science and Culture"
    (university course), 17
Sleep Revolution, The (Huffington),
    172–173, 201
Sleep Shepherd Biofeedback Sleep
    Hat, 206–207
sleep-talking, 101, 102
Sleep Thieves (Coren), 74

sleepwalking, 58, 73, 91, 99, 117
    devotional somnium, 106
    female sleepwalkers, 92, 100–
        102, 104, 105–115
"Sleep We Have Lost: Pre-
    Industrial Slumber in the
    British Isles" (Ekirch), 33
Smail, Daniel Lord, 207
smartphones, 203–204, 205
Smith, Mark, 123–124, 127
Smith-Rosenberg, Carroll, 181
Snow, John, 29
social change, 12, 196
socialism, 185, 187, 188
social justice, 137
social media, 10, 80, 203
Solve Your Child's Sleep Problems
    (Ferber), 163, 165
Some Thoughts Concerning Education
    (Locke), 146–147
somnambulism. *See* sleepwalking
Somneo Sleep Trainer, 209
spaceflight, 53–54
Space Works, Inc., 54
Spain, 201–202
sparrows, 208–209
Spencer, Herbert, 178
Spock, Benjamin, 153–154, 156, 164
Springfield Republican, 107, 108
squirrels, 44, 52, 54
State Lunatic Asylum (Worcester,
    Massachusetts), 110–111
Stearns, Peter, 158, 170
Steele, Richard, 76
steel industry, 39, 40, 204
Steel: The Diary of a Furnace Worker
    (Walker), 40
Stetson, Walter, 178, 180
Stevenson, Robert Louis, 159–160
stimulants, 208, 211
Stowe, Harriet Beecher, 134
stress, 34, 136, 164, 181, 190

Strong, George Templeton, 80–81
Sudden Infant Death Syndrome
    (SIDS), 166, 167
Sufis, 75
    supernatural abilities/events,
        104, 105
Swift, Taylor, 220, 222

technology, 5, 14–15, 16, 34, 59, 72,
        82, 118, 172, 173, 174, 192,
        194, 199, 200
    technological gadgets, 203,
        205–207, 222
telegraphy, 80, 180, 206
television, 200
Thatcher, Margaret, 212
Thompson, E.P., 144, 146
Thoreau, Henry David, 13–16, 57,
        91–92, 121, 135, 155, 191,
        193, 196, 203, 216,
        223–224
    brother John, 63, 64–66, 67, 68,
        74, 158
    cabin at Walden Pond, 69–70,
        223, 229
    as climate change scientist, 82
    and coffee, 74–75, 77, 78
    father of, 61–62, 87
    graduation speech at Harvard
        College, 66
    insomnia of, 64, 68, 84, 87, 88
    last days of, 88
    leaving Walden Pond, 87
    and nighttime, 85
    noticing details, 82
    and railroads, 72–73
    tuberculosis of, 60, 65, 66–67,
        87
Thoreau, John, 61–62, 87
time, 8–9, 14, 39–40, 40–41, 46, 58,
        70–71, 80, 81, 83, 84, 193,
        203

    globalization and, 205
    internal timing systems, 47–48
    measured by tasks, 144, 146
    railroads and sense of time, 72,
        73
    restructured experience of, 199
    time-management techniques,
        127
Tissot, Samuel Auguste David, 152
Tocqueville, Alexis de, 134
torture, 127
transportation accidents, 74
*Treatise of Cleanness in Meats and
        Drinks, of the Preparation
        of Food, the Excellency of
        Good Airs, and the Benefits of
        Clean Sweet Beds, also of the
        Generation of Bugs, and Their
        Cure, A* (Tryon), 27
Trump, Donald, 97, 220
Tryon, Thomas, 27, 122, 124, 125,
        172
tuberculosis, 67. *See also under*
        Thoreau, Henry David
Turner, Nat, 127–128, 132
*24/7: Late Capitalism and the Ends of
        Sleep* (Crary), 213, 214
Twin Oaks Community, 194–195

Uncle Tom's Cabin (Stowe), 134
US Commission on Industrial
        Relations, 136
Utica cribs, 116
Utopia (More), 174–175
utopianism, 155, 171–196, 212

ventilation, 28, 29, 30, 94
violence, 118, 124
*Vital Force: How Wasted and How
        Preserved*, 151
von Humboldt, Alexander, 82
vulnerability, 3, 18, 221, 229

Walden (Thoreau), 13–16, 57–58, 59, 62, 71–72, 81–82, 84, 86, 227
  different life forms in, 83
Walden House/Walden Pool communities, 194
Walden Pond State Reservation, 223
Walden Two (Skinner), 155, 191–195
Walker, Charles Rumford, 40
Warhol, Andy, 219
Watson, John, 158
Wear and Tear (Mitchell), 180
Week on the Concord and Merrimack Rivers, A (Thoreau), 65, 86
Wehr, Thomas, 34
Wesley, John and Charles, 98, 150
West, Kanye, 220–222
Wever, Rütger, 46–47
whales, 3
Where the Wild Things Are (Sendak), 168
Whitfield, George, 98
Whitman, Walt, 228
"Why I Wrote the Yellow Wallpaper?" (Gilman), 183
Wieden, Michael, 174
Williams, Simon, 211, 212
wine, 92, 208
winter, 41–42, 43, 44, 49, 52, 55, 61, 66. *See also* seasons
Wolf-Meyer, Matthew, 36, 45, 157, 211
women, 143, 175, 180, 181, 189. *See also* sleepwalking: female sleepwalkers; workers: female

Women and Economics (Gilman), 186
"Women's Labour, The" (Collier), 143, 146
Woodward, Samuel, 110, 111, 112, 114–115, 117
Woolf, Virginia, 57
workers, 8–9, 11, 12, 14, 28–29, 30, 31, 46, 58, 180, 185–186, 200
  blue-collar, 212
  in China, 204–205
  female, 81, 143, 175
  global workforce, 203
  knowledge workers, 130
  and long factory shifts, 39, 40, 62
  manipulation of sleep patterns of, 9, 38, 39
  midday sleep for, 172
  railway worker fatigue, 74
  and shift work sleep disorder, 37, 40, 209, 210
  sleeping car porters, 135–136
  See also industrialization; labor
Worster, Donald, 84
Worthman, Carol, 165

"Yellow Wall-Paper, The" (Gilman), 177–178, 181–183, 185
Yemassee, The (Simms), 129
Yemen, 75, 200
You Can't Sleep Here (Newhouse), 120
"Young Men's Early Rising Association," 150
youth movements, 169–170

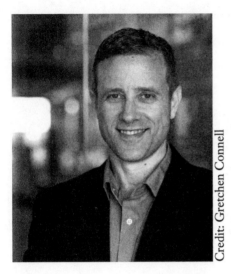

Credit: Gretchen Connell

BENJAMIN REISS is professor of English and co-director of the Disability Studies Initiative at Emory University. He is the author of *The Showman and the Slave: Race, Death, and Memory in Barnum's America* and *Theaters of Madness: Insane Asylums and Nineteenth-Century American Culture*, and he is the co-editor of *The Cambridge History of the American Novel* and *Keywords for Disability Studies*. A recipient of a fellowship from the John Simon Guggenheim Memorial Foundation, Reiss lives in Atlanta, Georgia.